Jane

you Are just
An AMAZing
woman

Sprend your
wings
And
fly

Love
Rob

Healing Psyche

Rob van Overbruggen Ph.D.

ISBN : 1-4196-4737-7

To order additional copies, please visit
http://www.createspace.com/3186766

Healing Psyche

Christiane Northrup, MD - Quite frankly, this book could save your life
"Healing Psyche is a treasure trove of rigorous research on the mind-body connection for cancer – all presented in practical ways that both doctors and their patients can access and implement easily. Quite frankly, this book could save your life."
Christiane Northrup, MD, author of Mother-Daughter Wisdom (Bantam, 2005), The Wisdom of Menopause (Bantam, revised 2006), and Women's Bodies, Women's Wisdom (Bantam, revised 2006)

Lothar Hirneise - I wish all oncologists would read this
"I am working for many years with cancer patients and over the years one get a feeling that our psyche plays a quite bigger role in cancer than most doctors knows. And it is no wonder that doctors know nothing about stress and cancer and psychological patterns and cancer - because they do not learn this at universities.

Even more the book from Dr. Rob van Overbruggen is so important because it is urgent needed that each therapist understands which role different psychological patterns are playing, not only for starting cancer, but also for surviving cancer.
I wish all oncologists would read this book."

Lothar Hirneise is a very knowledgeable advocate and writer on alternative healing who spent years traveling and searching for the most successful cancer therapies. He is the author of Chemotherapy Heals Cancer and the Earth is Flat).

Arielle Essex: encyclopedia of understanding
'Healing Psyche' provides such a complete and well grounded approach towards healing cancer, both patients and therapists will benefit from the careful explanations.
Up-to-date research findings, exploration of causes, handling the emotional aspects, useful question frames, comparisons of current treatment programmes, plus specific insights into the psychological approach are all combined in this easy-to-read book.

This useful resource is like an encyclopedia of understanding how to manage every aspect of treating cancer.

Dr. Van Overbruggen answers the questions every patient wants to know. He chooses to inform rather than prescribing one particular solution.
A must-read for every complementary therapist and every cancer patient.

Arielle Essex
Essex is a certified NLP Master Practitioner and Trainer with a broad background that includes osteopathy, naturopathy, kinesiology and psychology. She used NLP techniques to heal her own brain tumour.

Karen Simonton : Carl Simonton and Dr. Wirga are very impressed

Hello Rob,
I have yet to get my hands on your book as Carl has loaned it out to many and several people have orded it on Amazon. He and Dr. Wirga are very impressed with it and have enjoyed it very much.
I understand you site the Simonton work! But do know that he recommends it hightly.
Carl is in Japan and leave Monday.

We will be recommending the book in our next newsletter that will go out sometime the end of April.
Kind Regards,
Karen SCC

Ann Fonda - Extremely useful

I carried this book throughout my 9-day journey in Germany, continually fascinated and intrigued by the information within. Due to a terrifically busy schedule I rarely read an entire book, but this one is packed with the most interesting and comprehensive stories, tips, and much more. It has made me focus more fully on the mind-body connection, and given me a much stronger basis for understanding. In my work as an advocate for people with cancer, this is going to be extremely useful.
Thank you for the experience.
Ann F.

President, The Annie Appleseed Project
www.annieappleseedproject.org
A 501(C)3 corporation

DGEIM - deren Bedeutung überhaupt nicht überschätzt werden kann

DGEIM - Deutsche Gesellschaft für Energetische und Informationsmedizin:
Kein ganzheitlicher Krebskongress kommt um die Feststellung herum: Krebsheilung ist nur von der Psyche aus möglich. Und wie geht das, was bietet man dem Patienten an? Unübersehbar ist bereits jetzt die Zahl der spirituellen, psychotherapeutischen, psychologischen, psychoonkologischen etc. etc. Therapieansätze, aber der Überblick geht verloren.

Hier bietet das Buch von Rob van Overbruggen eine Hilfe an, deren Bedeutung überhaupt nicht überschätzt werden kann, die einfach klingt und unendliche Mühe erforderte: er hat sich über alle Verfahren informiert, sie beschrieben, gesichtet, geordnet und z.T. beurteilt. Wer immer in der unübersehbaren Szene für sich oder seine Patienten einen therapeutischen Ansatzpunkt sucht (und wer kennt sich wirklich aus?), braucht dieses Buch.

Dr. med. Hendrik Treugut, Chefarzt am Klinikum Schwäbisch Gmünd und Präsident der Deutschen Gesellschaft für Energetische und Informationsmedizin (DGEIM).

CONTENTS

SECTION A: HEALTH AND HEALING 1

1   INTRODUCTION 3
        1.1   Preface. 6
        1.2   Personal Background 7
        1.3   About this Work 10
        1.3.1   Overview 12
        1.3.2   Inclusion & Exclusion 13
        1.4   My Invitation 15
        1.5   Notes to the Reader 18
        1.6   Acknowledgements. .18

2   HEALTH AND HEALING 19
        2.1   Healing versus Curing 20
        2.2   Specialization. 21
        2.2.1   Medical Paradigm. 21
        2.2.2   Psychological Paradigm. 22
        2.2.3   Psychosomatic Paradigm 23
        2.3   Mind-Body Connection. 25
        2.3.1   Psychosomatic Medicine. 27
        2.3.2   Influence of the Mind 30
        2.3.3   Psychotherapy. 31
        2.3.4   History of Mind and Cancer. 33

3   CANCER. 37
        3.1   Benign vs. Malignant 37
        3.1.1   Benign. 38
        3.1.2   Malignant 38
        3.2   Classification 39
        3.2.1   TNM 39
        3.2.2   Staging System 40
        3.3   Normal Cell Growth. 41
        3.3.1   Growth Rate 43
        3.4   The Cancer Process 44
        3.4.1   Mutation 44
        3.4.2   Development. 47
        3.4.3   Immune System 47
        3.4.4   Survival. 50

SECTION B: PSYCHOSOMATIC MODEL 53

4 THE MODEL. 55
   4.1 Introduction. 55
   4.1.1 Stress. 55
   4.2 Psychosomatic Model. .57
   4.3 Events 62
   4.3.1 Life Change Units (LCU) 63
   4.3.2 Life Events and Difficulties Scales (LEDS) 64
   4.4 Perception 65
   4.5 Appraisal. 66
   4.5.1 Beliefs 68
   4.5.2 Conscious vs. Unconscious Beliefs 70
   4.5.3 Positive Thinking .71
   4.6 Coping. 71
   4.6.1 Development of Coping 72
   4.6.2 Coping Styles. 73
   4.6.1 Classification. 74
   4.7 Emotions 75
   4.8 Behavior 75

5 CONNECTIONS TO CANCER 77
   5.1 Events 77
   5.1.1 Experience of Loss 79
   5.1.2 Discussion 81
   5.2 Appraisal. 82
   5.2.1 Personality Traits 82
   5.2.2 Primary Appraisal. 85
   5.2.3 Secondary Appraisal. 87
   5.3 Coping. 93
   5.3.1 Emotional Repression 94
   5.3.2 Anti-Emotionality 97
   5.3.3 Social Support 98
   5.4 Emotions 99
   5.4.1 Emotions 99
   5.4.2 Emotional Cysts 103
   5.4.3 Depression. 106

SECTION C: CURRENT PSYCHOLOGICAL CANCER
         TREATMENT PROGRAMS 109

6   CURRENT TREATMENT PROGRAMS 111
6.1   Simonton Program 111
6.1.1   Results 112
6.1.2   Goals 112
6.1.3   Interventions........................... 113
6.1.4   Key Alements of the Approach 114
6.1.5   Program 115
6.1.6   Spiegel Program 117
6.1.7   Results 118
6.1.8   Goals 118
6.1.9   Therapeutic Overview.................. 119
6.1.10   Key Elements of the Approach 120
6.1.11   Program 121
6.2   Autonomy Training Program 122
6.2.1   Results 122
6.2.2   Goals 122
6.2.3   Key Elements of the Approach 123
6.2.4   Program 123
6.3   Cancer as a Turning Point Program.......... 124
6.3.1   Results 124
6.3.2   Goals 124
6.3.3   Key Elements of the Approach 125
6.3.4   Program 125
6.4   Type C Transformation Program 126
6.4.1   Results 126
6.4.2   Goals 126
6.4.3   Key Elements of the Approach 126
6.4.4   Program 127
6.5   Other Programs.......................... 128
6.5.1   Wellness Community Program 128
6.5.2   Exceptional Cancer Patients (ECaP)
             Program 128
6.5.3   Commonweal Cancer Help
             Program (CCHP) 129
6.5.4   Mind/Body Medical Institute (MBMI)
             Program 129
6.5.5   Fawzy Psychosocial Group Therapy
             Program 130
6.6   Summary and Overview.................. 131

SECTION D: PSYCHOSOMATIC MODEL APPLIED TO CANCER
TREATMENT 133

7   INTRODUCTION 135
        7.1   Psychological Therapy 136
        7.1.1   False Hope 137
        7.1.2   Benefits of Psychological Therapy 140

8   THERAPY 143
        8.1   The Process 144
        8.1.1   Timing 144
        8.1.2   Therapeutic Goal 145
        8.1.3   Presuppositions 149
        8.1.4   Coping with Recurrence 149
        8.2   The Therapist 150
        8.2.1   The Therapist's Beliefs 151
        8.2.2   Relationship with Clients 153
        8.2.3   Death 154

9   WORKING WITH EVENTS 155
        9.1   Diagnosis 155
        9.1.1   Questionnaire 156
        9.1.2   Creative Listing 158
        9.2   Therapy 158
        9.2.1   Evasion 158
        9.2.2   Desensitization 159

10   WORKING WITH PERCEPTION 161

11   CHANGING THE APPRAISAL PROCESS 163
        11.1   Diagnosis 164
        11.1.1   Life Events 165
        11.1.2   Determined from Emotions 166
        11.1.3   List of Beliefs 166
        11.1.4   Behavior 168
        11.1.5   Imagery 168
        11.1.6   Pitfalls 174
        11.1.7   Healthy and Unhealthy Beliefs 175
        11.2   Therapy: Generic Appraisal Interventions ... 176
        11.2.1   Mapping Across Sub-modalities 177
        11.2.2   Rational Emotive Therapy (RET) 177
        11.2.3   Reframing 178
        11.2.4   Imagery 179
        11.2.5   Changing History 179
        11.2.6   Installing Useful Beliefs 181
        11.3   Therapy: Specific Appraisal Interventions ... 182
        11.3.1   Personality Traits 182

11.3.2   Primary Appraisal. 192

11.3.3   Secondary Appraisal. 208

11.3.4   Secondary Gain 224

12   EMOTION-FOCUSED COPING 233

12.1   Diagnosis 234

12.2   Therapy. 234

12.2.1   Emotional Expression 234

12.2.2   Anti-emotionality. 243

13   EMOTIONS 247

13.1   Diagnosis 249

13.2   Therapy: Generic Emotional Interventions . 249

13.2.1   Relaxation, Meditation, Hypnotic Trance 250

13.2.2   Physical Exercise 252

13.2.3   Selective Support System 253

13.3   Therapy: Specific Emotional Interventions . 254

13.3.1   Distressing Emotions 254

13.3.2   Comforting Emotions 259

SECTION E: DIRECT PSYCHOLOGICAL INFLUENCE ON PHYSIOLOGY 265

14   INTRODUCTION 267

15   INFLUENCING PHYSIOLOGICAL SYMPTOMS . . 269
15.1   Conditioning 269
15.2   Hypnotic Suggestions 271
15.2.1   "Towards" or "Away From" 272
15.2.2   Treatment of Warts 275
15.3   Communication with Symptoms 276
15.4   Imagery................................. 279
15.4.1   Types of Imagery 281
15.4.2   Elements of Imagery 285
15.4.3   Applications 289
15.4.4   Common Problems in Imagery 294

16   INFLUENCING PAIN 297
16.1   Imagery................................. 298
16.2   Communication with Pain 299
16.3   Secondary Gains from Pain................ 301
16.4   Creating Pleasure 302
16.5   Changing Focus 302
16.6   Hypnotic Pain Management 303

SECTION F: CONCLUSIONS AND RECOMMENDATIONS 305

17   RECOMMENDATIONS FOR FURTHER RESEARCH. 307
    17.1   Mind-Body Connection 307
    17.2   Psychological Markers of Cancer Clients 309
    17.2.1   Metaprograms 309
    17.2.2   Organ Language 310
    17.2.3   Combined Psychological Markers 312
    17.3   Specific Cancers 313
    17.4   Interventions 314
    17.4.1   Conditioning 314
    17.4.2   Hypnotic Suggestions 314
    17.4.3   Imagery 315
    17.4.4   Regression 317

18   CONCLUSIONS 319
    18.1   General Conclusions 319
    18.1.1   Psychotherapy Plays an Important Role in Cancer Treatment 319
    18.1.2   There is Much Information, But Less Hard Data 320
    18.1.3   One Should Use "Complementary" as a Descriptive Term 321
    18.1.4   There is Always Hope 322
    18.2   "Fundamental Image": A New Psychosomatic Model 322

19   ABOUT THE AUTHOR 327

APPENDIX 329
    Diagnostic Belief list 331
    Healthy Beliefs 333
    Imagery Scripts 335
    Healing Psyche Online Resources 337
    FREE Companying Audio Programs 339
    Bibliography 341

Section A

Health And Healing

1

Introduction

Personally, I remember that when I first heard the story of Mr. Wright, it had a great impact on me. Although the story is well-known, it has so much impact that it bears repeating. The following was reported by psychologist Bruno Klopfer.

Tumors That Melt Like Snowballs on a Hot Stove
Mr. Wright, a client of psychologist Bruno Klopfer in 1957, had far-advanced lymphosarcoma. All known treatments had become ineffective. Tumors the size of oranges littered his neck, armpits, groin, chest and abdomen. His spleen and liver were enormously enlarged. The thoracic lymph duct was swollen closed; and one to two quarts of milky liquid had to be drained from his chest each day. He had to have oxygen to breathe, and his only medicine now was a sedative to help him on his way.

Despite his state, Mr. Wright still had hope. He'd heard of a new drug called Krebiozen, which was to be evaluated at the clinic where he lay. He didn't qualify for the program, because the experimenters wanted subjects with a life expectancy of at least three, and preferably six, months. Wright begged so hard, however, that Klopfer decided to give him one injection on Friday, thinking he would be dead by Monday and the Krebiozen could be given to someone else. Klopfer was in for a surprise:

"I had left him febrile, gasping for air, completely bedridden. Now, here he was, walking around the ward, chatting happily with the nurses, and spreading his message of good cheer to any who would listen. Immediately I hastened to see the others...No change, or change for the worse, was noted. Only in Mr. Wright was there a brilliant improvement. **The tumor masses had melted like snowballs on a hot stove,** *and in only these few days, they were only half their*

original size! This is, of course, far more rapid regression than most radio-sensitive tumors could display under heavy X-ray given each day. And we already knew his tumors were no longer sensitive to irradiation. Also, he had had no other treatment outside the single useless "shot."

This phenomenon demanded an explanation, but not only that, it almost insisted that we open our minds to learn, rather than try to explain. So, the injections were given three times weekly as planned, much to the joy of the patient.....Within 10 days he was able to be discharged from his "deathbed," practically all signs of his disease having vanished in this short time. Incredible as it sounds, this "terminal" patient gasping for his last breath through an oxygen mask was now not only breathing normally, and fully active, he took off in his own plane and flew at 12,000 feet with no discomfort.

*Within two months, conflicting reports began to appear in the news, all of the testing clinicians reporting no results...This disturbed Mr. Wright considerably...He was... logical and disturbed in his thinking, and he began to **lose faith** in his last hope...After two months of practically perfect health, he relapsed to his original state and became very gloomy and miserable.*

But Klopfer saw an opportunity to explore what was really going on---to find out, as he put it, how quacks achieve some of their well-documented cures. (Remember, all healing is scientific.) He told Wright that Krebiozen really was as promising as it had seemed, but that the early shipments had deteriorated rapidly in the bottles. He told of a new super refined, double-strength product due to arrive tomorrow.

*The news came as a great revelation to him, and Mr. Wright, ill as he was, became his optimistic self again, eager to start over. By delaying a couple of days before the "shipment" arrived, his anticipation of salvation had reached a tremendous pitch. When I announced that the new series of injections were about to begin, he was almost ecstatic and **his faith was very strong**.*

With much fanfare, and putting on quite an act... I administered the first injection of the doubly potent, fresh preparation---consisting of fresh water and nothing more. The results of this experiment were quite unbelievable to us at the time, although we must have had some suspicion of the remotely possible outcome to have even attempted it at all.

*Recovery from the second near-terminal state was **even more dramatic** than the first. Tumor masses melted, chest fluid vanished, and he became ambulatory, and even went back to flying again. At this time he was certainly the picture of health. The water injections were continued, since they worked such wonders. He then remained **symptom-free for over two months**. At this time the final AMA* announcement appeared in the press: "Nationwide tests show Krebiozen to be a worthless drug in treatment of cancer."*

*   **Within a few days** of this report, Mr. Wright was readmitted to the hospital in extremis; his **faith was now gone**, his last hope vanished, and he **succumbed in less than two days**. [emphasis mine]*

*American Medical Association
Siegel (1986[1])

This story both shocked and awed me, and it still does when I contemplate the implications.

When I first heard this story, I was stunned, perplexed and didn't believe it, but my interest was born. From that moment on, I was tuned to the workings of the mind in relation to the cancer process.

Researchers are experimenting with meditation, imagination and biofeedback to align the parameters of the mind to assist in healing. This relatively new field, called PsychoNeuroImmunology (PNI), focuses on the mental and emotional effects on the immune system. Studies suggest that long-term, unresolved negative emotions weaken the immune system, while positive emotions strengthen the immune system.

Currently, no studies have scientifically proven that patients can control the course of their cancer with their mind. On the other hand, no study has scientifically proven that the course of their cancer cannot be influenced by the mind. There are many documented cases of patients who, against all odds, went into remission. The question if the attitude or mental state aided their healing cannot be answered scientifically. Science cannot deal with such mental aspects, because the human mind is not an entity that succumbs to the "Scientific Method", which, as one knows requires experimental repeatability, and rigorous standards of experimentation.

- What if we could find patterns among these remarkable cases, the patterns and structure of spontaneous remission?
- What would happen if the influence of the mind acted as the final blow to cancer already undergoing medical treatment?
- What would happen if it were possible to use the mind to influence the course of the disease, or even heal patients?

Simonton works with medically incurable patients, and has shown that half of these people were outliving the statistics after receiving psychological treatment in addition to medical treatment.

Example:
I was out of the country when my granddad (84) developed severe lung cancer. According to the doctor, he would die any minute. I immediately returned to my home country, even though the doctor said it was probably too late. I spent two weeks at home, and every day the doctor said that my grandfather would probably be dead by tomorrow. The two weeks I spent with him were great; we had a wonderful time. Every morning the doctor was surprised that my grandfather was not dead yet. As soon as I went abroad again, his condition got worse, and he died within a week.
He died 4 weeks after the first time the doctor said he would not live through the night. This is my personal experience with a man the doctor predicted would die on a specific day, who didn't listen to the doctor.
What caused him to continue living? And what happened that made his condition deteriorate so quickly after I left?

1.1   Preface

Faced with the diagnosis of cancer, patients enter an emotional roller coaster and come into contact with many different treatment methods and viewpoints. Many specialists arrive on the scene with advice on specific treatments ranging from medical treatments such as surgery, radiation and chemotherapy, but dietary restrictions and psychotherapy are also suggested. It all depends on the specialist at hand. For patients, the complexity increases. The multitude of options makes it hard to decide.

Besides medical treatments, there has been much development in the field of complementary treatments. A study published by the New England Journal of Medicine (1993[2]) showed that a third of American cancer patients now use complementary therapy, often without their physician's knowledge.

Complementary cancer therapy is a multibillion-dollar business lacking regulation and scientific evidence. Each day, we are bombarded by the media claiming to have the ultimate solution to cancer therapy. Sometimes it is a new medicine, a new radiation technology, dietary restrictions, meditation or psychotherapy. New mainstream and complementary therapies are invented and promoted on a daily basis. Some of these are based on scientific research, while others are based on a single case history.

Popular psychological literature is particularly given to propagating simple solutions to the complex cancer question. Some of these claims are hardly backed by any research. Many of the remarkable claims about mind-body effects are distorted, inflated or go far beyond what has been researched. Some studies have been fully adopted and complete therapies are based on a single case history. Other claims are based on a more solid scientific foundation. In this study, I would like to provide the scientific evidence on which many therapies are based.

Not all therapies can be underpinned in this way, but even without science knowing what is going on there are some miraculous things happening. The results of research and case histories cannot be denied. O'Regan et al. (1993[3]) collected over 1700 accounts of spontaneous remissions, the disappearance of a malignant tumor without a curative medical intervention. The story of Mr. Wright, whose tumors disappeared spontaneously, is probably the most famous. Several other cases of disappearing tumors were reported by Carl Simonton, Michael Lerner and Lawrence LeShan, to name only a few. Too many cases exist to dismiss them as hoaxes. There must be something of value in these cases.

"I have met with cases in which the connection appeared so clear that I have decided questioning its reality would seem a struggle against reason."
- Walter Hoyle Walshe -

1.2   Personal Background

My therapeutic education consists of Neuro Linguistic Programming (NLP) and hypnotherapy. While studying these fields and reading about all the ideas and historical works, I gradually changed many of my beliefs about what is possible and what is not. I used to believe that something has to be proven before it is true. This belief not only limited me in many ways, it is also absurd. The spectrum of human knowledge is only a very limited part of the full spectrum of reality. Reality is not created upon what has been proven. Reality is just "as is." To deny the potential reality of something just because one cannot devise a method of proof is a very narrow and false stance to take. My old belief gradually evolved to "Everything is true, unless proven otherwise." This new belief is scientifically just as correct (or incorrect) as the one I used to have, but it grants me more possibilities, and widens my view.

I also have a formal education in software engineering and mathematics, finding and creating patterns and, when something is not functioning properly, investigating the patterns to discover where the real cause lies. Fixing a software program is a complex issue. One needs to find the root cause, because when the fix is applied to the symptoms, the program becomes unstable and its overall behavior gets worse. The problem is hidden rather than eliminated, and other problems will be harder to detect and fix. When a possible root cause is found, one must ask oneself how it came about. Maybe there was a certain reason for the programmer to do it this way because it serves another, larger purpose.

After repairing the root cause, one needs to decide on the solution. The consequences for the rest of the system must be investigated. It could be that the solution creates problems in other areas of the program. Although it can take a lot of time and effort, debugging a piece of software is relatively easy. Technical systems can be reset into a default/normal state. When the end state is not what was expected, one can go through step-by-step from the initial state to the end state. This way, the bug can be tracked down.

Finding the root cause in the minds of people is much harder. There is no way of going through the mental processes one step at a time, and the mind cannot be reset to the initial state. This makes it hard to find causes in diseases (either mentally or physically). When we notice symptoms, we know there is something going on, but we cannot go back in time to discover all the changes in the mind and body.

When I first heard stories of people who were recovering spontaneously from cancer, I was interested. I wanted to find out how they recovered and how this could be applied to others.

When the symptoms disappear, we assume it is caused by the interventions, but we are not sure! It is a pretty good guess that the sudden disappearance of the symptoms is caused by the interventions, but we cannot be certain. Something else might also have caused the change. Reproducing the symptoms and applying the same interventions would allow us to conclude whether the interventions were the cause of the change or not.

Example:
I had a headache and ate a bar of chocolate, and 5 minutes later the headache was gone. I would then assume that the chocolate caused my headache to disappear.
In order to prove this, we need to prove several other things too.

Suppose we want to prove the assumption "Eating chocolate causes a headache to disappear in 5 minutes." For the sake of argument, we will call this assumption 1.

To validate assumption 1, we need to be sure that the headache would not disappear anyway in these 5 minutes. So, in order for assumption 1 to be true, assumption 2, "Not eating chocolate will cause the headache to disappear in 5 minutes," must be false.

The human body is in a constant state of change, so we can NEVER prove assumption 1 and assumption 2 with the same starting point. There is no way back. When my headache is gone, I cannot go back to the same state (i.e. the same headache) that I was in before I ate the chocolate. The only thing that can happen is that I get a similar headache, but there are always differences, even as small as the belief that "The previous time the chocolate worked."

Example:
The closest thing to the computer debugging process is systematic and statistical animal research in which animals are bred in such a way that they resemble each other as much as possible (cloning would be ideal, as their physiology would be the same). Then there is a need to systematically induce the headache, so that all the animals have the same headache. Finally, you could feed one animal the chocolate and feed the other nothing.
When measuring the headache, if ALL the mice that did not eat chocolate still have the headache, and NONE of the chocolate-eating

mice have a headache, you could reasonably conclude that "Eating
chocolate causes the headache to disappear," but only for that specific
headache, and only for mice.

The fact that physiology and psychology cannot be reset to their
initial state like a computer, together with the many variables inherent
in physiology, makes research into these areas very complex. Sometimes
these variables were not even considered to exist or have influence
before.

> **Example:**
> *In one case, there was an experimental setup consisting of two groups*
> *of mice. One group had medication administered and the other group*
> *did not. When the experiment was over, the conclusions were the*
> *opposite of what the researchers expected. They expected one group*
> *of mice to have certain results compared to the control group. They*
> *noticed that the results for that group were the opposite of what they*
> *expected. They had expected the health of the mice to deteriorate, and*
> *instead their health had improved.*
> *The researchers were investigating all the variables that could have*
> *caused the deviation, but could not find the cause. Finally, they noticed*
> *that the only difference was that the lab assistant for one group only*
> *fed the mice, while the assistant for the other group fed the mice and*
> *gave them attention and petted them for a while. The attention and*
> *petting by the assistant was shown to be the cause of their increase in*
> *health.*

An undefined number of variables and the inability to reset one's
physiology and psychology make it almost impossible to debug a person.
With my experience in finding patterns, I was able to combine many
scientific studies into a comprehensive whole.

1.3   About this Work

When I heard the story of Mr. Wright, I was very interested in
what had happened. The therapist in me wondered how I could use this
to aid people in their healing process. The software developer in me
wanted to find out what mental processes were running. My ultimate
goal was to find the patterns present with Mr. Wright, and then apply
these principles to cure cancer patients. In this regards I agree with
Walt Disney who said:

"It's kind of fun to do the impossible."
- Walt Disney -

With the help of psychotherapy, I wanted patients to be hopeful and fighting to regain their health. There is always hope of a spontaneous remission, which could be instigated by psychotherapy. Over the course of this study, I realized that increasing the quality of life of the patients was the ultimate goal.

During this process, the following questions came to mind:
- Why do some people die while others experience a spontaneous remission after the same diagnosis?
- What is the pattern of spontaneous remission?
- How important is the role of the mind in healing cancer?
- How can psychotherapy aid people in healing their cancer?
- Can psychotherapy induce spontaneous remission?
- What are the optimal therapeutic interventions for assisting cancer patients?

My desire to answer these questions prompted me to choose this as the subject of my study. The topic of my dissertation was easy, although much harder to realize than I had imagined. In retrospect, if I had known all this in advance, I might have chosen another subject. Writing this piece brought me a little closer to life and living, and became a truly personal development plan, in accordance with the rest of my efforts in life. I hope this study will contribute to an increase in the body of knowledge and acceptance of complementary psychological cancer treatment (CPCT), actual usage in therapy, and acknowledgement from the mainstream medical community.

The goal of my dissertation is to present an accessible, manageable and coherent model for therapists and patients that combines many insights from the field of complementary psychological cancer treatment (CPCT). This model includes the psychological elements of influence on the cancer process, and makes the subject of psychotherapy for cancer patients easy to understand.

This has led to the overall question of: "How can the therapeutic process be organized, and what elements does it contain to aid cancer patients in regaining health and well-being?"

1.3.1   Overview

This complementary study focuses on the psychological processes that could aid in healing. Elements of dietary and medical interventions are left out.

The study is divided into six sections:

Section A is an introductory section, explaining my views on health and healing and discussing the issue of cancer from a medical perspective. It also provides a more realistic notion of cancer. Cancer federations around the world are shifting their attention to life after cancer. Like the slogan of the Dutch Cancer Federation, "Cancer is not always the end," this section will focus on the reality of cancer and survival.

Section B discusses my psychosomatic model, which I based on Folkman's model and how it relates to cancer development. This model is used to provide the reader with an overview of the relationship between various psychological processes, and is used to structure the psychological elements. First I will explain the psychosomatic model, after which I will continue with the different components and how they relate to cancer development.

Section C discusses the most widely known complementary psychological cancer treatments and their elements of success.

Section D is about the therapeutic applications of the elements found in Section B. It provides guidelines for the therapeutic process, and will list interventions that have been used with cancer patients. These interventions are structured according to my psychosomatic model, as in Section B. This section also includes those psychological interventions that deal directly with symptoms, without going through the psychosomatic model.

Section E discusses several psychological interventions to directly influenced by the physiology of the client.

Section F presents my recommendations for further research and finally my conclusions.

1.3.2 Inclusion & Exclusion

Many researchers have studied the effects of specific psychological markers or psychological therapy on the progress of cancer. Some concluded that the intervention positively influenced the prognosis, while others concluded that there was no measurable effect. When researchers try to reproduce a study described by others, they do not always produce the same results. The most common conclusion that they reach is that the original study was flawed. This is only one of the conclusions that one can draw, and a limited one at that.

In his review of articles concerning psychological factors in cancer development, Garssen (2004[4]) concluded that most factors which were proven in studies present fundamental flaws in their research design.

The influences of the psychological factors are minimal. Although some studies show promising results, others fail to replicate the same conclusions.

When the reproduction does not yield the same results, other conclusions can also be drawn:
- The original study was wrong.
- The original description was not complete.
- The reproduction of the study was incorrect.

Spiegel (2002[5]) conducted a review of 10 studies on the effects of psychosocial interventions and survival time. Some of the studies concluded that survival time was enhanced, while others were unable to produce similar results. However:

> *"It is worth noting that there are no published trials that show that psychosocial intervention significantly shortens survival time. If the results of the ten trials were merely random variation, it would be expected that as many trials would show adverse effects on survival time as positive effects."*

Spiegel thereby concluded that it is never counterproductive to perform psychosocial interventions, and in half of the studies an improvement in survival time was indeed observed.

Example:
Suppose, for example, that a study is published stating that when a person jumps into a creek, they will become wet.

Someone else tries to reproduce the study and concludes that when a person jumps into a creek, they will not get wet every time. The result is conflicting.

If my wish is to get wet, the research is inconclusive, and I have no way of obtaining my goal. However, if I take a close look at the original study and do whatever they did, I have a good chance of achieving the desired results.

The most interesting question concerns the working elements of the original study. This is a fundamentally different approach. Instead of only looking at studies which are conclusive, I look at the studies that produced results. These successful studies are the most valuable in determining the elements that can be used with patients.

Working in this manner is all about how successes are created, and not about what hypothesis is true. I will not look at ways to prove or disprove a method, but how it can be used to create new successes. Instead of looking for the perfect therapy, I will look at different therapies and distill their successful interventions.

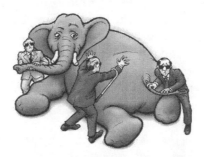

Example:
Six blind men are researching an object and describing it to each other. The first man describes it as "Much like a wall," the second says that it's "A lot like a spear," and others describe it as "Kind of like a snake," "Like a tree," "A lot like a fan," and "Similar to a rope." Based on their research of the object, they argued about who was right, and how the others could not be right.

In reality, they were all right, but only for the part they researched!

Some researchers promote active, aggressive fighting positions, while others advocate acceptance and denial. By combining all of these conclusions, one all-encompassing model can be developed. This model can be applied to therapeutic interventions. The therapist can decide which element to place the most emphasis on at a given time. The implications for this study are that I focused on those elements that have a proven relationship to cancer prognosis.

In the upcoming chapter on the development of cancer, I will discuss the surveillance theory. This theory is based on research showing that there are always some cancer cells present in the body. There is nothing that creates a first cancer cell; rather, the cancer is spread or contained by the body. Considering this, there is no need to make a distinction between research on the cause or the progression of cancer. Therefore, I will not differentiate between the psychological variables related to the cause or progression of cancer, as I have included both.

Social Support

Research on social support suggests that there is a strong connection between such support and the development of the disease. In my opinion, the working elements of social support have more to do with patients' beliefs and coping with their emotions than actually participating in a support group. One can have a strong social support network and still feel alone. On the other hand, one can have only one friend, and feel supported. It is not the social support that aids a person towards health, but the perception of support that is helpful. This perception can be worked through individually. This is why I devote little attention to social support. What I do explore in greater depth is how the translation is made from social support to the individual handling or requesting of support.

1.4   My Invitation

Like most adults, I am conditioned to expect certain things when I look. This conditioning restricts my perception and prevents me from looking objectively.

Example:
Take out 6 coins and put them in the order shown below.
You need to form 2 rows of 4 coins by only moving one coin.[6]

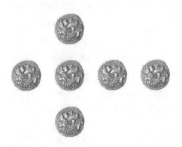

This illustrates that we are conditioned to look for a specific solution and that we often find it hard to think outside our preconceived notions. My conditioning (formal education) is in computer science, not medicine or psychology. I have no conditioned expectations about what is possible and what is not, and this is my strength. It allows me to think outside the paradigms of medicine and psychology.

Many people formally educated in one field or another cannot think outside their paradigm. Having accepted that a specific disease cannot be cured tends to limit their thinking. Possible cures are overlooked.

> *"When LeShan received a research grant in 1952 to start investigating if there were personality factors that could influence the presence and development of cancer , he heard a shocking and rather honest reply from one of the chief surgeons "Even if you prove it, I won't believe it"*
> *- Lawrence LeShan -*

Many miraculous cures are reported, and many people claim that they healed themselves by changing their attitude. Whether these claims are true or false is not the issue; the fact remains that they were sick and are now well. This was a result of their medication, a placebo, an attitude change or even prayer, but the bottom line is that these people are healthy again.

> *"Miracles happen, not just in opposition to nature, but in opposition to what we know of nature."*
> *- St Agustine -*

Such people did not fit into any theory about healing, so I think the theory on how cancer is healed should be changed to make room for the facts we have observed in spontaneous remissions.

Although it might seem trivial, one can observe this frequently. People heal spontaneously from certain conditions, which was not supposed to be possible. The conclusion is usually that the diagnosis was wrong, or that they are not really healed. In some way, the possibility that the person healed without knowing how is overlooked. This is an example of a fixed paradigm in which possible solutions are not recognized.

"When the facts do not concur with your model, change the model, not the facts."

One of the examples in this case is also the work of Einstein. In one of his calculations, he predicted an expanding universe and black holes. He came to a conclusion that was so absurd that it must be impossible. Something else must be going on. Years later, evidence of what Einstein had predicted was found, and he was forced to change his model to leave out the corrections he had made earlier to concur with his preconceived notions.

In science, there is a tendency to lose sight of plain observations. When people are cured from cancer without medical intervention, it is called spontaneous remission. These observations are real and should be studied intensively.

"You cannot scientifically prove that God exists, but you cannot prove that God doesn't exist either."

Some time ago, there were bold statements that almost nobody believed could be true, until they were proven right. This was the case, for example, with the statement that the earth was flat; that one could never run a mile in less than a minute; that no one can stand on the moon; that the earth is not the center of the universe, and many others.

The statement that the mind influences health was once just as bold. It is now becoming more widely accepted.

My invitation to you is: Wonder what could be possible!

1.5   Notes to the Reader

In this study, I speak of therapists when I am actually referring to all psychotherapists, hypnotherapists, life coaches, and people assisting clients psychologically with their healing processes. To keep this study readable, I use the male form when discussing clients; by no means am I implying only male clients. In the first sections, I will mention patients, and in the last ones I refer to them as clients. The rationale is discussed in the section on therapy.

The overall goal of this dissertation is to present a model which can be used as complementary therapy in addition to traditional medical treatment.

I am not a medical doctor, nor do I possess any specialized medical knowledge, therefore I cannot prove or even question the medical terms and theories that are discussed. This is not my focus of expertise, and this lack of expertise might be my strength in this case. If you are looking for specialized treatment, you will not find it here, as I am not a doctor. What you will find are some ideas on what a complementary psychologically-based treatment could look like.

In the event of any illness, always consult your physician and follow his or her advice.

1.6   Acknowledgements

I would like to thank the following people for assisting me in completing this work. First, I would like to thank Dr. Tad James for his inspiring training, which led me to study this topic. Dr. Alex Docker supported me in my research and the completion of this work. I would also like to thank the following people for supplying information and research papers: the Institute of Noetic Science for their complimentary copy of their work on spontaneous remissions; Dr. Spiegel for his therapeutic programs on breast cancer; Dr. Ephraim Lansky, Dr. Eveline Bleiker and the Helen Dowling Institute. In addition to these people, I would like to thank Hanny van Overbruggen for helping me to create structure and consistency. She helped me to make my work readable and comprehensible, and without her help I wouldn't be able to finish this. This was a large task, for which I am grateful. I would like to thank Tania Tate for correcting my English spelling and grammar throughout the process. There were many times when I just wanted to quit, but I am glad I pulled through.

2

Health And Healing

The word "health" originates from the Greek word *holos*, meaning "whole" or "complete." Healing therefore means to make whole again. It implies that something is "broken," which can be on the physical or mental plane.

The World Health Organization has defined health as follows:

"Health is a state of complete physical, mental and social well-being
and not merely the absence of disease or infirmity."
- World Health Organization – (1948[7])

This definition merits a closer look. The World Health Organization recognizes that health is not only a state of not being sick, but includes a mental and social state of well-being. Wholeness or health is not equal to being happy or living a life without pain or handicaps. Wholeness applies to the integration of physical, mental and social well-being, which can be fully achieved in the presence of a disease.

This study is about working towards health with psychological interventions. In this way, patients not only increase their health and well-being, but also grow as people. This is what Karl Menninger meant with his conclusion that patients who included psychological interventions to overcome their diseases became "weller than well." They not only overcame their diseases (physical), but grew psychologically and spiritually. These three aspects were geared towards well-being. During this process, patients learned valuable lessons for living and experienced more control over their destinies. This increased their feeling of well-being more than simply being cured of the disease.

2.1   Healing versus Curing

Depending on the area of expertise, someone is healed or cured. Curing is reserved for physicians, and healing is mostly used by complementary approaches. Healing and curing are often used interchangeably, but there are important distinctions.

Curing focuses on creating a physical state where disease is not present (or cannot be detected.) This is based on an outdated definition of health: "The absence of disease." Typical interventions remove all symptoms and evidence of the disease. This allows patients to extend their lifetimes, and to live just as happily and healthily as before the disease. Patients who are cured do not show symptoms, but they might not be at ease with the situation. People can be cured of a disease and still have trouble with it. An illustrative example of this is phantom leg pain. The actual leg is physically removed, and yet patients continue to have pain in that leg. They are cured but not healed.

Healing refers to becoming whole again. It is focused on creating wholeness where physical, mental, and social elements are in balance. When people are healed, they experience a heightened state of well-being. They experience a state of physical, mental and social well-being. A person who is healed might still display symptoms, but they feel healthy. In the definition of healing there is no reference to the absence of disease, but only to a state of well-being. This definition thus agrees with the current definition of the World Health Organization.

Example:
My grandmother's friend had all kinds of medical conditions, pains, ulcers and a heart condition. She walked funny and had to take 12 different medications a day. When asked how she felt, she replied: "I feel fine and healthy."

Another person had a slight cold. When asked how he felt, he said: "I feel sick."

Healing requires a different field of expertise than curing. Curing is focused on the physical body, and requires detailed medical knowledge. Healing takes place on the psychological, physical and spiritual planes. When struggling with a disease, people should make an effort to be cured and an effort to be healed.

2.2   Specialization

There have always been people who were specialized in healing others.

Up to the time of Hippocrates (460-370 BC), healing was a combination of science and rituals. When Hippocrates founded western medicine, his assumption was that "Nature is the healer of disease." He was convinced that health could only be present in those people whose minds were in balance. A healthy body can only exist with a healthy mind.

With the advancement of science, people began specializing. Some people were more concerned with the body, while others were more concerned with the mind.

In reality, no clear distinction can be made between body and mind, but for the sake of clarity I will discuss them separately and in extremes.

2.2.1   Medical Paradigm

Science in western cultures evolved with research into the anatomical composition of the physical body. Scientists investigated an object that was broken down into many other sub-objects. With the use of autopsies, researchers discovered the different parts of animals and humans and what their functions were. We are now able to identify all parts of the body. We know how a healthy part looks, and can identify a diseased or malfunctioning part.

The human body consists only of a limited set of parts that work together. Nothing else comprises the body. If one part is malfunctioning, it needs to be cut out, replaced or fixed, just like any machine would be repaired. The body metaphorically represents a machine. Patients are also just a set of parts. This paradigm is still present in present-day medical practices. Medical students are schooled in those parts of the body.

Example:
Extending this paradigm, it would be possible for us to bring our body to the "body shop," go shopping and come back to pick it up when it is fixed.

A disease can be seen as a car with bad tires. Most people bring the car to the garage to have it fixed.

This primary focus on the body led to the alarming development of doctors treating their patients in an objective manner. The person is objectified. There is a body that needs to be fixed. If the disease cannot be cured with the interventions at hand, the person is considered to be having "complications" or "bad luck." The procedure is correct, but for some mysterious reason it doesn't catch on. People who are cured without medical interventions are assumed to be falsely diagnosed or not cured at all. Within this paradigm, there is no room for other healing practices besides the known medical interventions.

Example:
A disease can be seen as a car with bad tires.
Medical paradigm: People bring the car to the garage to have it fixed, and have new tires put on.

2.2.2   Psychological Paradigm

While some people began specializing in the workings of physiology, others specialized in psychology, or people. Psychology and psychiatry were born. Practitioners in this field are mainly concerned with the psychological state of well-being without worrying about the physiology.

The development of psychology is more recent than medicine. Before 1800, there was barely any consistent psychological research. The serious science of psychology started around 1850. In the early years, the primary focus was on gaining basic knowledge. Interventions for psychotherapy were being developed. Psychological interventions or theories that could deal with physical illness were not taken seriously, and were discarded.

Descartes concluded in the seventeenth century that the mind and body were separate entities and should be treated separately (this was called "the Cartesian Split"). Medical doctors worked with physical ailments. Psychologists or psychiatrists worked with mental ailments.

In the beginning of the 20th century, scientists discovered that there was a relationship between the mind and the body. Numerous observations linked psychological states to physical illnesses. Scientists were convinced that the mind could influence the body. Although the mind was considered totally separate from the body, the two did influence each other. Without detailed knowledge, this conclusion led to interesting quotes.

> *"Persons, who, during a small-pox epidemic, are in constant dread of "catching" the disease, are extremely liable to contracting the disease upon exposure. Abundant proof of this has been furnished. The mind has been so concentrated upon the subject and upon the symptoms of the disease that there exist no longer resistive powers."*
> *- WM. Wesley Cook (1901), A.M. M.D.-*

The lack of specific psychological interventions to help people limited the researchers in their efforts to gain more insights into how the mind and body were interconnected.

With new research, a new paradigm arose: the psychological paradigm. It assumes that a physiological ailment is purely psychological. The initial paradigm considers some physical ailments as being a manifestation of a psychological conflict. Based on these notions, the quote "Mind over body" became popular. The mind is stronger than the body.

Example:
A disease can be seen as a car with bad tires.
Psychological paradigm: The driver is investigated regarding his/her driving style.

2.2.3   Psychosomatic Paradigm

Now there are two incompatible paradigms. The psychological paradigm uses psychological interventions to alleviate physical symptoms, and the medical paradigm uses biological interventions to alleviate the same symptoms. These paradigms led to many controversial discussions. Instead of appreciating what the other viewpoint has to offer, many discussions were going on about who was right! Both the medical and psychological paradigms fight for their truth, and yet neither are completely correct.

> *"The more that is being discovered about psychosomatic diseases, and in general about the extremely complex two- way traffic between the brain and the rest of the body, the more obvious it has*

become that too rigid a distinction between mind and body is of only limited use of medical science, in fact can be hindrance to its advancement."
- Nikolas Tinbergen -

This fight gave birth to a new paradigm that combined the medical and psychological viewpoints. This psychosomatic paradigm assumes that the medical paradigm and the psychological paradigm are correct. The body is considered an integrated system of psychological and physiological processes that fit together like a jigsaw puzzle. When one piece is missing, the entire puzzle ceases to function properly.

Example:
When considering the bad tires on the car:
Psychosomatic medicine would recommend bringing the car in for new tires, and at the same time going to driving school to learn better driving techniques.

In this combination of the human body and mind, it would be illogical to say that everything is caused by the mind. This would ignore the body. It would be equally illogical to say that everything is caused by the body, because that would ignore the mind.

"The mind influences the body and the body influences the mind. You need to treat the whole person in order to achieve healing."

	Medical	**Psychological**	**Psychosomatic**
Considered cause	Body	Mind	Body-Mind interaction
Interventions	Biological	Psychological / Social	Biological and Psychological / Social
Patient's Involvement	None	Maximum	Maximum
Treatment	Fixing body	Fixing mind	Fixing the body and the mind

Table 1: Medical-Psychological-Psychosomatic paradigm

Sometimes symptoms are caused by a broken part, and sometimes by the entire system. When the part is broken, one should replace or repair it. When the system is tuned incorrectly, one must retune it with a medical intervention, a psychological intervention, or both.

Example:
If I break my leg, I will have it fixed by a physician so it can heal.
If I have an infection, I take antibiotics. If I suffer from depressive
feelings, I will visit a psychotherapist. However, if my leg is not healing
the way it should, or I have a disease physicians cannot explain with
a "broken part theory," then I will seek help somewhere else.

Physicians are specialists in the workings of the body; unfortunately, not all are specialists in communication or in handling emotions. There should be a team of specialists working towards health, including a medical staff and a psychological staff. This team must work together to promote health. This ensures that the specialists work in their area of expertise and leave the other areas to other experts.

"In a tight election, 10% can make all the difference in the world."
- Ken Wilbur -

Temoshok (1992[8]) explains that when the psychological component in healing is only a small fraction of the entire healing process, it could make the difference between health and disease. It is therefore worthwhile to investigate.

Example:
In almost every house, there is a multitude of chemicals present to clear and do all kinds of specific tasks. These chemicals are designed to be used in a specific way. In and of themselves, they are relatively harmless, but mixed in the right combinations and amounts; they could form dangerous combinations and even explosives.
Only when mixed properly, and with all the right elements, is the mixture dangerous. If we leave one element out, the mixture remains harmless.
The reaction between all elements is what it makes it explosive.

2.3 Mind-Body Connection

Making a separation between mind and body is useless, as no disease can be termed as solely physical or solely mental. The body affects the mind and the mind affects the body, and vice-versa (The National Institutes of Health 1995[9]). Activities that seem solely physical, such as walking, massage, dance or sports, have been proven to have healthy effects on the body as well as the mind. Some activities that seem solely psychological, such as meditation, imagery and suggestion, have proven to have healthful effects on the body as well. The thoughts and emotions that one has influences one's physical well-being. The fitness of the body also influences one's psychological well-being.

Researchers in biofeedback have demonstrated that every physiological process can be controlled with volition. Autonomous bodily reactions can be measured and the subject can learn to influence them. Subjects were connected to a monitor that measured their heart rate, for example. They noticed that certain thoughts influenced their heart rate. They only had to repeat the thoughts to influence their heart rate, and were thus able to control it. Other reported changes involved muscle tension, sweating and skin temperature.

Example:
Like children learning what happens when they press the remote control for the TV, and discover that a certain button corresponds to a certain reaction. A certain thought also corresponds to certain reactions by the body.

Green et al. (1977[10]), pioneers in the field of biofeedback, have reported incidents where people where even able to control the activity of a single nerve cell.

"Every change in the mental emotional state, conscious or unconscious, is accompanied by an appropriate change in the physiological state and conversely."
- Elmer Green and Alyce Green-

Example:
Think clearly and most vividly about a piece of lemon, the color, the structure, the juices flowing out... and now take a big bite....
Most people experience changes in their saliva production.

Mind and body cannot be separated and their communication seems instantaneous. As soon as there is a psychological change, a physical change can also be observed, and vice-versa. Based on the work of David Bohm in quantum mechanics, I came to the conclusion that the mind and body are not interconnected, but in fact are just different manifestations of the same thing. The mind is just one aspect of the whole, just as the body is one aspect of the whole. Change the whole and both will be different.

Example:

The images below (W.E. Hill, 1915) illustrate the interconnectedness. There is an old woman and a young lady visible in the image. Depending on your preferences and conditioning you see either one of them (but you can change focus to see the other).

When you take a pencil and change the image of the young woman, the image of the old woman changes at the same time (on the right). They cannot be changed independently of each other.

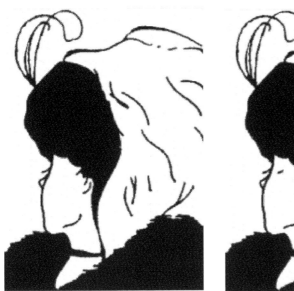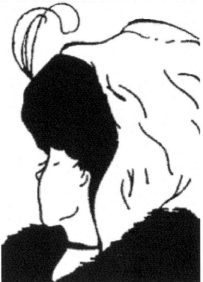

"The human body is the best picture of the human soul"
- Ludwig Wittgenstein -

2.3.1 Psychosomatic Medicine

Psychosomatic medicine often comes to mind when people discuss the issues of mind and body healing. It started out as a proper descriptive term of the connection between psyche and soma (body). The actual medical definition is a "disorder which persists in the absence of organic pathology." A psychosomatic disorder is where the broken "part" cannot be found. The symptoms and the distress of the patients are real. The disease is real. The only issue is that the specialists haven't found an organic cause. The absence of an organic cause often led to the false conclusion that "It is all in the patient's head" or it is not real. The treatment often consisted of the advice to "stop whining." The symptoms were often disregarded and diagnosed as an imagined illness.

The inability to find an organic cause does not make the disease less real.

Example:
I feel dizzy because I have been turning around very fast in a merry-go-round. Nobody can find the cause of the dizziness by examining my body; however, it is real and it bothers me.

"Psychosomatic" actually implies that the pain and distress are real, and that it could have a psychological origin or is amplified by psychological stress.

Tension and anxiety tend to leave stomach acid in the stomach longer because of the sympathetic activity of the nervous system. When this acid stays too long in the same place, it affects the stomach lining. A compromised stomach lining is one of the factors that could aid an ulcer in its development. The physical elements caused the ulcer. Tension and anxiety caused the acid to stay in the stomach for a prolonged period of time. The ulcer is real. The symptoms are physiological but the cause is partly psychological.

The following case, written up in "Mind as a Healer, Mind as a Slayer" by Kenneth Pelletier, gives a clear example of how a physiological problem can be caused by psychological issues.

Example:
"This pattern is illustrated by the case of a young physician who was admitted to a psychosomatic-medicine clinic presenting symptoms of extreme muscular tension in the neck, back, and buttocks. Pain from this tension had become so great that the patient was unable to sit down on anything other than a very soft cushion. After a period of therapy involving clinical biofeedback, it became evident that during the process of breathing the physician would thrust his shoulders forward just prior to exhalation and thrust them back immediately before inhalation. This bellows motion created a great deal of

unnecessary tension in his back muscles, which radiated upward into the neck muscles and downward into the buttocks and quadriceps. In the course of therapy the patient became aware of his unusual manner of breathing, and remembered that at age fourteen he had been punched in the stomach by his father and tried to recover his breath by flexing his shoulders in this bellows like fashion. Under the circumstances, the maneuver worked very well. However, after the incident and into adulthood, every time the young man was under stress he would automatically shift into the bellows breathing pattern, and the results were deleterious. This manner of breathing no longer produced the desired end of helping him catch his breath and ultimately relax; the effect was just the opposite. This behavior contributed to his anxiety by increasing the tension in the muscles of his back, and what was once a perfectly functional response had become chronically dysfunctional. In effect, an expedient positive choice became an increasingly negative behavior, leading to extreme tension. In therapy the young physician came to realize his responsibility, and in a relatively short period of time was able to rectify the dysfunctional way of breathing by substituting a normal respiration pattern."
(Pelletier 1992[11])

Many researchers agree that there are psychological factors of importance in the causes of high blood pressure, heart attack, migraine, headaches and certain skin disorders. The diseases are real and observable. The psychological processes simply initiate the diseases or make the symptoms worse.

> *"The question is not if the mind modulates in healing, but how we can deploy the mind to aid healing."*

Psychological intervention cannot cure the disease, for example, but it can be helpful in addition to other treatments.

Example:
- *Taking tennis lessons is no guarantee that you will win that championship, but it surely helps.*
- *Finishing a university degree is no guarantee that you will find a job, but it surely helps.*
- *Laughing will not guarantee that your illness will be gone, but it is more fun than being depressed, and it surely helps.*

2.3.2 Influence of the Mind

There are many examples in our daily lives where we can recognize that our mind influences our physiology. Getting sexually aroused is a mental state that has many physiological effects. Most heart attacks are on Monday mornings when the new work week starts. People tend to get sick when there is "time to get sick." Small business owners do not get sick unless they are on holiday. These are only a few of the many examples in our day-to-day lives where our mindset influences our body.

Cohen et al. (1991[12]) published a study in which the direct link between the mental state and the susceptibility to the common cold virus became apparent. In this study, they injected subjects with 1 of 5 different strains of the cold virus or a dummy. As they expected, some of the subjects contracted the cold while others did not. Statistically, the risk of getting ill was directly related to the amount of stress they had experienced in the past year. Stress was the only determining factor in getting ill.

Research has proven beyond any level of doubt that changes in the mental state are always accompanied by changes in physiology. There is no longer any debate on this. The debate has shifted to the extent to which the mind influences the body, and to what extent psychological interventions are helpful in healing physiological diseases. In PsychoNeuroImmunology (PNI), there is proof that the immune system can be conditioned. The debate now concerns whether the mind can influence the immune system *enough* for a disease to evolve or a healing to occur. Ader, one of the leading experts and founders of PsychoNeuroImmunology (PNI), says that the reaction of the scientific community towards PNI shifted from "It is impossible" to "We knew it all along." This shift followed the path of truth as defined a long time ago by the philosopher Schopenhauer.

"All truth passes through three stages. First, it is ridiculed. Second, it is violently opposed. Third, it is accepted as being self-evident."
- Arthur Schopenhauer -

Dramatic examples of how the mind and body influence each other come from the field of Multiple Personality Syndrome. Although discussing Multiple Personality Syndrome (or Dissociative Identity

Disorder, as it is called nowadays) is outside the scope of this work, it does illustrate the dramatic effects and the speed at which the mind-body connection functions (more on this subject is discussed in the section on research recommendations).

Example:
After a change in mindset, researchers reported a change:
- *In dosages of tranquilizer for it to have an effect.*
- *In dosages of anesthetic to get the patient "under."*
- *From drunk to sober.*
- *In allergic reactions.*

Understanding the healing power of the mind is one of the most fascinating fields in human performance today. We know from many research projects in the fields of hypnotherapy, psychoneuroimmunology, meditation, biofeedback, and many others that the mind is capable of doing extraordinary things. Understanding and utilizing this power may be the key to solving the riddle of "incurable diseases."

"When I examine myself and my methods of thought, I come to the conclusion that the gift of fantasy has meant more to me than my talent for absorbing positive knowledge."
- Albert Einstein -

2.3.3   Psychotherapy

Psychotherapy is derived from the Greek words meaning "Healing the soul," meaning to heal the mental and emotional "parts" of clients. This is not the only application of psychotherapy. Mind and body are one system and psychotherapy can be a valuable intervention to complement the traditional treatments.

Psychological treatment has indirect effects on physical health as well. Researchers already know that stress suppresses the body's ability to protect itself. What they now suspect is that the coping skills that psychologists teach may actually boost the immune system's strength. In one well-known study, for example, patients with advanced breast cancer who underwent group therapy lived longer than those who did not. Research also suggests that patients who ask questions and are assertive with their physicians have better health outcomes than patients who passively accept proposed treatment regimens.
APA (1997[13])

Eysenck (1991[14]) compared survival times after different types of interventions. When no medical or psychological intervention was performed, the median survival time was 11 months for women with advanced breast cancer. When there was only a chemotherapy intervention, the median survival time increased to 14 months. A median survival time of 15 months was reported when the only intervention was psychotherapy based on the methods of Grossarth-Maticek (1985[15]; 1995[16]). However, when receiving chemotherapy and psychotherapy, the median survival time increased to 22 months, almost a third longer than a single medical or psychological intervention. They concluded that psychological intervention was effective due to the involvement of the immune system in the healing process.

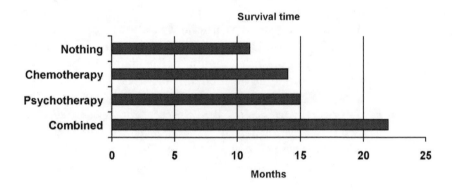

Table 2: Survival Times with Different Therapies

Healing should be a team effort involving medical and psychological experts. As Eugene Pendergrass told the American Cancer Society:

Presentation:
Now, finally, I would like to leave you with a thought that is very near to my heart. Anyone who has had extensive experience in the treatment of cancer is aware that there are great differences among patients...
I personally have observed cancer patients who have undergone successful treatment and were living and well for years. Then an emotional stress, such as the death of a son in World War II, the infidelity of a daughter-in-law, or the burden of long unemployment, seemed to have been precipitating factors in the reactivation of their disease which resulted in death... There is solid evidence that the course of disease in general is affected by emotional distress... Thus,

we as doctors may begin to emphasize treatment of the patient as a whole as well as the disease from which the patient is suffering. We may learn how to influence general body symptoms and through them modify neoplasm which resides within the body. As we go forward in this unrelenting pursuit of the truth to stamp out cancer... searching for new means of controlling growth, both within the cell and through systemic influences, it is my sincere hope that we can widen the quest to include the distinct possibility that within one's mind is the power capable of exerting forces which can either enhance or inhibit the progress of this disease.
(Pendergrass 1959[17])

In cases of physiological symptoms, psychotherapy is viewed as a supplement to traditional medicine. Cancer, for example, is a physiological disease which can be treated very well with traditional medicine in most cases. Psychotherapy can aid patients during the healing process.

In the literature, additional therapies are usually called alternative or complementary therapies. It is important to make a distinction between these two. An alternative is to use something "instead of" something else. Although some practitioners work this way, I strongly disagree. True healing occurs with medical and psychological interventions, not just one or the other. Healing is the integration of psychological and physiological health and well-being.

Complementary therapy (not to be confused with complimentary = free of charge) is a much better description. This indicates that it is used in addition to other therapies. Traditional medicine is accompanied by psychological treatment. Both work at the same time to assist patients.

2.3.4   History of Mind and Cancer

Reports about the connection between cancer and the mind date back a long time. Prior to 1900, the common thought was that cancer was very much influenced by the mind. Reports from that era are illustrative of the general thinking, but lack psychological interventions and details. Between 1900 and 1950, things were pretty quiet in this area of investigation. Scientists focused on medical interventions and made tremendous progress with that. Around the 1950s, more research became available on the additional psychological issues that might play a role in the development of cancer.

Bahnson (1980[18]) reported that the first known connection between the psyche and the development of cancer was made by Galen (130 AD). In his work "De Tumoribus" Galen noticed that breast cancer was more common in depressed women than in cheerful women.

Women who experienced serious depression and high levels of anxiety had, according to Gendron, a higher probability of cancer. He noticed that cancer occurred in those people who experienced "disasters in life," such as much trouble and grief. He wrote up the following case:

> *Example:*
> *"Mrs. Emerson, upon the Death of her Daughter, underwent Great Affliction, and perceived her Breast to swell, which soon after grew Painful; at last broke out in a most inveterate cancer, which consumed a great Part of it in a short Time. She had always enjoyed a perfect state of health."*
> *(Gendron 1759[19])*

Burrows (1783[20]) was convinced that cancer was caused by chronic stress: "...the unease and passions of the mind with which patients are strongly affected for a long time..."

Nunn also connected the development of cancer to the patient's emotional state.

> *Example:*
> *"With a shock to her nervous system caused by the death of her husband. Shortly thereafter, the tumor again increased in size and the patient died."*
> *(Nunn 1822[21])*

Walter Hoyle Walshe (1846[22]) concluded: "There is a connection between cancer and the influence of mental misery, sudden reverse in fortune and habitual gloominess of temper." He believed that cancer was caused by genetic predisposition and long-term psychological stress. Amussat (1854[23]) attributed cancer to the appearance of grief. Willard Parker (1855[24]) wrote about his 53-year experience as a surgeon operating on breast cancer. He concluded that grief and great mental depression play an important role in the development or growth of cancer.

Sir James Paget (1870[25]) wrote in Surgical Pathology:

> *"The cases are so frequent in which deep anxiety, deferred hope and disappointment are quickly followed by the growth and increase of cancer that we can hardly doubt that mental depression is a weighty additive to the other influences favoring the development of the cancerous constitution."*
> *- Sir James Paget -*

Watson (1871[26]) believed that both genetic predisposition and mental stress were highly influential in the cancer process.

> *"Great mental stress has been assigned as influential in hastening the development of cancerous disease in persons already predisposed. In my long life of experience, I have so often noticed this sequence that I cannot but think the imputation is true."*
> *- Sir Thomas Watson-*

Snow (1893[27]) noticed that 156 of 250 patients reviewed with cancer of the mammary or uterus had experienced trouble, such as the loss of a near relative. Snow (1893[28]) also agreed that the incidence of the connection of cancer to depression was much too common to be a coincidence. He wrote:

> *"...malignant disease of the breast and uterus follows immediately antecedent emotion of a depressing character..."*

Evans (1926[29]) concluded, in her study of one hundred patients, that many patients lost or disrupted a major relationship that was very emotional prior to the development of cancer.

The general tendency in those days was to think that there was no doubt that emotional life history plays a major role in the development of cancer.

3

Cancer

Before I continue to explore the psychological issues of cancer, I would like to discuss some physiological issues.

Cancer is not a single disease; it is a category of diseases with certain commonalties. Cancer consists of more than 200 different diseases. Each disease has its own symptoms, its own prognosis and its own treatments, and yet they are all called cancer. The symptom that they all have in common is an uncontrolled growth of abnormal cells.

It occurs in different types of people, of different races and at different ages. There are no vaccinations, and no proven preventive methods. Cancer can be diagnosed in almost any organ or tissue in the body.

The real cause of cancer is still unknown, but related factors have been identified.

- Smoking is connected with lung cancer, but not all smokers get lung cancer, and not all lung cancer patients are smokers.
- Spending too much time in the sun is connected to skin cancer, yet not all people who spend long periods of time in the sun will develop skin cancer. Others who have not spent so much time in the sun have developed skin cancer.
- Being exposed to asbestos is connected to cancer, yet not all people who are exposed at the same level develop cancer. Some get cancer without being exposed.

3.1 Benign vs. Malignant

The reproduction of cells is a normal and healthy process that takes care of growth in the body and repair of damaged tissue. Reproduction is carefully monitored so that it only takes place when needed. When there is a cut in the skin, the body begins reproducing skin cells to repair the cut. The reproduction stops when the skin is repaired.

A cancerous cell reproduces continuously, without stopping. After a while, there are so many cells in that specific area that they form a lump that can be felt. However, not all of these lumps are dangerous tumors.

3.1.1   Benign

Benign tumors are lumps that have been created by an accumulation of cells; however, the multiplication has stopped and they are contained. Contained lumps are harmless, and usually require no intervention. Examples of such benign tumors include moles, freckles and fatty lumps in the skin. They always remain in the same place, and do not spread or destroy other tissue. They have well-defined borders and present no danger.

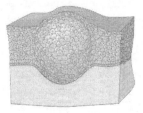

Figure 1: Benign Tumor[30]

3.1.2   Malignant

Malignant tumors are lumps of cells that do not stop reproducing. They are not contained, and have no defined borders. These tumors are called cancer. The abnormal growth eventually begins pressing against other organs and interfering with vital bodily functions. If the growth does not stop, it will eventually block many vital functions.

These malignant tumors have three characteristics:
- They spread and invade surrounding tissue.
- They have no borders.
- They have the ability to spread to other parts of the body, where they could form a new tumor (metastasize).

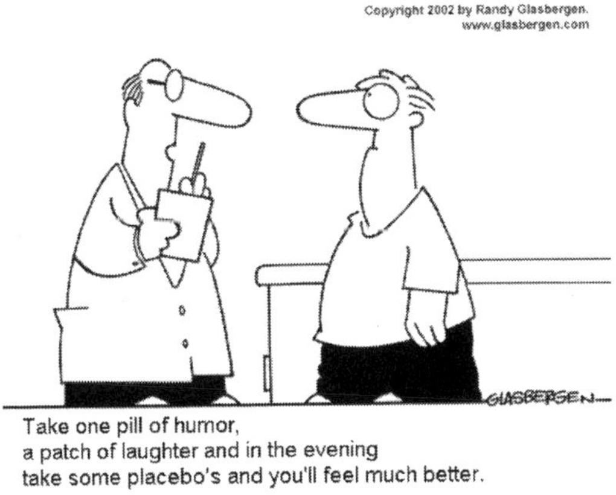

Copyright 2002 by Randy Glasbergen.
www.glasbergen.com

Take one pill of humor,
a patch of laughter and in the evening
take some placebo's and you'll feel much better.

Figure 2: Malignant Tumor[31]

These types of lumps are dangerous because:

- They overcrowd other cells so that they cannot perform their functions.
- They steal nutrients from other cells. The other cells die of starvation.
- They intrude upon organs and reproduce themselves from within those organs. Eventually, the organs are replaced by the cancer.
- They press against nearby organs and tissue, thus inhibiting their functions.

3.2   Classification

In order to define the current state of a tumor, several classification codes have been developed. A classification code provides a common terminology for the different stages of cancer, making discussions about proper treatment and prognosis possible.

The two most commonly used systems are the TNM (Tumor, Nodes, and Metastasis) and staging systems. TNM is a very complex system, with many different categories. The staging system groups the TNM categories into stages. This leads to a more comprehensive (and therefore less detailed) system.

3.2.1   TNM

The TNM (Tumor, Nodes, and Metastasis) system is the most commonly used classification. It consists of three separate values combined into one code. The T stands for the size of the tumor, whether it is large or small. The N stands for the number of lymph nodes affected. The M indicates whether or not the cancer has metastasized to other areas. The higher the number, the more serious the cancer.

Tumor
- T0 means that there is no tumor, or the entire tumor has been cut out.
- T1 indicates the smallest tumor size.
- T4 indicates the largest tumor size, which may have set roots in nearby organs or tissues.

Nodes
- N0 means that nearby lymph nodes are tumor-free.
- N1-3 indicates an increase in the number and location of affected nodes.

Metastasis
- M0 means that no metastasis has been found.
- M1 indicates that metastasis has been detected.

This system seems quite simple, but is actually a bit more complex because the classifications differ for each type of tumor. Depending on the location of the cancer, a size of 3/4" indicates a large or small tumor. The same size might be classified as a T3 (large tumor) if the tumor is found in one specific location, while the same tumor size in another location might be classified as a T1, or very small tumor.

Example:
Breast Cancer:
- *$T^1N^0M^0$ is a small tumor, with no affected lymph nodes and no metastasis.*
- *$T^2N^1M^0$ is a fairly large tumor affecting some lymph nodes, but there is no metastasis.*

3.2.2 Staging System

This system is easier to use because it groups several TNM categories into one stage. Four stages have been defined. The higher the stage number, the more serious the cancer. For each cancer location, the possible TNM values have been grouped in such a way that Stage 0 is harmless, while Stage IV is very serious. Each stage consists of multiple TNM values.

The staging system is easier to use in communication, and for recognizing the seriousness of the patient's condition.

Example:
Breast Cancer:
- *Stage I: $T^1N_0{}^oM^o$*
- *Stage II: $T^oN^1M^o$ or $T^1N^1M^o$ or $T^2N^oM^o$*

Lung Cancer:
- *Stage I: $T^1N^oM^o$ or $T^2N^oM^o$*
- *Stage II: $T^1N^1M^o$ or $T^2N^1M^o$*

3.3   Normal Cell Growth

When the sperm cell meets the egg cell, they merge to form a single cell at the moment of conception. If we define this cell as human, this is a one-celled human being.

This single cell contains all the information needed to grow into a human being featuring millions of cells and thousands of different types of cells. Every single cell in the human body is developed from that one cell.

This cell divides, creating two identical cells with exactly the same genes. These basic cells are called stem cells. The time it takes for one cell to divide is called doubling time. In this phase of human development, every cell division creates an exact duplicate. This process of cell division will continue for a while to form a cluster of cells called a blastocyst.

After a while, these stem cells activate certain genes. Some cells activate the specific genes for the nervous system. These cells will grow into nerve cells. Other stem cells activate the specific genes for the skin. These cells will grow to form skin cells. The differentiation of cells begins. Just as clay can be shaped into any kind of sculpture with the right actions, stem cells can be made to form any kind of cell by activating the right genes.

All of the information present in the stem cells is also available in the specialized cells. These specialized cells continue to multiply until they form the fully grown organ.

Example:
An analogy for this process could be a typewriter. The typewriter is the original stem cell, which contains all of the information, or DNA (keys). What comes out depends on which keys are pressed. When a specific set of keys is pressed, a word is formed. When you activate other keys, another word appears. The potential of the typewriter is unlimited; it all depends on which keys are activated.

From the moment of conception, the cells begin multiplying rapidly. This happens so quickly that one cell forms an entire human child in a period of only 9 months. This is a highly complex and perfectly orchestrated process. For the next 15 to 17 years or so, the human organism will continue to grow.

When the organism is damaged, it repairs the damaged tissue through the use of cell division. The body quickly begins to create new replacement cells. Rapid cell growth is a normal function we need to develop as an organism. Without it, we would not be able to grow into an adult, or repair our body quickly enough for the survival of the organism.

In addition to developing and repairing itself, the body also replaces old cells. By replacing old cells, the body remains in a constant state of renewal. The old cells die and are replaced by new ones. This is like rebuilding a house by removing one brick and replacing it before going to the next brick. Most of this renewal takes place within one year. A year from now, your body will be almost entirely replaced by new cells that did not exist a year ago. It takes 30 days to replace the entire skin, and every six weeks the liver is replaced.[32] The body is never the same as it was some time ago.

"You cannot step into the same river twice."
- Heraclitus-

When the body is fully grown, all damage has been repaired, and old cells have been replaced, the division of cells stops. It stops just as quickly as it started when there was damage to be repaired. It almost seems like there is an on-off switch for cell division.

When cancer develops, cells continue to divide without stopping.

The switch seems to be stuck, or something "forgot" to turn it off. The body has kept itself in perfect harmony for many years, starting and stopping rapid cell division when needed. Suddenly it forgets to switch it off, or cannot stop the rapid growth. At the same time, other processes in the body continue to run in perfect harmony, including the starting and stopping of cell division.

3.3.1   Growth Rate

Every cancer starts with only one cell, which cannot or will not stop dividing. After the first multiplication, there will be two cells. After the second multiplication, there are four cancer cells. Then there will be eight, and so on. The time that it takes to divide a cell is called the doubling time, or the time it takes to make double the amount of cells. Sometimes one doubling can take weeks or even months. Typically, a "fast-growing" cancer doubles itself within one to four weeks. A "slow-growing" cancer doubles itself in two to six months[33].

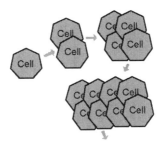

Figure 3: Cell Doubling

The time between the first mutant cell and a detectable cancer is called the silent period. This silent period can last many years. For a tumor to be seen on an x-ray, it must be at least ½" (=1cm) in diameter. Newer detection technologies (CT scan, PET scan or MRI) may detect smaller tumors. A tumor that is ½" in size contains about 1 billion cells, which equals roughly 30 doubling times. (2^{30} cells is slightly more than 1 billion cells.)

After 30 doublings, the first lump is detectable by x-ray. It could take many more doublings before symptoms appear. At 40 doublings, the tumor weighs about 2 lbs (1 kg). At 41-43 doublings, the tumor is so large (4-16 lbs/8 kg) that it leads to death.

Example:
On average, the doubling time for breast cancer is 4 months.[34] *This means that it takes 4 months for one tumor cell to divide. It takes about 30 doubling times for it to become detectable. In this case, the time it takes to form a detectable tumor would be 4x30 = 120 months (= 10 years).*

If it is a fast-growing tumor, it could have a doubling time of only 2 months. Then the time it takes to form a detectable tumor would be only 2x30=60 months (5 years).

If it is a slow-growing tumor with a doubling time of 2 years, it would take 60 years before the tumor could be detected.

The growth rate and the associated prognosis depend on the doubling time. Typical doubling times differ for each type of cancer, for each person, and over time for the same person. This makes reaching a prognosis very difficult.

3.4   The Cancer Process

When we examine the causes of cancer, there are a few aspects we need to consider. Cancer is an uncontrolled multiplication of cells. The first cell somehow mutates and begins dividing uncontrollably without the body being able to stop it. In this section, I will discuss how cancer is formed, what the body does to prevent it, and what the current survival statistics are.

3.4.1   Mutation

There are many factors that could cause a cell to mutate and become cancerous. Evidence indicates that there are a multitude of influences that can individually or jointly cause the first cell to mutate.

There are a number of different theories about the causes. Excessive food intake has been identified as a possible cause, but so has a deficiency in food intake. The intake of toxic substances (uranium, asbestos, nickel, smoke) has been identified as causing cancer. Another cause could be the external influence of radiation (sun, x-rays, etc.) Certain hormones or drugs could be a cause. Viruses or bacteria are of influence, or it can be inherited from parents. Those substances that could mutate a cell are called carcinogens (cancer-inducing agents).

Carcinogens have been proven capable of inducing cancer in some situations. Extremely excessive smoking could cause cancer, although this is not guaranteed. When exposed to carcinogens, some people stay healthy while others get cancer. Being exposed to carcinogens or having parents with cancer increases the statistical risk of developing cancer. Such a "risk factor" means that a person is statistically more likely than someone else to develop cancer sometime in his life. When cancer is diagnosed in a person with a certain risk factor, people tend to say that it is due to the risk factor, but this relationship is not carved in stone. There is no way to determine what actually caused the cancer. The bottom line is that we do not know what really causes cancer; we know more about how it develops. The exact cause of cancer is still a mystery.

3.4.1.1 Genetics

There are several debates going on about what is encoded in our genetic information. Some things are clearly encoded in our genes, while there is much debate about whether others are genetically determined at all.

If something has a large genetic component, it means that the children will probably inherit that variable. Blood type is an example of something that is clearly noted as being genetic, which means that the children will inherit the same blood group as one of their parents. Height is an example of a variable that has a large genetic component.

There is much controversy about whether the susceptibility to certain diseases has a genetic component, and how dominant that component is in contracting the disease. Some people believe that there is a large genetic component in Alzheimer's, Multiple Sclerosis (MS), and Diabetes. Others believe that they have no genetic component whatsoever. Genetic components need to be activated to be of influence. If this "cancer gene" is not turned on, it cannot do its work.

There is only a genetic component in 5% to 10% of all cancers. This does not mean that they are genetic, only that there is a predisposition for contracting the diseases. The gene must still be activated.

In experimental studies, researchers bred mice with genetic cancer, or cancer-prone mice. These mice were genetically more susceptible to getting cancer. From this batch of mice, bred by Dr Vernon Riley

(1975[35]), 80% were supposed to develop cancer. He divided the mice into two groups, and placed one in a stress-free environment and the other in a highly stressful environment.

- 92% of the mice in the stressful environment actually developed cancer, which is 12% higher than expected.
- Only 7% of the mice in the stress-free environment developed cancer, which is 73% lower than expected.

All of the mice were genetically predisposed to develop cancer. Statistically, 80% should have developed the disease. The mice in the stress-free environment somehow beat the odds. The element of stress created a deviation of 85% from the statistics. This is a clear example of how genetic predisposition is not the only determining factor, and how stress is a mediating factor.

3.4.1.2 Oncogenes

The body consists of many organs and tissues. Every part of the body is made up of cells. A cell contains all the genetic information present. The cells themselves are made up of forty-six chromosomes. Each chromosome contains thousands of genes. These genes carry all of the genetic information.

The theory of oncogenes suggests that somehow normal genes can be transformed into genes that promote tumor growth. These genes can be seen as promoters of cancer. Besides oncogenes, there are tumor suppressor genes, whose task is to prevent oncogenes from having an effect on the cell.

Example:
Think of a cell as a multinational company. This company, "BabyCell, Inc.", is a merger of two other companies. A couple of years ago, there was a company called "MomCell, Inc.", with 23 divisions, and thousands of people working in each division. The director went to talk to the director of "DadCell, Inc.", which also had 23 divisions, to discuss a merger. The merger received the code name "baby." When the merger was successful, "BabyCell, Inc." was introduced to the public. Within this company, there were now 46 divisions, and each division had thousands of people working for it.

"BabyCell, Inc." is a healthy company, but for some reason there was one person somewhere in some division who was not happy with the situation. This person turned against the multinational and was able

to turn the healthy company into an unhealthy one - just this one person, oncoperson.

Within every division of "BabyCell, Inc.", there are also people whose job is to make sure that everyone works with satisfaction. Whenever there is an unhappy person in the division, this satisfaction engineer makes sure that this person becomes happy, or is removed from the company.

Cancer can only develop when a gene is transformed into an oncogene, and the tumor suppressor gene is unable to do its job.

3.4.2 Development

Once there is a mutated cell, cancer can develop. To be able to develop, this cell must remain alive and be given the opportunity to grow and divide. This opportunity must be kept in place for a long time. (It could take decades for one initially mutated cell to become a problem.)

For a cancer cell to grow into a tumor, there are a few conditions:
1) Normal functioning of the body includes replacing every single cell occasionally. Unhealthy or old cells are replaced. The cancer cell must be replaced by another cancer cell or not be replaced at all for the cancer to develop. If the cancer cell is replaced by a healthy cell, the disease will never develop.

2) The immune system guards the body against harmful intruders. When there are bacteria entering the body, the immune system kicks in. It prevents these bacteria from doing any harm. For cancer to develop, the immune system must leave the cancer cell intact.

If one of these conditions is not met, the first mutated cell will never have the opportunity to develop into a problem.

3.4.3 Immune System

The development of cancer seems to be related to the workings of the immune system. The job of the immune system is to recognize and neutralize any foreign invaders, including cancer cells. In the case of diagnosed cancer, the immune system seems to have failed in recognizing and neutralizing the cancer cell.

Many studies have shown that when the immune system is impaired, cancer gains a stronger foothold for growth.

So, how does the immune system tie into the cancer process?

3.4.3.1 The Surveillance Theory

The surveillance theory of cancer basically assumes that everyone has cancer cells in their body. They are present in many places, and in many organs and tissues. Each day, many of these cells die and many new cancer cells are created by whatever cause. When these harmful cells flow through the body, the immune system recognizes and eliminates them. The immune system is always on the lookout for these cancer cells, hence the name "surveillance theory." According to this theory, cancer cells are not a problem unless the immune system is not doing its job.

> *Example:*
> *Our bodies can be compared to a large city with many individual people and organizations which have their own specialties. Some of the individuals misbehave and form groups of organized crime. As long as they are only small groups, they will hardly be noticed at the city level. However, as they grow, more people will get scared. If nothing is done, the city will eventually collapse.*
> *Fortunately, there is a police force, an organization geared towards detecting criminals and criminal organizations. They continuously patrol the city to detect and eliminate criminals.*
> *New criminals arrive for whatever reasons, and the police force keeps them from doing harm.*

The effect of the immune system is illustrated in the case study presented by Glasser in his book, "The Body is the Hero." The study is about rare incidents of transplanted cancerous kidneys. Before the actual transplants took place, all necessary precautions had been taken to ensure that the kidneys did not contain cancerous cells. No cancer cells were detected because the cancer was still in its silent period, but the cells were present. After the new kidneys were transplanted, the patients received immunosuppressant drugs to prevent their bodies from rejecting the new kidneys. The patients kept using this medication so that the new kidneys would be accepted.

> *Example:*
> *Within a few days, the kidney began to enlarge and the x-ray revealed*

a new tumor that had not been there four days ago. When another tumor appeared in the patient's other lung, they decided to operate. A biopsy indicated that the new kidney was now full of malignant cells, so the doctors concluded that the tumors had metastasized from this kidney tumor. The speed at which these tumors had developed was staggering, considering that it would normally take years for them to grow to such a size, and they had developed in a few days.

Because of the critical situation, the doctors decided to stop the immunosuppressant treatment and let the body's immune system take over. A rejected kidney was better than the situation at hand, so they were forced to take the patient off the medication.

The immune system was working again within a few days, and immediately began to fight. Almost immediately, the tumors in the lung and kidney began to shrink. Eventually, the kidney was removed and the patient never showed any evidence of cancer [emphasis mine].

(Glasser 1976[36])

The immune systems of the patients and the donor had kept the cancerous cells in check. When the immune system was suppressed, the cancerous cells were given free rein to grow and become a problem.

Another study followed a large group of women diagnosed with carcinomas, confirmed with a pap smear test and a biopsy. West (1954[37]) reported that although they did not receive treatment, the carcinomas disappeared in 80% of the women. West also reported several other cases in which the cancer spontaneously disappeared. This backs up the existence of the surveillance theory (Barrios 1961[38]).

Rossi (1986[39]) wrote about the discovery that the presence of neuroblastoma (cancer cells) in babies is higher than one would expect from the statistical evidence of the disease. Furthermore, almost all autopsies performed on men over 50 showed evidence of prostate cancer, yet statistics of the incidence of prostate cancer did not concur. This indicates that there are always cancer cells present in the body. The body keeps the cancer cells in check for healthy people.

The surveillance theory illustrates that the presence of cancer cells, or how they are formed, is not of great importance. The real issue is how the body handles the cancer cells that are present.

3.4.4   Survival

Cancer is currently the second leading cause of death in the US. The final age-adjusted data for 2001 indicates that heart disease accounts for 29% of all deaths in the US, while cancer accounts for 23% (Arias et al, 2003[40]).

Although these are the hard facts, people tend to be more afraid of cancer than of heart disease. One clear illustration of this is a conversation I overheard: "...Your disease is not what you feared. It is not cancer." In the same breath, this doctor told the patient that the diagnosis was something else, and that he would die within a few weeks.

Every year, many people are diagnosed with cancer. Everyone probably knows someone who has died of cancer. One might also know someone who was cured of cancer. The stories of people dying seem to outnumber those of people who are recovering. The reality is that many people die from cancer, but many are also cured and live happy lives afterwards.

3.4.4.1 Curing

The question of how many people are cured is difficult to answer because there is no unified definition of "cured from cancer." When considering a broken leg, it is easy to x-ray the bone and diagnose the fracture. If you x-ray the leg again 6 weeks later and the bone appears whole, you can say for sure that the bone is cured. In the case of cancer, researchers use the "5-year survival" criteria. This means that if the person is still alive after 5 years, they are cured. There is, however, always a possibility that the cancer will return (or that new cancer will develop in the same place). Steward (1925[41]) wrote about a patient of his who had a recurrence of breast cancer after 31 years.

A cultural belief has manifested itself that cancer is equal to death. This is a fatal misconception. There are many people who die from cancer, and there are also many people who are cured of cancer. With the many advances in diagnostics, medicine, surgery and radiation, the cancer survival rate has increased tremendously.

Medical science has evolved into an era in which many cancer patients can be successfully treated, and can live normal lives afterwards.

Some people are even cured without knowing how - the so-called spontaneous remissions.

When people were diagnosed as having cancer In the early 20th century, there was not much hope for a cure. In the 1930s, people had a 25% chance of being cured of the disease. In 1997, the 5-year survival rate went up 56% (American Cancer Society 2002[42]), which means that one has a higher chance of being cured than of dying from cancer. Today, the 5-year survival rate is 62% for all cancers combined. These figures have been adjusted for normal life expectancy, including factors such as dying of heart disease, accidents, and the diseases of old age (American Cancer Society 2002[43]). The trend is that since 1991, the cure rate has increased by 1.8% per year. Contrary to popular belief, two-thirds of all cancer patients get cured.

5-year overall survival rate

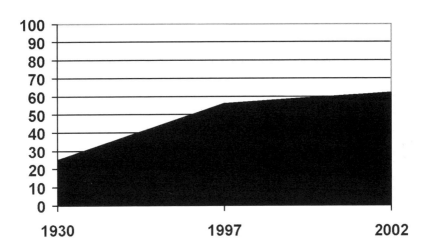

An important note here is that all of these statistics are based on people who were treated at least eight years ago, so these numbers do not reflect new advances in treatment.

You are more likely to survive than to die from cancer!

The most common forms of cancer are (American Cancer Society 2004[44]):

Incidences:

Prostate (33%)

Lung & bronchus (13%)

Colon & rectum (11%)

Urinary bladder (6%)

Melanoma-skin (4%)

Survival:

Prostate (98%)

Lung & bronchus (15%)

Colon & rectum (62%)

Urinary bladder (82%)

Melanoma-skin (90%)

Incidences:

Breast (32%)

Lung & bronchus (12%)

Colon & rectum (11%)

Uterine corpus (6%)

Ovary (4%)

Survival:

Breast (87%)

Lung & bronchus (15%)

Colon & rectum (62%)

Uterine corpus (84%)

Ovary (53%)

SECTION B

PSYCHOSOMATIC MODEL

4

The Model

In an early work on psychological factors and the onset of cancer, Blumberg et al. (1954[45]) concluded that intense emotional stress profoundly influences the growth rate of cancer in men. At the same time, they hypothesized that cancer could be explained in terms of coping with stress caused by emotional events. They discussed emotions and made conclusions about coping. Folkman (1997[46]) created a model of psychological processes on which my model is based. In this section, I will use my psychosomatic model to explain the different sub-processes. In later sections, I will discuss each of these sub-processes in more detail and how they relate to cancer.

4.1 Introduction

The purpose of this chapter is to identify the psychological processes that take place from the moment an event occurs until a reaction to the event is produced. This can be a feeling of distress or the development of a psychosomatic illness.

The connection between stress and illness has been investigated and confirmed by many observers. Concepts of stress are important in understanding psychosomatic models.

4.1.1 Stress

The impact of stress on psychosomatic issues has been studied intensively. Most authors agree that elevated levels of stress are not healthy, and can stimulate illness. The main problem with these studies is that "stress" is defined differently. Definitions range from the event experienced by the subject (life event or stressor), to the feeling of being overwhelmed (distressing emotion), including the reaction to the event, or coping with stress.

When people talk about stress, they generally mean one of two things. They are either referring to the situation (stressor) or their reaction to it (stress response). The stress response can be either biological, psychological, or both. Hans Selye (1956[47]), a pioneer in stress research, defined stress as the physical reaction to a disturbing event. If we consider this, the term "stress response" is more suitable. Others define stress as an event that causes an undesired physical response. Such events are better described by the word "stressor."

The following are several authors' definitions of the term "stress response":
- Selye (1956[48]): "A non-specific outcome (either physical or psychological) of any demand made upon the organism."
- Lazarus (1976[49]): "Stress occurs when there are demands on the person which tax or exceed his adjustive resources."
- Vingerhoets et al. (1994[50]): "Stress is the condition that results when an individual perceives a discrepancy – real or not – between the demands of a situation and his/her capacities to deal with those demands."
- Dept. of Medical Oncology at the University of Newcastle: "The sum of the biological reactions to any adverse stimulus, physical, mental or emotional, internal or external, that tends to disturb the organism's homeostasis. Should these compensating reactions be inadequate or inappropriate, they may lead to disorders."[51]

Lazarus mentions that the stress response will occur when the person cannot adapt to the situation, i.e., does not have the coping mechanisms to release the tension. Vingerhoets makes an important distinction in his definition, in that it is the person's perception that makes the difference. Whether or not the person has the coping styles is not as important in this case as his perception of whether he can cope with the situation. The University of Newcastle brings into focus that the stressor can also be internal, i.e. perceived stressors, which could eventually lead to disorders.

By combining the above into one all-encompassing definition, I arrived at the following:

"The stress response is the sum of all the biological and psychological reactions to any stimulus, physical, mental or emotional, internal

or external, real or imagined, which is perceived as a discrepancy
– real or not – between the demands of a situation and the person's
perceived capacities to deal with those demands. Should these
compensating reactions be inadequate or inappropriate, they may
lead to disorders."

I will refrain from using the word "stress," which will be replaced with the following, more descriptive, terms:

- Stressor: A stimulus (real or imagined) that causes a stress response.
- Stress response: A pattern of physiological, behavioral, emotional, and cognitive responses to a real or imagined "stressor."
- Distress: Pain or suffering affecting the body, a bodily part, or the mind.

The early research on stress focused mainly on the effects of an external stressor on the internal system of the animal or human. The subjects were exposed to a certain stressor, and the changes in their physical functions were then measured. The conclusion reached by Basowitz et al. (1955[52]) is of interest:

*"In future research... we should **not** consider stress (reaction) as*
***imposed** upon the organism, but as its **response** to internal or*
external processes which reach those threshold levels that strain
its physiological and psychological integrative capacities close to or
beyond their limits." [Emphasis mine]
- Harold Basowitz -

4.2 Psychosomatic Model

Many researchers have discussed different psychological sub-processes that take place in reaction to a stressor. Reid (1948[53]), Fritz (1957[54]), and Lazarus et al. (1957[55]) wrote that emotional experiences are also regulated by the expectations, perceptions and values that one places upon the event.

Vingerhoets et al. (1994[56]) added that perception, personality, coping and previous experiences determine to a large extent whether an event results in a feeling of distress or a challenge.

Howard (1994[57]) combined the work of Thompson (1988[58]), Plutchik et al. (1989[59]), and Lazarus (1991[60]) to establish a series of sequential sub-processes that eventually determine the result of a stressor.

The processes identified were:
- Event
- Perception
- Appraisal
- Coping
- Emotions

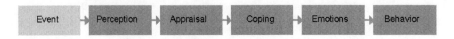

Figure 4: Simplified Psychosomatic Model

Folkman (1997[61]) expanded and revised this model, particularly in the area of coping. He incorporated "making meaning," and included several feedback loops from emotions to events, in which emotions function as new events.

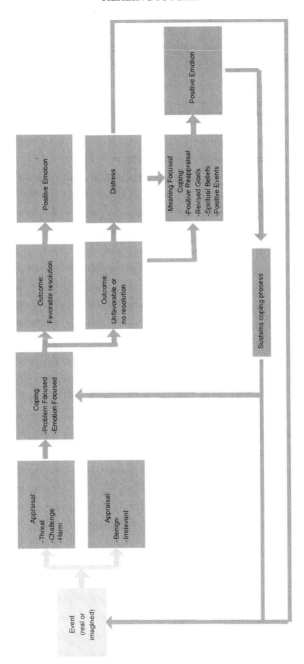

Figure 5: Folkman Model
During his lifetime, every individual develops a set of personal
values, beliefs, goals, and self-image. These will gradually change, but

most are consistent over time. Folkman calls these "global meanings." When a major event occurs, like a diagnosis of cancer or the loss of a loved one, these global meanings are confronted with the meaning of the particular event ("situational meaning").

Coping is geared towards reconciling the global meaning with the situational meaning of the event, through appraisal and reappraisal, problem solving, emotional control, and "meaning making."

The goal is to achieve a new balance. This might include a change in values, beliefs, self-image and/or life goals.

To illustrate this, Folkman uses the following example:

Example:
A young distance runner has had a leg amputated due to osteosarcoma. The runner must reconcile the loss to fit his lifelong goals, or alter his global meaning to incorporate the loss.

In this case, the runner must change his goals to accommodate the reality of the missing leg.

For this study, I extended this model with the behavior and health implications resulting from the outcome. Meaning-focused coping ("making meaning") is included because it is always present as one of the coping styles available to a person. Every process that the person is conscious of also constitutes an event. Everything is therefore fed back as an event. For the sake of clarity, I have removed the feedback lines and created the following psychosomatic model:

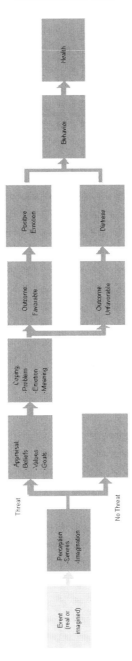

Figure 6 : Psychosomatic Model
In the next chapters, I will discuss each process individually, and its connection to illness in general. In upcoming sections, I will discuss how these processes relate to cancer specifically.

4.3   Events

Events can be experiences, situations, thoughts, emotions, or anything real or imagined that triggers psychological processes. These events can be positive or negative. Typically, such negative events are called stressors. Some events are external to the person, like the weather or winning the lottery. Other events are internal, like feeling angry or thinking happy thoughts. Some are real, while others are only imagined.

> *"Experimental and clinical psychologists have proved beyond a shadow of doubt that the human nervous system cannot tell the difference between a 'actual' experience and an experience imagined vividly and in detail."*
> *- Maxwell Maltz -*

Many different terminologies are used. In stress research, an event is usually called a stressor. In behavioral and cognitive therapy, an event is called a trigger. A trigger initiates a process or reaction, and is therefore more neutral than a stressor. Because "trigger" implies action, I will continue to use it to denote the stressor.

The entire process starts when a particular event occurs. This can be any event, positive or negative.

While events make up only a small portion of the entire model and are highly individual, the topic of events could be an important starting point for therapeutic interventions.

Since the early days of medical research, physicians have noticed relationships between life's misfortunes and the onset of illnesses. There are many quotes from physicians who observed a connection between certain triggers and the onset of disease. Many pointed to a relationship between stressors and illness. Wolff (1953[62]) was one of the first who systematically researched the relationship between triggers and disease. By observing a patient's triggers, emotional states and illness, he was able to conclude that stressors play a causative role in the disease process.

Example:
What might occur is the following. A certain event is happening to

*you, and has some kind of relevance to you. Say there is a car rushing
towards you at 100 mph.*
*Under normal circumstances, you react in some way to the event.
In this case, you would probably jump away because this event
constitutes a threat.*

Everything in life causes some level of arousal, some level of tension
or excitement, whether it is a "good" trigger or a "bad" trigger. Triggers
also have an effect on how we arrange our lives, and changes might be
needed.

Traumatic experiences, such as facing death or losing a close friend,
trigger psychological processes, but daily issues like small conflicts with
co-workers or children also trigger processes. Happy things might also
trigger these processes.
    A trigger in and of itself is not positive or negative; it just contains
facts.
    Any trigger – good or bad- that brings some level of excitement or
tension could be a potential stressor. Every trigger has some impact,
large or small, on our lives. The intensity of that impact varies with every
person: one may be devastated, for example, while another, experiencing
the same situation, feels challenged and is stimulated positively.

Much research has been conducted on the diversity of events
and the onset of disease. Some studies focused on the physical effects
of exposing animals and humans to certain triggers. The actual
psychological processes were ignored (Selye 1956[63]). Other studies
focused on the triggers and the onset of disease later in life. Holmes et
al. (1969[64]) were the first to quantify triggers and determine how they
influence health.

This chapter will discuss the major findings concerning the
influence of events on disease. It will also describe the two most widely
used scales, developed by Homes et al. (1967[65]) and Brown et al. (1989[66]),
for determining how many events a person has experienced. Other
scales less commonly used in research, such as Cochrane (1973[67]), Rahe
(1973[68]) and Mattila (1977[69]), will not be discussed.

4.3.1   Life Change Units (LCU)

In their research, Homes et al. (1967[70]) concluded that the effect
of any trigger was not dependent on the kind of stressor per se. The

effect was related to the amount of change that the person was required to undertake. The more changes were required, the higher the stress response, and the greater the chance of disease. Based on their research on more than 5000 people, they created a list of situations that require changes.

They used situations that had a significant impact on the current situation in the lives of the subjects. Their assumption was that the tension resulting from the need to change was associated with disease.

This led to the development of the Social Readjustment Rating Scale (SRE), which rated each situation depending on the number of changes required to deal with it. This rating was termed "Life Change Units (LCU)." Some events required more life changes, and therefore received more LCU points than others.

They did not differentiate between commonly accepted "good" or "bad" situations, as both require changes. The list was validated using double-blind studies to avoid the self-fulfilling prophecy phenomenon in the onset of illness.

With LCU points attributed to events, they were able to calculate the subjects' "scores" in order to measure how much tension they had encountered.

Retrospective studies have shown a strong connection between the intensity of adaptation and the onset of serious diseases. Of the subjects scoring more than 300 points, 49% reported an illness during the study, while only 9% of those with scores below 200 reported an illness during the same period. They concluded that anyone who scored 150 LCU points or more would have a 50% chance of experiencing a significant negative health change. People who scored more than 300 LCU points had a 90% chance of suffering a serious health change.

4.3.2   Life Events and Difficulties Scales (LEDS)

Although the most widely known scale is the Social Readjustment Scale, the one most used in research is the "Life Events and Difficulties Scales" (LEDS) (Brown 1989[71]). This scale focuses on different loss events and the emotions that these events trigger. The test consists of 38 classes of triggers involving changes in the subjects' lives.

The Social Readjustment Rating Scale can be self-administered; the LEDS scale depends on the skills and sensitivity of the interviewer. Events are treated in the same way for each individual. For example, a divorce is always treated as a major form of loss, even though the participant might feel released from constraints, and experience the event as a happy one.

Brown acknowledges that this is a limitation of his test.

4.4   Perception

For the trigger to set off a series of internal processes, the person must be aware of it. This awareness is the perception of the trigger. Through the use of the five senses, the trigger is perceived. Pure perception is like a video camera. There is neither evaluation nor personal bias in the perception.

Symington et al. (1955[72]) noted that the stress response only occurred when the subjects were conscious and able to perceive the threat. As long as patients were unconscious, no stress response could be measured in the body. Patients who were conscious did show a physiological stress response.

They concluded that the stress response was only present in those who were conscious of their approaching death.

Example:
Before you perceive the car, nothing special is happening - you are just walking happily across the street. As long as you continue to not perceive the car, you go on doing what you are doing. When the car enters your perception through sight, sound, smell, touch or taste, psychological processes will be triggered.

Imagined Triggers

Studies show that there is no difference between real and imagined stressors. Whether a stressor is real or imagined, the same physical reactions can be noted.

Shannon et al. (1963[73]) demonstrated this with dental injections. The physical reactions were the same for the injection and the anticipation of the injection. Epstein (1967[74]) noted a marked physiological stress response prior to a jump by a skydiver. Physiological stress responses were also measured in people when there was no real stressor associated. They were watching a movie inside a theater (Birnbaum 1964[75]; Nomikos et al. 1968[76]), and displayed physiological stress responses.

The mind does not seem to differentiate between real and imagined triggers.

Example:
This can be recognized when walking in a dark alley after watching a scary movie. Some people imagine bad things happening to them, and experience emotions and thoughts stemming from that fear. They might then run through the alley, which is a behavioral reaction to the imagined event of bad things happening there.

4.5   Appraisal

> *"It is not the things themselves that confuse people, but their judgment of those things"*
> *- Epictetus - "The Enchiridion" (100 AD)*

Once the event (real or not) is perceived by the person, they will interpret and evaluate the situation according to their personal view of the world.

This interpretation is the appraisal process, as described in the model.

The appraisal process determines coping activities and the emotional reaction to a trigger (Lazarus et al. 1970[77]). The core components of the entire process are the beliefs patients hold. These beliefs influence whether or not the appraisal results in a feeling of threat or irrelevancy. The level of distress is determined by the outcomes of the appraisal process (Lazarus et al. 1952[78]; Arnold 1960[79]; Lazarus 1966[80]).

Distress will only occur when the trigger is interpreted as a threat (Appley 1962[81]). This high level of individuality is found in several studies (Goldstein 1959[82]; Eckerman 1964[83]). Depending on the meaning that one attributes to the trigger, it either elicits the stress response or a response of excitement.

> *"One man's stress is another man's excitement."*
> *- Unknown -*

Selye (1956[84]) demonstrated that the body produces the same symptoms when confronted with a daily psychological trigger (such as being scolded) and a physiological threat to life (such as an immediate, life-threatening danger). The psychological trigger is interpreted as a life-threatening situation. This study also makes it clear that there is no difference between a truly dangerous situation and the feeling that a situation is dangerous, even when it is not.

Example:
Some people show similar physical symptoms when doing a presentation as they would if threatened in a dark alley.

Example:
When a person gets married and is happy, there will be no stress response. If he evaluates marriage as something that ties him down, he could develop a stress response.
A divorce can potentially be stressful. When a person evaluates the situation as hopeless and feels helpless, this event is highly stressful.
If a person evaluates the situation as a relief, and feels that he now has the time to make a life-long wish come true, then it is probably less stressful.

Lazarus (1991[85]) divided the appraisal process into two different sub-processes, or primary and secondary appraisal filters. When a certain trigger is evaluated, it will first be evaluated by the primary appraisal filter, and then by the secondary appraisal filter.

Primary Appraisal Filters
Primary appraisal filters evaluate the trigger based on the relevance of its impact on the person's major goals. This process is based upon three pillars:

1) Goal relevance: How important is the trigger in relation to clients' wishes to reach their major life goals?
2) Goal congruence: How much is the trigger helping or preventing the client from reaching their goals? When the trigger prevents clients from reaching their major life goals, their distress will be very high.
3) Goal content: How many emotions will clients experience? Do they feel guilty or not? How does it influence their self-perception in the areas of self- and social esteem, moral values, ego ideals, meanings and ideas, persons and their well-being?

Secondary Appraisal Filters
Secondary appraisal focuses on how responsible clients think they are, and whether they can handle the situation.

1) Source: Do clients feel responsible, or do they blame others?
2) Coping Potential: Do clients think they can handle the situation, or is it too much for them to handle?
3) Future Expectations: What do clients believe about the future? Will things get better or worse?

4.5.1   Beliefs

"Men are disturbed, not by things, but by the principles and notions which they form concerning things."
- Epictetus - "The Enchiridion" (100 AD)

The appraisal process is determined by the beliefs people have. These expectations people have about life, disease, treatment, progression of disease, and themselves have been shown to influence the healing process. Believing that one will die a horrible death and that the disease will worsen often increases the chance of a poor prognosis. At the same time, believing that one will overcome the disease and live a long and happy life is often associated with a positive prognosis.

One of the key areas for researching the effects of beliefs is the placebo effect. A placebo is a dummy treatment that does not contain any actual medical interventions for clients' illnesses or complaints. The placebo effect occurs when this dummy treatment improves the clients' health. The placebo effect works on the clients' beliefs. When they strongly believe in some effect of the dummy treatment, this belief will usually manifest itself. It can be directed towards healing or illness. Usually, when the effect is in the direction of healing, it is called a placebo (Latin for "I shall please"). If it is in the direction of disease, it is usually called a nocebo (Latin for "I shall harm").

"The placebo is the doctor who resides within."
- Norman Cousins - (1979)

Volgyesi(1954[86])notedamarkedincreaseinimprovementaftergiving patients with a bleeding peptic ulcer the suggestion "This injection will cure it." After a year, 70% of those patients still showed improvement.

Of those patients who were told "The injection is experimental, with undetermined results," only 25% showed improvement after a year.

In his review of 15 double-blind studies of the placebo effect, Beecher (1959[87]) concluded that 35% of the patients found relief through the placebo. Evans (1985[88]) confirmed these findings in another review of 11 double-blind studies. Evans also found that 36% of the subjects found at least 50% relief from the placebo. In a surgical procedure to relieve chest pain, Beecher (1961[89]) noticed that just opening the chest without performing any surgical intervention caused as much relief as the actual operation.

Brehm et al. (1964[90]) and Wrightsman (1960[91]) investigated patients' reactions to painful injections. They noticed that the feelings and behaviors of patients could be better predicted based on their expectations, rather than the actual injections.

It has even been observed that administering a drug designed to induce vomiting actually reduced the tendency to vomit after patients were told that it would stop vomiting (Wolf 1950[92]). In these cases, the clients' beliefs actually overruled the pharmacological effect of the medication.

Rossi (1989[93]) concluded that the placebo effect counted for 55% of any healing, regardless of the disease. Goleman (1993[94]) concluded that in almost all diseases, a third of all symptoms can be improved by giving patients a placebo instead of medication.

The effects of nocebos are less widely investigated, but could be important. A nocebo typically causes an increase in symptoms based on the patients' beliefs.

Fielding et al. (1983[95]) reported hair loss, nausea and vomiting in the group that received the nocebo. Another extreme example of the effects of nocebos is "voodoo death." Victims believed so strongly that they were under a spell and would die soon that they actually died. Cannon (1942[96]; 1963[97]), who studied the physiology of voodoo death extensively, concluded that the victims' actual deaths were caused by prolonged exposure to the distress of believing themselves to be under a spell. The actual physiological cause of death was an over-activated sympathetic nervous system, caused by their belief that they were going to die.

4.5.2   Conscious vs. Unconscious Beliefs

Clients are not always aware of all of their beliefs. Some beliefs are known by clients, while others are unconscious to them. Sometimes unconscious beliefs contradict conscious beliefs. Both conscious and unconscious beliefs influence health and well-being.

L. W. Simmons recorded the following anecdote about a Hopi Indian in the western United States. This story illustrates the power of (un)conscious beliefs, and the persistence of such beliefs.

Example:
The traditional belief in the tribe was that when a person steps on the tracks of a snake, his ankles get sore. The Hopi Indian has to go to a medicine man to perform certain healing rituals so that the pain will disappear. A well-educated modern man left the Hopi traditions and beliefs and moved to another culture. For him, the medicine man had no added value compared to a medical doctor. Despite this, the man did get sore ankles after treading on the tracks of a snake. Only the medicine man could alleviate the symptoms.
(Simmons 1947[98])

Despite all of the man's conscious effort to adopt new beliefs, his old beliefs were still present and effective.

The effects of beliefs were also noted by Simonton et al. (1978[99]). They treated middle-aged Japanese men with standardized radiation therapy. The men started to suffer from unknown side effects which could not be explained. After talking to a Japanese major, they noticed that the men all had expectations about radiation based on stories of Hiroshima. Simonton et al. concluded that these men had beliefs that created the side effects. These beliefs did not show up after talking to the patients themselves.

These stories illustrate an important issue when working with belief systems. It is not the beliefs that are *uttered* by patients that are of importance, but the beliefs that are present at the unconscious level that influence the body. It is therefore important to find methods of discovering these unconscious beliefs, and begin working from there.

*"The greatest discovery of my generation is that human beings can
alter their lives by altering their attitudes of mind."*
- William James -

Clients might say that they really need a vacation, yet not get around to taking one. In many cases, there is a difference between what clients say and their true beliefs. This is also illustrated by the Hopi Indian story. The man does not think he believes that stepping on snake tracks will give him sore ankles, and yet it does. The old unconscious belief system is still present, and affects his ankles.

When discussing beliefs, it is important to talk about clients' unconscious beliefs, not just what they claim they believe.

4.5.3 Positive Thinking

There is a tendency to emphasize positive thinking. Particularly in the case of complementary medicine, therapists often force the client into a positive mindset. This thinking is based on over-generalized interpretations of studies on the effects of positive thinking. There is a widespread rumor that one must think positively in the face of illness or death. Culturally, it is almost not accepted to express negative beliefs about the disease or progression.

There is a difference between expressing a positive outlook on life and actually having one. Clients could express positive beliefs, and at the same time experience negative beliefs. A positive expression might be a cover-up (conscious or unconscious), to avoid receiving too much pity or attention.

Research indicates that a positive outlook is associated with better health, but research also shows that holding back one's true feelings is associated with poorer health. Having a positive outlook is healthy, but only when the positive outlook stems from one's unconscious beliefs.

4.6 Coping

Once clients have interpreted the trigger during the appraisal process, the process of coping begins in order to deal with the situation at hand.

Example:
In the case of the rapidly approaching car, the emotional coping is

probably an emotion of fear, and the cognitive response is something like "Get the heck out of here!" Then comes the behavioral response of jumping away.

Coping is how people react to the trigger in order to control, discard, reduce or accept the situation. In this section, I will discuss the process of coping that is how a person tends to cope with different situations that occur in life in relation to illness.

The definitions of Oosterwijk (2004[100]) and Folkman (1997[101]) can be combined into the following definition of coping:

> *"Coping is the behavioral, cognitive or emotional effort that one makes to control, discard, reduce or accept the demands by others, oneself or the situation."*

4.6.1 Development of Coping

Most people's current behaviors and the way they react to situations are habitual. They have responded in the same way for a long time, and still do so without questioning the effectiveness of their behavior.

During childhood, most people tried new behaviors. When certain behaviors did not yield the results they wanted, they tried others until they found some that did produce the desired results. This way, children developed a set of behaviors they could rely on. Over the years, we tend to favor certain behaviors over others. Other behaviors that were learned are never applied again, such as crying and yelling when we can't have candy. Only a limited set of behaviors survives into adulthood.

In some situations, people have a wide range of behaviors to choose from in order to respond. In others, they have a limited set of behaviors available.

Example:
When we wanted a cookie in early childhood, we tried asking, yelling, demanding, crying and stealing until we found a method that worked for us and did not get us punished later.
If crying was successful every time we used it, we would not have a need to create alternative reactions, such as asking, which leaves us with a limited set of choices. If we wanted something later in life and

crying was not an option, we would not have an alternative, and would not be able to cope with the situation.

4.6.2   Coping Styles

There are many different styles of coping. Some people meditate to relieve tension, and some take medication. Others run away from the event, physically or through denial, or see only the positive side. Still others seek support from loved ones.

There are basically three ways of coping with a situation. One can cope with the event itself, one's response to it (Mechanic 1962[102]), or one's interpretation of it (Folkman 1997[103]).

- **Problem-focused coping**: Eliminating or reducing the intensity of the cause of the trigger. When this coping style is applied, clients do something with the situation itself. This style includes actions such as ending a relationship, quitting a job, moving to a different city, skipping an exam, and getting help from other students. This style will be discussed further in the sections on events.
- **Meaning-focused coping** (Folkman 1997[104]): Changing the interpretation of the event. Examples of this coping style include seeing the positive side and attributing meaning to the event itself. This will be further discussed in the section on appraisal.
- **Emotion-focused coping**: Regulating the distress itself. This type is focused on reducing the emotions. Examples of this coping style include taking one's mind off the situation, relaxing, or taking tranquilizers. This style of coping will be the primary focus of the coping section.

Example:
When you face an exam in 10 minutes and feel stressed because this is the one exam you failed last time, you have several options for coping with this exam:
a)   You can run away and skip the exam (problem-focused coping).
b)   You can take a moment to relax (emotion-focused coping).
c)   You can remind yourself that passing or failing this exam is not a life-threatening issue (meaning-focused coping).

The most effective coping style depends on the situation. In some cases, problem-focused coping is the most efficient. In others, emotion-focused or meaning-focused coping will be more suitable.

> *Joke:*
> *A man goes to a psychoanalyst's office and describes his problem: "Doctor, whenever I'm in bed, I'm convinced there's someone under my bed, and whenever I'm under my bed, I'm convinced someone is on my bed. Can you help me?" The doctor answers, "Sure, if you come into analysis with me for 2 years, once a week for $200 a session, you'll get over it." "I'll think about it," says the man, and walks away.*
> *A couple of weeks later, the man runs into the psychoanalyst on the street. "How is it going with your phobia?" asks the doctor. "The bartender solved my problem for only $50," says the man. "How?" asks the analyst. "He told me to saw the legs off the bed."*

4.6.1   Classification

Different coping styles can also be classified in a hierarchical structure. Menninger (1954[105]) suggests a classification of coping, and draws a parallel with bodily homeostasis. His classifications follow a continuum on which each order overlaps the next. First-order coping styles are simple "count to 10," "don't worry," and denial procedures. Fifth-order coping strategies include rage and violent behavior. Higher orders correspond to more destructive behaviors.

The chosen coping style depends on the intensity of the perceived threat. Minor triggers are met with a first- or second-order style. Major triggers are met with a fifth-order style.

When the chosen coping style does not alleviate the distress, another must be chosen. This new coping style might even belong to a higher order. Eventually, the chosen coping style is the best available option for maintaining mental homeostasis with a minimum of loss (Menninger 1954).

> *"Disease may be seen ... as a positive expression of the survival efforts of the organism, inept and costly as they may be."*
> *- Karl Menninger -*

When people have only a limited number of behaviors to choose from, they move to a higher order sooner. People with a large number of behaviors to choose from take another style from the same order, and do not have to opt for destructive styles. Those with a larger set to choose from will be healthier in handling different situations than those with only a limited set of coping styles at their disposal.

4.7 Emotions

Patients eventually experience some kind of emotions as a reaction to the outcome of their psychological processes. These emotions differ among people and triggers. Depending on the preceding processes, patients will experience strong or weak emotions that they may or may not like.

Some emotions relate directly to the experienced event, while others trigger past experiences at the same time.

Example:
If there is a car approaching me at 100 mph, I experience emotions of fear. If someone cuts in front of me at the supermarket, I might get angry. These emotions are directly related to the event.

If someone cuts into line and I get furious, this emotion relates to more than just the immediate event. I have probably experienced similar emotions of anger, which have been building up over time.

Emotions, such as anger, anxiety, loneliness and hopelessness, influence the health of patients. Several researchers have found a relationship between the experience of these emotions and a higher incidence of illness and cancer. The accumulation of distressing emotions has been recognized by many authors as a factor in the development of diseases and the prevention of healing. These emotions tend to shut down the immune system.

Researchers have also found that desired emotions, such as fun, laughter, love and support, have a healing effect.

4.8 Behavior

Behavior has been shown to influence health in numerous ways. Behaviors such as smoking, overeating, and overwork have been shown to increase the chance of disease. Physical exercise and a healthy diet have been shown to increase health. However, such healthy behaviors are outside the scope of this work.

5

Connections To Cancer

In an earlier chapter, I discussed the surveillance theory. This theory explains that there are always cancer cells present in the body. The immune system is on guard and destroys those cancer cells before they form a tumor. The presence of cancer cells does not mean that a malignant tumor is present or being formed. This makes it less pressing to discover what causes normal cells to become cancerous. Where healing cancer is concerned, the focus must be on helping the body fight the existing cancer cells, slowing down their growth rate, or stopping the division of the cells.

Many biological variables influence the growth rate of cancer, the division of cells, and the body's ability to heal from cancer. In addition to biological variables, psychological variable are also of influence, such as beliefs, coping styles, and emotions.

The psychological elements that have been proven to influence the progression or remission of cancer are the topic of this section. This section will identify and summarize these psychological factors. The next section will focus on how these elements can be used in the therapeutic process.

5.1 Events

People's experiences, and how they relate to the development of cancer, have been the topic of many studies. These experiences are referred to as events or, in some cases, life events.

Gendron (1701[106]) was probably one of the first to relate cancer to life events. He connected the "disasters of life" to the onset of cancer. One of his illustrative examples that are still used today is the following:

Example:
One woman suddenly developed breast cancer after the death of her daughter. She had always enjoyed perfect health. Another woman developed breast cancer suddenly after her husband went to prison. She had never experienced any problems with her health.
(Simonton 1978[107])

These examples are anecdotal at best, but underline the results of recent research. Most research in the area of life events and cancer is focused on the issue of loss. These loss events include not only the death of a loved one, but also divorce and retirement (the loss of a job).

Ramirez et al. (1989[108]) studied 50 women who were in remission when they experienced the first recurrence of breast cancer. They found a correlation between the recurrence of the disease and the events the women had experienced. The women suffering from recurring cancer showed a higher incidence of major life-changing events. No difference was observed in minor triggers.

"These results suggest a prognostic association between severe life stressors and recurrence of breast cancer, but a larger prospective study is needed for confirmation."
- A.J. Ramirez -

Geyer (1991[109]) compared the experiences of 39 women suffering from breast cancer with those of 58 women diagnosed with benign disorders, using the Brown and Harris scale. He found that the women with breast cancer had experienced significantly more severe life events in the eight years prior to the diagnosis, compared to the other women.

Life-changing events, emotions and psychological traits were also investigated by Forsen (1991[110].) He studied 87 breast cancer patients and a control group. The number of events, and especially those related to loss, were significantly higher in the breast cancer group. Those events involving broken relationships or long-term, continuous distress in relationships were of particular importance. After eight years, he conducted a follow-up study. He noticed that when clients experienced major life-changing events during the twelve months prior to the onset of cancer, their survival chances were reduced.

Cooper et al. (1993[111]) studied 2,163 women who entered the hospital for a routine breast screening. They noted that the women diagnosed with breast cancer had experienced the most life changing events during the previous two years. They noticed that the experience of a single major event was more damaging than regular exposure. This led them to conclude that those patients with more experience in handling stressors might be less physically affected by the event.

Prior to a biopsy and diagnosis, Chen et al. (1995[112]) interviewed 119 women who had undiagnosed lumps in their breasts. They used the standardized life events schedule (LEDS) to structure the interviews. Women who had experienced severe life events over the previous five years had a substantially higher chance of being diagnosed with cancer, compared to those women interviewed who had experienced milder life events.

Goodkin et al. (1986[113]) observed a noticeable connection between life-changing events and cancer progression, especially in those cases where clients displayed hopelessness. Goodkin suggested that clients who experience severe life events, and interpret them in such a way that they find themselves hopeless, have a higher probability of developing cancer.

A meta-review by Garssen (2001[114]) of 5 studies on the effects of life events and the disease-free interval displayed inconsistent results. He concluded that the discrepancies could be attributed to the differences in the duration of the follow-ups. The studies that did show a correlation conducted follow-ups covering seven to twenty years, while those showing no correlation conducted follow-ups spanning less than six years.

5.1.1 Experience of Loss

Many researchers have invested time and effort into finding the connection between specific life events and the onset or progression of cancer. Although the specific life events have not been identified, other interesting correlations have been found. Those life events involving the loss of an important relationship have been proven, in multiple studies, to have some connection to the development of cancer.

Herbert Snow (1893[115]) noticed that a high proportion of cancer patients had lived a difficult life and recently experienced a traumatic event, particularly the loss of a loved one. The Jungian psychoanalyst Elida Evans (1926[116]) noted, in a group of 100 patients, that many had lost an important emotional relationship (personal or job-related) prior to the onset of the disease.

Greene (1954[117]) noted a high degree of consistency between those people who had experienced the loss of a significant person or life goal and the development of a malignancy. The experience of loss could be related to a specific person or life goal that must be relinquished. The experience eventually leads to depressive feelings. According to Greene, the greatest loss was the death (or threat of death) of a mother, or a mother figure such as a wife. Other major events that were of influence included the loss of a job (including retirement), or a change of home.

LeShan (1956[118]; 1977[119]) studied 400 patients with cancer. He noted that 72% of them had experienced the loss of someone close to them just prior to the diagnosis. Only 10% of the control group had experienced the same kind of loss. His conclusion was that the risk of cancer was heightened by the loss of a loved one. Other characteristics included the inability to express hostility, feelings of unworthiness, and tension over the relationship with one or both parents.

Experiences of loss were most widely investigated as a result of the death of a spouse due to natural or unnatural causes. Evidence is also available relating cancer to losses due to retirement or divorce. Divorce puts people at an even greater risk of developing cancer than the death of a spouse (Pennebaker et al. 1988[120]; Holland 1990[121]).

LeShan (1989[122]) noted, based on statistics, that the peak period for cancer occurrence was just after retirement.

"...This was even true for the former Nazis who, in 1946-1947 were forced to retire from the German bureaucratic service at 35 or 40."
- Lawrence LeShan - (1989)

Cooper et al. (1993[123]) noticed a relationship between events of loss or bereavement and the development of breast cancer.

Kiecolt-Glaser et al. (1994[124]) noted that the results of different studies regarding life-changing events and cancer are "remarkably consistent across populations and kinds of events." They also concluded that the most influential events are those involving the loss of an important relationship due to death or separation.

Martikainen et al. (1996[125]) noted a correlation between the death of a spouse and subsequent cancer death. This correlation was the strongest in the first six months after the death of a spouse. They also noticed a differentiation between younger and older people. The relationship observed was more pronounced in the younger generation. The authors suggested that older people were better at handling such events. This connection between the death of a spouse and subsequent cancer death was absent in cases of stomach and breast cancer.

Booth (1969[126]) provided a psychoanalytical perspective on these relationships. He explained that people with cancer are characterized by a need to exercise control over chosen objects, people or relationships. Such people depend on their power to maintain their relationship to the chosen object. This makes them so rigid that when the object is lost, they are unable to replace it with something else. They end up in a state of psychological stalemate.

5.1.2 Discussion

Those researchers who studied the connection between life-changing events and the onset of cancer used different techniques with different ratings. Some used checklists that were specifically designed for their form of research (Greer et al. 1975[127]), while others used a standard scale, such as Homes et al. (1967[128]) and Brown et al. (1979[129]). Although both methods have their advantages and disadvantages, this makes it difficult to compare them and draw conclusions.

Specifically designed checklists make it harder to compare different studies, but easier to answer a certain research question. Standardized checklists make it more difficult for anyone to include their own opinions about a situation, but comparisons with other studies are relatively easy.

When checklists are used, individual interpretations of the event are ignored.

Among the participants in a study, each will have their own interpretation of the words on the checklist. One person's "severe life event" is not another person's "severe life event."

Such personal differences also hold true for events of loss. The actual perception of the event is based on the psychodynamics of the person, and not on the event.

> *"...it pointed to the fact that the specific life event may not be as important as the person's reaction to that occurrence."*
> *- David M. Kissen - (1967[130])*

5.2   Appraisal

When an event is perceived, it is interpreted through the appraisal process. The appraisal process is based on the beliefs people have. Based on their beliefs, people make interpretations about the situation, themselves and the prognosis in the event of illness.

Researchers make a distinction between a specific interpretation of an event and characteristic interpretations. Characteristic interpretations are typical for a person *regardless* of the situation. These characteristics or traits are discussed separately as personality traits. Specific interpretations are based on the type of event and the impact it has on the person. These are handled by the primary and secondary appraisal filters. The primary filter evaluates the impact of the situation on the client's goals. The secondary filter, which comes after the primary filter, evaluates whether and how clients can handle the situation.

In this section, I will discuss the different beliefs and personality traits that have been shown to influence the prognosis of cancer. A combination of personality traits and primary and secondary appraisal filters determine what emotions will surface. Although these processes cannot be separated, I will discuss them separately the sake of clarity.

5.2.1   Personality Traits

When people react in the same way regardless of the situation, we tend to speak of personality traits. Some of these personality traits have been identified as having some connection to the growth of cancer.

Research on personality traits and cancer has shown several links. These are discussed separately, as each may require different therapeutic strategies.

5.2.1.1 Self-image

LeShan et al. (1956[131]) found a connection between the lack of self-worth and the presence of cancer. In a study of 250 people, he noticed that the key characteristics of cancer patients were that they displayed feelings of unworthiness and self-dislike. The control group lacked these feelings.

This was later confirmed by Simonton et al. (1975[132]), who noticed that cancer patients often displayed a poor self-image. They displayed this feeling much more than the control group.

5.2.1.2 Assertiveness

Being assertive means expressing what one wants and being confident. This includes speaking one's own mind and not relying on socially accepted answers.

Blumberg et al. (1954[133]) was able to predict tumor growth based on personality traits. They noticed faster-growing tumors in patients who were always trying to make a good impression, and in those who rejected affection even when they wanted it.

They concluded that the extreme desire to make a good impression blocked patients' emotional outlets, and therefore resulted in faster-growing tumors.

In a study by Jansen et al. (1984[134]), subjects were asked to write a self-descriptive text. The researchers compared the texts written by 69 women with breast cancer, 82 women with benign breast disease and 71 healthy women. They found that the different groups of subjects used different wording in their descriptions of themselves. The breast cancer group was remarkably different from the other groups, and used words such as timid, non-assertive, calm, easy-going and likely to hold back anger.

Stavraky et al. (1988[135]) interviewed lung cancer patients and classified their personalities. Those patients who were described as having a reserved personality with a high need for sympathy showed a threefold increase in their risk of mortality from cancer.

Kune et al. (1991[136]) studied the personalities of 637 patients and 714 control subjects. They noticed that the tendency to show socially acceptable reactions to events was one of the distinctions between the cancer group and the control group. The avoidance of conflict and a preference for socially acceptable reactions to avoid offending others were both associated with poor prognosis.

Petito (1993[137]) bred unaggressive, socially inhibited mice. They were bred to avoid any conflict. These mice showed a greater susceptibility to cancer and lower levels of natural killer cells than the more assertive group.

5.2.1.3 Pleasing Others

One aspect that is closely related to assertiveness is the notion of pleasing others. This could also be viewed as a combination of the lack of assertiveness and the lack of self-worth. Those who tend to please others usually find others more important than themselves. This type of belief is closely associated with making the other person their primary goal in life, which could set them up for extreme experiences of loss.

LeShan et al. (1956[138]) noted the typical behavior of constantly pleasing others in cancer patients. These patients were described by their friends as being exceptionally fine, thoughtful, uncomplaining and almost "too good to be true."

Brémond et al. (1986[139]) noticed that cancer patients were very committed to social norms. They felt a strong desire to be viewed as "nice" or a "good person."

In her description of the Type C personality, Temoshok (1987[140]) pointed out that the cancer patients had been completely devoted to pleasing others. They felt almost compelled to please their spouses, parents, siblings, friends, co-workers, and even complete strangers. They tended to take more care of others than of themselves. Their identity seemed to be based upon others, avoiding conflict and maintaining an appearance of niceness and self-sacrifice. Temoshok noticed that the cancer patients had the distinct personality traits of stoicism, niceness, sociability, and conventionality.

Pleasing others can also take the form of feeling responsible for the other. Simonton et al. (1978[141]) noticed that cancer patients often take responsibility for the emotions and wants of others.

People who are concerned with pleasing others will not easily express their own emotions or needs. Based on their belief systems, their emotions and needs are not relevant. Bahnson et al.(1966[142]; 1969[143]), Temoshok (1987[144]) and LeShan (1989[145]) pointed out that cancer patients have often lost awareness of their own needs and wishes.

5.2.2   Primary Appraisal

The primary appraisal filter is based on how important an event is to people's life goals, and how their egos are involved. People react more strongly and with more emotion when the issue is more important to them.

Many researchers noted that the loss of one's life goals was a clear sign of a poor prognosis. This sign often emerged when patients had lost an important relationship that served as their primary purpose in life.

The Jungian psychoanalyst, Evans (1926[146]) studied 100 cancer patients. She noted that they had often lost an emotional relationship prior to the onset of cancer. The patients had a strong identification with this relationship, which could be personal or work-related. The connection became particularly apparent when the patients had only a few resources for coping with the loss.

In his 15-year study, Greene (1954[147]) noticed a consistency among leukemia and lymphoma patients. All patients had experienced a (perceived) separation from a significant person, or the loss of a major goal.

LeShan (1977[148]; 1989[149]) noted that feelings of hopelessness often emerged when patients had lost their main way of relating and expressing themselves. The loss of a relationship could be due to death, divorce, retirement, a move, or even a child leaving home. Patients often referred to this relationship as their primary reason for living. During the 12 years LeShan worked in Revici Hospital, he noticed that the majority of these patients lost their hope of ever achieving the life they wanted. They lost their hope for a deep and satisfying, meaningful life, and their appetite for life itself. This lack of hope often emerged after loosing an important relationship, and not finding a substitute object for relating or expressing themselves.

Bahnson et al.(1966[150]; 1969[151]) and Newton (1982[152]) noticed that many cancer patients displayed behavior suggesting that they wanted to die.

> *"A large segment of cancer patients' population consists of individuals whose behavior strongly suggests that they truly do not want to live."*
> *- Newton -*

Example:
A patient canceled his session because someone came to buy his lawnmower.

This patient clearly demonstrated that the session was not important for him. This behavior suggests that this patient does not want to get well.

Some of their patients came only a few times because they felt they had no control over the situation. Their lives had lost their meaning; they had nothing to live for. When clients think this way, the existing pain and discomfort actually increases. Behavior that is traditionally interpreted as a resistance to treatment or lack of compliance could have a death wish at its foundation.

The clinical observations made by LeShan (1989[153]) concur with mortality statistics. Such statistics show that widowers with children have a lower mortality rate then those without children. He reasoned that this could be explained as children being a part of their primary relationship. Further study led him to conclude that when these patients lost another important relationship, their children would replace it.

Within relationships, many people begin idolizing their spouses and make them their primary reason for living. By taking care of their spouses, they create meaning for their own lives. When the spouse falls away, through divorce, separation or death, they lose their way of giving meaning to their own lives. When this relationship is not replaced by another, the risk of cancer is increased.

The observation recorded by LeShan (1989[154]), that the highest occurrence of cancer in men takes place just after retirement, can be explained. This observation also applied to those men who retired at age 35-40. For men, a job is often a primary relationship. They attribute part of their purpose in life to their jobs. When the job falls way, their purpose in life disappears.

LeShan (1977[155]; 1989[156]) noticed three elements associated with cancer development:

- Feelings of hopelessness: the belief that there will be no positive future.
- Losing a major way of relating and expressing oneself.
- Absence of a substitute relationship to replace the lost one.

5.2.3   Secondary Appraisal

The outcomes of the secondary appraisal filters are based on beliefs about whether one can handle the situation, and expectations of processes and outcomes. Several authors noticed connections between these secondary appraisal filters and prognosis. Coping potential and expectations of outcomes were most widely investigated.

5.2.3.1 Coping Potential

Coping potential is the belief patients have that they can handle the situation. This belief is different from their actual way of coping, or coping style. This chapter is about patients' belief that they can cope with their situation. In a later chapter, I will discuss several coping styles and their effects on prognosis.

Those people who believe that they influence their world are said to have an "internal locus of control." The source of control lies inside the person. People who believe that they cannot influence their world are said to have an "external locus of control." In this case, the source of control lies outside the person. An internal locus of control is the belief that one has control over one's own destiny. An external locus of control is the belief that one is destined to be, and can exercise no influence on one's own destiny. Some authors refer to this internal locus of control as "fighting spirit."

Visintainer(1982[157]) injected a group of mice with a solution that would lead to the development of a tumor. There were three groups of mice: one that was subjected to an inescapable shock, one that could escape from the shock, and one group that was not subjected to a shock at all.

The group that could not escape the shock developed 36% more tumors than the group that received the same shock, but could escape from it. Both groups received identical amounts of the same shock. The latter group, however, experienced some control over the shock.

Of the group that had no control, 73% developed a tumor. In the group that could control the shock, only 37% developed a tumor. The only difference between these groups was that the latter believed they were in control of the shock; the amount and intensity of the shock was the same among both groups.

A year earlier, Sklar et al. (1981[158]) wrote about similar findings. They noticed that those mice that did not experience control over their destinies died faster of cancer. The ones that did experience control lived longer.

Greer (1982[159]) analyzed verbatim statements by patients and noticed that those who displayed stoic acceptance, helplessness, or hopelessness had the least favorable outcomes, compared to those with a fighting spirit. Temoshok (1987[160]) even noticed that stoic acceptance actually made it possible to predict the progress of the tumors over the next 18 to 29 months.

Another interesting experiment resulted in the coining of the term "learned helplessness" (Peterson et al. 1987[161]). A group of dogs was subjected to an inescapable electric shock in the floor. The next day, the dogs were placed in a box with a small barrier in the middle. They could easily escape the shock by jumping over the barrier. They did not. The dogs sat passively enduring the shock. Another group of dogs, who were subjected to a shock that was escapable by pushing a lever, did jump over the barrier the second day.

The first group of dogs learned that they were helpless. They learned that they could not escape the shock in the first instance, and then when a new situation arrived, they believed that they could not influence the shock. The other dogs believed they could influence their situation, and did so by jumping the barrier.

Shavit (1990[162]) studied the effects of the perceived level of control on the development of tumors. He noted that when animals were given the ability to control events, their immune system was enhanced and tumor development diminished. Conversely, the inability to control events decreased immune function and increased tumor development.

Wiedenfeld et al. (1990[163]) noted an enhanced immune function when patients thought they had control over the situation. They observed that a rapid increase in perceived self-efficacy seemed to predict a rapid increase in immune function. Blancy et al. (1992[164]) noted that those patients who felt they were in control of their lives had an enhanced immune system (T-Cell activity).

Peterson et al. (1993[165]) conducted an experiment in which students were exposed to a loud noise. One group was told they could stop the noise by pressing a button, and the other group was told nothing. The group who believed they were in control performed better, regardless of whether or not they actually used the button. They concluded that the belief of being in control was important, whether or not control was exercised.

> *"...exposure to uncontrollable shocks, but not to controllable ones,*
> *can suppress immune functioning and increase susceptibility to*
> *tumor growth"*
> *- Peterson – (1993)*

Grossarth-Maticek et al. (1995[166]) interviewed participants in 1973 to assess their level of "self-regulation." Self-regulation is defined as people's ability to notice the results of their behavior and correct it to achieve their goals. By definition, self-regulation can only take place when people have an internal locus of control. Fifteen years after the initial interview, they conducted a follow-up study to assess the participants' health status. Of those who scored in the lower section of the test, only 2% were still alive. Of the participants who initially scored in the higher regions, 81% were alive.

Those patients who actively sought solutions displayed more favorable outcomes than those who were passive in their coping (Goodkin et al. 1993[167]; Visser et al. 1998[168]).

Breast cancer patients' quality of life improved and their fear was reduced when they were able to co-decide on the time and type of medical follow-ups that they would undergo (Anderson et al. 1999[169]). Being actively involved in decision-making about treatment increases the patient's quality of life. Paul Martin (1999[170]), in his book "Healing Mind," concludes:

> *"Tumors develop sooner, grow faster, reach a larger size and are more likely to prove fatal in animals subjected to uncontrollable stressors, compared with animals subjected to identical amounts of controllable stressors (or no stressors at all)."*

Example:
When skydivers jump as a tandem master they feel less fear than when they jump as a passenger on a tandem jump. In that case, they feel out of control.

Cunningham et al. (2000[171], 2000[172], and 2002[173]) found a significant connection between the degree of involvement in psychological work and survival. Patients were classified as showing high, moderate, or low involvement in their psychotherapeutic processes. Patients who were categorized as "highly involved" devoted several hours daily to self-help strategies such as relaxation, mental imaging, meditation, cognitive monitoring and journaling.

Their conclusion supports clinical observations that those who are dedicated to their own therapeutic processes live longer than those are not.

There is quite a bit of evidence suggesting that those patients who believe they can control the situation, and actively seek solutions, have a much better prognosis than those who do not.

5.2.3.2 Expectations About Processes and Outcomes

> *"Anyone who doesn't believe in miracles is not a realist."*
> *- David Ben-Gurion -*

Expectations can be broadly divided into two different groups. One set of expectations covers the beliefs that people have about the outcome of something. The other set of expectations covers what people believe about how the process will be until that outcome is reached.

Example:
My outcome expectations about my vacation are that I will be
spending time in the mountains and feeling relaxed.
My expectations about the process are that I will be bored during the
10-hour drive to the mountains.

Patients all have ideas about what the outcome of their disease will be, and whether they will get over it or die. They have expectations of what a possible disease and dying process will be like. Everyone has preconceptions (conscious or unconscious) about these issues. Some of these expectations are associated with a good prognosis, others with a poor prognosis.

"Whether you believe you can or you believe you cannot, either way
you are right."
- Henry Ford -

Where cancer is concerned, most of the stories that circulate and the news that is broadcast are about horrific effects. These stories promote the idea of a horrible disease that cannot be cured. The beliefs that these stories support are scientifically wrong, and no doctor will support them fully. This is only one side of the story. There are also many stories around from survivors who are living happily now; however, these rarely show up in the media.

The stories that circulate influence the beliefs people have.

Example:
If we know ten people who have died from breast cancer, we might
come to believe that breast cancer means death. On the other hand, if
these people have survived, we might come to believe that the disease
is quite curable.

These beliefs influence the disease process.

"Good news travels fast; bad news travels much faster."

Fortunately, there is a change taking place in this field. The media is paying more attention to the possibility of health, and the fact that a cure is possible in many cases.

Many people have similar sets of expectations concerning their disease. They regard it as a very strong, deadly disease that is difficult or almost impossible to combat. Based on their general expectations, these people also have similar sets of beliefs. Simonton et al. (1978[174]) summarized some of the commonly held beliefs of the seventies:

- Cancer is synonymous with death.
- Cancer is something that strikes from without and there is no hope of controlling it.
- The treatment is drastic and negative and frequently has many undesirable results.
- Cancer is a strong and powerful enemy and is able to destroy the entire body.

These beliefs about the process and outcome have not been proven to be associated with a poor prognosis of cancer. However, as one can imagine, they definitely do not promote health or well-being. These beliefs promote helplessness and hopelessness. They are based on the medical knowledge of that time (1978), but are no longer scientifically accurate. For example, nowadays many people recover from cancer and live a happy life. (See the section on cancer and survival.)

Effects of Expectations

In their study of 152 patients at the Travis Air Force Base, Simonton et al. (1978[175]) noted the effects of positive and negative expectations on the disease process. The patients' responses to treatment depended on their expectations. When patients expressed a positive attitude towards treatment, their responses were positive. When they expressed a negative attitude, their responses to treatment were negative.

The researchers found that the patients' attitudes served as a predictor to the disease prognosis. A positive attitude was associated with a good response to treatment. In their book, "Getting Well Again," they did not specify what a positive or negative attitude comprised.

Patients with positive beliefs and a severe prognosis did better and experienced fewer side effects than patients with negative beliefs and a less severe prognosis (Simonton).

Cunningham et al. (2000[176]) asked patients to rate on a five-point scale how strongly they believed that psychological interventions would affect the course of their disease. A strong connection was noticed between this rating and actual survival.

"No one really knows enough to be a pessimist."
- Norman Cousins -

Greer (1979[177]; 1990[178]) and Dean (1989[179]) concluded that the belief that one will overcome the disease has a positive influence on health and increases survival time. Minimizing the impact of the disease was associated with longer survival times in patients suffering from metastatic melanoma (Butow 1999[180]) and metastatic breast cancer (Butow, 2000[181]).

In her dissertation on the cognitive strategies of breast cancer patients, Oosterwijk (2004[182]) concluded that those patients who minimized or denied the seriousness of the disease were better off. Although she did not indicate any link to the disease prognosis, she did indicate that such denial enhanced the quality of life for the patients.

It should be noted that minimization, or denial of the seriousness of the disease, is not the same as denial of the disease itself. Minimizing, or denying the seriousness, means expecting that one will heal and lead a happy life afterwards. These are examples of positive outcome expectancy. On the other hand, denial of the disease is a coping style of repression, which is associated with a poorer prognosis. This is illustrated by Cooper et al. (1993[183]). They concluded that those people who used denial as a coping mechanism when confronted with major stressful events were more at risk of contracting breast cancer.

"Don't deny the diagnosis. Try to defy the verdict."
- Norman Cousins -

5.3   Coping

In a previous chapter, I discussed the three different categories of coping: problem-focused coping, meaning-focused coping, and emotion-focused coping. The problem-focused coping style has already been discussed in the chapter on events, and meaning-focused coping has been discussed in the chapter on appraisal. In this section, I would like to discuss emotion-focused coping separately.

People handle their emotions in many different ways. Some people express their emotions, while others deny or repress them. This chapter explains different ways of coping with emotions, and how they relate to cancer. A later chapter will discuss the actual emotions associated with poor prognoses.

5.3.1   Emotional Repression

One of the most frequent connections found between cancer development and the handling of emotions is non-expression. Non-expression can occur through suppression or repression (Bleiker 1997[184]; Temoshok 1985[185]). Suppression is when clients hold back the emotions they are aware of. Repression is a psychological defense mechanism whereby clients do not consciously know what emotions are present. Emotions are signals; repressing them is like ignoring the message.

> *Example:*
> *An ostrich puts its head in the sand when a hunter approaches. Somehow it thinks the danger will go away. The danger will actually increase as the ostrich ignores it, in which case it makes itself an easy prey for the hunter.*

Repressing emotions does not make them go away; on the contrary, their toxicity increases. Pert (1997[186]) suggests that when emotions are repressed or suppressed, they will eventually blow up in our system and become dangerous. She argues that all emotions are represented by peptides in the body. When we repress or suppress these emotions, they form a cluster of peptides in the body, a kind of emotional cyst.

Pert mentions in Moyers (1993[187]) that emotions play a key role in disease, and that emotional repression could even be causative of disease. She also relates this idea to the healing practices of native cultures that include a complete release of emotions. Positive thinking only assists in healing when the person actually believes it, rather than merely doing it. Otherwise, it could mask the emotions.

> *"Positive thinking could mask the emotions and help to repress them, if it denies the truth."*
> *- Candace B. Pert - (1993)*

Temoshok (1985[188]) made a clear distinction between the expressed emotions (real or faked) and the emotions that were actually present.

She studied the influence of coping styles on the prognosis of malignant melanoma. By comparing the expressed anxiety to a physical, electrical skin response, she found a correlation. The melanoma patients were repressing their anxiety more than the control groups (of heart patients and healthy people).

She also found that patients who were expressing anger and sadness had a higher lymphocyte count. (In other words, more lymphocytes were attacking the tumor.) Those who were repressing anger and sadness displayed a higher rate of mitosis (cancer growth). Patients who kept their emotions private had a slower recovery rate than those who were more expressive with their emotions. A higher degree of perceived stress and anxiety contributed to melanoma progression. Expressing these emotions can decrease the progressive effects of the stress.

Example:
A high degree of consciously perceived stress subjectively experienced as anxiety, distress, and/or dysphonic emotion, contributes significantly to melanoma progression.
It is possible that coping with this stress by expressing the emotion will buffer these otherwise negative effects.

In 1940, Wilhelm Reich proposed the model that cancer results from a failure to express emotions, especially sexually-related emotions (Pert 1997[189]). He suggested that through parental or social punishment, people had learned to repress their emotions.

Blumberg (1954[190]) noticed that patients with fast-growing tumors tried to make a good impression on others, compared to those with slow-growing tumors. The patients with fast-growing tumors had difficulties expressing their emotions because of their (obsessive) desire to make a good impression.

"It seemed that the emotional outlets were blocked by an extreme desire to make a good impression."
- E.M. Blumberg -

LeShan (1956[191]; 1977[192]) concluded in his study that one of the differentiating factors between cancer patients and non-patients was the ability to express anger and hostility. These emotions were "bottled up" by the patients. Goldfarb (1967[193]) summarized many studies on the psychological testing of cancer patients. He concluded that one of the main characteristics of patients with malignancies was that they were unable to express hostility. This confirmed the results obtained by LeShan.

Kissen (1966[194]), from the University of Glasgow, noticed that smokers who developed lung cancer had "poorer outlets for emotional discharge" than those who did not develop lung cancer. Smokers who had normal outlets for emotional discharge were much less likely to develop the disease.

Dattore (1980[195]) studied approximately 3000 male veterans and noted that those with cancer showed a significantly higher degree of emotional repression (measured by the Byrne's Repression-Sensitization scale), compared to the non-cancer group.

Watson (1984[196]) noticed that among the 57 patients investigated, the group with cancer showed a higher tendency to control emotional reactions and repress emotions. This was particularly true of emotions such as anger and hostility.

Greer et al. (1975[197]; 1978[198]) found a correlation between the suppression of emotions (especially anger) throughout the patient's adult life and the diagnosis of breast cancer. Their conclusions were later confirmed by Bagley (1979[199]). Greer et al. noticed that women with breast cancer never lost their tempers. To measure the expression of anger and other feelings, they developed a structured interview, and conducted this interview with 160 women. Associations between poor emotional expression and cancer development were found by Tarlau (1951[200]), Reznikoff (1955[201]), Schonfield (1975[202]), and Brémond (1986[203]). Connections to the development of breast cancer were found by Weihs (2000[204]). Links to lung cancer were found by Ganz (1991[205]), Thomas (1974[206]), Bieliauskas (1982[207]), Jensen (1987[208]), and Weihs (1996[209]; 2000[210]).

Gross (1989[211]) reviewed 18 studies concerning the effects of emotional expression on the development of cancer. Although there are some differences in the definition of emotional expression, the consensus is that the non-expression of emotions "may be directly involved in cancer onset and progression."

Cooper (1993[212]) noted that women diagnosed with breast cancer tended to bottle up their emotions. Those experiencing a stressful event who were unable to express themselves faced the highest risk. The ability to express anger seemed to decrease the risk of cancer.

A meta-analysis by Garssen (2000[213]) concluded that those patients who did not express their emotions (so-called "repressors") showed a negative progression in their cancer. Although negative emotions might be unhealthy, expressing them is healthier than non-expression. Garssen (2001[214]), Reynolds (2000[215]), and Hislop (1987[216]) showed that more expression and less suppression of emotions resulted in longer survival times.

Pert (1997[217]) provided a theoretical background of why the repression of emotions might have the effect that many researchers observed. She explained that emotions are always tied to a specific flow of peptides (molecules). Repressing these emotions represses the peptides, so that they are stored in the body (or "bottled up"). Eventually, these stored peptides disturb the body's natural healing processes.

In situations where people are diagnosed with cancer, many emotions will surface, including emotions such as fear and feelings of depression. Expressing these emotions may be highly appropriate, rather than a sign of helplessness (Garssen 2002[218]).

5.3.2   Anti-Emotionality

Anti-emotionality (or rationality), as defined by Bleiker (1995[219]), is "an absence of emotional behavior or a lack of trust in one's own feelings." Cancer patients typically displayed a tendency to rationalize their emotions (Wirsching 1985[220]), or to control their emotional reactions (Watson 1984[221]). Emotional repression involves not showing emotional reactions, and pushing away emotions. Anti-emotionality is not recognizing and not acting upon one's own emotions.

Example:
When making decisions, many people have an instinctive feeling of what to choose. Anti-emotionality is when they need fundamental, rational reasons for their choice, and ignore their feelings.

Grossarth-Maticek (1985[222]) conducted a prospective study of personality and cancer among more than 1300 people. He noted that those who scored high on anti-emotionality and rationality faced the highest risk of cancer later in life. He also found that a specific type of behavioral therapy, geared towards changing this attitude of anti-emotionality, resulted in a reduction of risk.

Temoshok (1992[223]) noticed a commonality among cancer patients in that they displayed a high level of self-denial and unawareness of their own emotional needs. Those patients had larger tumors and weaker immune systems compared to other patients.

In a large-scale, controlled study involving more than 9000 participants, Bleiker (1996[224]) noticed a small increase in cancer occurrence in those women whose behavior was the least influenced by emotions, and who tended to mistrust their emotions. Women who scored high on anti-emotionality had a higher chance of developing cancer later. Their degree of emotionality was measured by questions about whether or not they trusted their emotions, responded emotionally to people, and whether their behavior was influenced by emotions.

5.3.3   Social Support

Hislop(1987[225]) and Waxler-Morrison (1991[226]) studied social support issues in cancer patients. They concluded that expressive social activities with social support were associated with longer survival times. The most important variable was not just the social support network, but how patients interacted with their contacts. These social interactions created situations where patients were able to express their emotions, and at the same time learn new ways of handling their feelings.

Reynolds(1990[227]) demonstrated that women with few relationships, especially few friends, and those experiencing social isolation had a higher chance of developing cancer.

Maunsell (1995[228]) followed 224 women with breast cancer over a period of seven years. He concluded that those women who had at least one trustworthy person, someone they could discuss their problems with confidentially, had a longer survival rate than those who did not. Of the women who had a support person, 72% were still alive, compared to 56% of those lacking such a person. This indicates that being able to talk about problems is related to extended survival.

5.4 Emotions

As discussed in the psychosomatic model, the appraisal process leads to coping styles which trigger emotions and, finally, result in behaviors. These emotions are often an indicator of how the appraisal and coping mechanisms have worked and the underlying beliefs behind these processes. Research has indicated that certain emotions are associated with poorer health outcomes. This chapter is about those emotions.

Some of the emotions discussed are related to the news of the diagnosis. Other emotions were already present in the lives of the patients. Some emotions were already present, and are aggravated by the diagnosis.

All emotions influence the immune system directly, with the help of peptides Pert (1997[229]). Emotions cause certain peptides to flow through the body. These peptides can be seen as the chemical representations of those emotions. The immune system receives the peptides and changes its workings.

In this chapter, I will discuss research on singular emotions and emotional cysts. Singular emotions are emotions that are directly related to the event or situation. Emotional cysts usually begin in childhood. During the patient's life, similar emotions come together to form a metaphorical cyst.

5.4.1 Emotions

5.4.1.1 Anxiety

When diagnosed with cancer, many people interpret this as a death sentence, for which there is no hope. This interpretation used to be accurate, but it no longer is. Many people are cured of cancer and go on to live healthy, active, and productive lives.

Although statistically there is a higher chance of survival than of dying from cancer, people most often experience anxiety after hearing the diagnosis. This anxiety is usually very persistent. Even after patients are cured, the fear of recurrence can persist. Research has shown that high levels of anxiety are associated with poorer health outcomes.

Gilbar (1996[230]) interviewed 40 breast cancer patients. After eight years, eight of the patients had died of cancer. Those patients who died had also shown much higher levels of anxiety in the initial interview than those who survived. Gilbar concluded that elevated levels of anxiety in the initial interview may predict survival times.

Weihs (2000[231]) noticed that patients with low levels of anxiety also showed a lower mortality rate. However, those people with a low level of anxiety and a high level of emotional repression showed a higher mortality rate. High levels of anxiety were associated with higher mortality regardless of the emotional expression. He concluded that the restriction of emotions was one of the elements that predicted mortality from breast cancer. This is particularly true when it is combined with anxiety.

5.4.1.2 Anger and Hostility

When comparing cancer patients with non-patients, LeShan (1956[232]; 1977[233]) noted that one of the main differences was the ability to express emotions of anger and hostility. Patients tended to bottle up these emotions, while non-patients did not experience these emotions as much.

Goldfarb (1967[234]) reviewed many studies on the psychological testing of cancer patients. He concluded that one of the characteristics of cancer patients was their inability to express hostility. This was again confirmed by Greer et al. (1975[235], 1978[236]), who studied this trait in 160 women. The women were interviewed regarding how they handled life. Those women with cancer tended to suppress their anger throughout their lives, whereas the others did not. These findings were also confirmed in a study by Scherg (1981[237]), of 2026 women, and Watson (1984[238]); Jansen (1984[239]) Bremond (1986[240]).

Simonton (1975[241]) argued that the tendency to harbor resentment and the inability to forgive are characteristics of cancer patients. Cooper (1993[242]) noted that the ability to express anger reduced the risk of cancer. Garssen (2002[243]) concluded that cancer patients could be characterized by the non-expression of emotions, and especially the non-expression of anger.

These studies show that there is an increased risk of cancer when people repress their anger.

5.4.1.3 Hopelessness and Helplessness

The issues of hopelessness and helplessness have been briefly discussed in the chapter on beliefs. Hopelessness is often an emotional expression of the belief "The future will be worse." Helplessness is often an emotional expression of the belief "I cannot do anything about it." Hopelessness and helplessness denote a tendency towards negative moods and outcomes; therefore they are sometimes referred to as "pessimism" (Garssen 2004[244]).

Schmale (1971[245]) observed that female cancer patients often expressed feelings of hopelessness towards a surrounding conflict. They saw no solution for the conflict, and showed behaviors indicative of "giving up." The conflict had often occurred six months prior to the diagnosis of cervical cancer. Based on the level of helplessness that patients expressed, Schmale was able to predict, with 73.6% accuracy, who would develop cancer and who would not.

Temoshok (1987[246]) noted that helplessness or hopelessness where predicting factors for melanoma in men. States of helplessness or hopelessness were often observed in men 18-29 months prior to the actual diagnosis. She found similar patterns for cervical and uterine cancer, and for cancer in general in men. These patterns were also noticed by other researchers, such as Goldfarb (1967[247]), Thomas (1974[248]), Bahnson (1980[249]), Jensen (1987[250]), Everson (1996[251]), Schulz (1996[252]), Molassiotis (1997[253]), Watson (1998[254]), and Garssen (2000[255]; 2001[256]).

Example:
The Type C individual may be seen as chronically hopeless and helpless, even though this is not consciously recognized, in the sense that the person basically believes that it is useless to express one's needs: the needs cannot, or will not, be met by the environment.
(Temoshok 1987)

Watson (1999[257]) investigated the psychological responses of 578 women with breast cancer. In a follow-up study 5 years after the initial interview, a correlation was observed between feelings of hopelessness or helplessness and an increased risk of relapse or death from cancer.

Greer (1979[258]; 1982[259]; 1991[260]) investigated the psychological response to breast cancer during the 3 months after surgery. A follow-up study conducted 5 years later indicated that those with the poorest prognosis initially showed feelings of hopelessness and helplessness, prior to or just after the surgery. These findings were confirmed in a 10-year and 15-year follow-up study (Greer 1990[261]).

Everson et al. (1996[262]) investigated the link between hopelessness and cancer occurrence among 2428 participants. In their 6-year follow-up study, they noticed that those who received moderate or high scores on the initial hopelessness scale had a mortality rate three times higher than those with low scores, or those in the control group. They also noticed that hopelessness increased the risk of cancer itself. Grossarth-Maticek (1985[263]) concluded that long-standing hopelessness was associated with a higher risk of developing cancer.

5.4.1.4 Bereavement and Grief

A study by Barthrop (1977[264]) focused on 26 people who just had lost their spouses. This bereaved group showed a significant decrease in immune function compared to the control group, who had not been bereaved during the previous two years. The lymphocyte function (which plays an important role in the natural healing response to cancer) of the bereaved group was significantly depressed. This decrease in immune function lasted for a long time, and was even measurable several weeks after the spouses had died.

Jasmin et al. (1990[265]) performed a double-blind experiment in which 77 women were interviewed before undergoing a breast biopsy. Patients and interviewers were unaware of the diagnosis. They concluded that women with unresolved recent grief were more likely to develop breast cancer.

Cooper et al. (1993[266]) concluded that the combination of bereavement and emotional suppression increased the risk of breast cancer.

5.4.1.5 Loneliness

Many articles have been written about loneliness, isolation, and the development of cancer. Loneliness is the personal experience of being alone. Some people can feel alone in a crowd, while others live on their own and never go out, but do not feel that they are lonely.

Glaser et al. (1985[267]) found that students who scored high on the UCLA loneliness scale also had a depressed immune system compared to those who scored normally on the loneliness scale. According to Kieholt-Glaser (1984[268]), those students who felt alone were having more trouble producing plasma cells, which are needed to create antibodies required during the healing process.

Reynolds et al. (1990[269]) reanalyzed the data presented by Berkman et al. (1979[270]), and confirmed the original conclusion that those who felt socially isolated were substantially more at risk for cancer mortality. They analyzed 6928 adults. Those with few social contacts who felt isolated were twice as likely to die from cancer as those who did not.

Ell et al. (1992[271]) associated emotional support with longer survival times in breast, colorectal and lung cancer patients. It must be noted that even with emotional support, people can feel lonely and isolated.

"In particular expressive-social activities and social support,
not merely extraversion, have been found to be related to longer
survival time."
- David Spiegel -(1997[272])

In a seven-year follow-up study, Maunsell (1995[273]) noted that women with no confidants during the first few months after surgery had a death rate almost twice as high as those who did have a confidant. The confidant could also be a physician or a nurse.

Hislop (1991[274]) discovered six elements of social relationships that were significantly associated with longer survival.
Those elements were:
- Marital status.
- Support from friends.
- Contact with friends.
- Total support from friends.
- Relatives and neighbors.
- Employment status.
- Social network size.

5.4.2   Emotional Cysts

When similar emotions build up and combine, they can form some kind of connection. This connection can be seen as an emotional cyst.

Usually a trauma leads to the formation of a cyst. Similar unresolved emotions are linked to the original trauma and increase the size of the cyst. Several researchers discovered a relationship between the presence of such an emotional cyst and the later development of cancer. A trauma could lead to an emotional cyst, and the cyst could increase the risk of cancer.

This configuration could have started many years ago, and is sometimes defined as an emotional "Gestalt." The Merriam-Webster Online Dictionary for 2004 defines it as "a structure, configuration, or pattern of physical, biological, or psychological phenomena so integrated as to constitute a functional unit with properties not derivable by summation of its parts."

Some authors have noticed a pattern of emotional trauma in groups of cancer patients that was absent in the control groups. LeShan (1989[275]) reviewed the literature from 1800 to 1900 and concluded that almost all studies mentioned the patients' emotional life histories. The presence of traumas was important in assessing the risk of cancer, and the possibility of a poor prognosis. In his study of 250 patients diagnosed with a malignancy, LeShan (1956[276]) noted that a childhood trauma was present in 62% of the cancer patients, and in only 10% of the control group. He concluded that an early emotional trauma increased the risk of cancer later in life. Such trauma would supposedly lead to an increase in tension towards one or both parents. Later, LeShan included the presence of a childhood trauma as one of the psychological indicators for predicting cancer development.

Later, LeShan (1977[277]) reconfirmed his initial findings. He studied the life histories of 500 patients. One of the typical patterns identified was a childhood trauma. Such trauma included feeling of isolation, neglect, difficult, dangerous or intense interpersonal relationships, parental deprivation, and coldness. He noticed that 76% of the cancer patients showed such patterns in their past, and had also recently experienced an emotional loss. Traumatic patterns were relived through the recent emotional loss, which influenced cancer growth.

"The result was despair, as though the "bruise" left over from childhood had been painfully struck again.... The growing despair

that these people faced appears to be strongly connected with the loss
that each suffered in childhood."
- Lawrence LeShan - (1977)

Kissen (1967[278]) studied 366 male patients with lung cancer. The patients were characterized by a "childhood trauma resulting from death or absence of parents or chronic friction between them." Kune (1991[279]) noticed that cancer patients showed a higher incidence of childhood unhappiness than those without cancer.

Thomas (1974[280]) conducted a prospective study of 1337 medical students. Medical students who graduated between 1948 and 1964 were interviewed and followed later in life. Those students who developed cancer later had also scored the lowest on the closeness-to-parents scale during the initial interview. This lack of closeness to one or both parents was believed to have a predictive value for the onset of cancer later in life. Lack of closeness to a parent and emotional deprivation were particularly present in relation to the mother. Shaffer et al. (1982[281]) later reported the prognostic value of closeness to the father (for cancer in men). They followed people for 16-32 years. Those who later developed cancer had scored lower on the closeness-to-father scale during the initial interview than the control group.

Bahnson (1980[282]) claimed that the main psychological differences between patients and non-patients were the loss, despair and disappointment they had experienced with regard to their parents during childhood. For cancer patients, relationships with parents were dependent and conflicting in nature. They were unsatisfying, particularly with regards to the mother. It was a huge effort for the children to sustain these relationships. Later in life, when such patients experienced a separation, they would feel severe deprivation. They would go to great lengths to replace that emotional relationship with another relationship or with an object of adoration (person, work, etc.) Such patients would have to conquer their learned mistrust and hostility towards the new relationship. Once the relationship had been established, the childhood losses would be out of sight. If the relationship broke up, the original childhood despair would return and intensify. The patients had never really learned to handle their emotional pain, but had covered it up with new relationships. This increased their mistrust and hostility every time they experienced a similar emotional separation. This could eventually lead the patients to give up all hope of ever achieving a worthwhile relationship.

Example:
When a child is bitten by a dog at a young age, a (minor) trauma can emerge. When the same person is confronted with a dog later, they are cautious of the interaction. If they work hard to trust the dog, they can put aside their fear and mistrust, which were learned during childhood. They can even create a meaningful relationship with the dog. However, if the dog bites them after they put aside their fears, the trauma which was present is reactivated and intensified. This is a normal reaction towards learning.

Bahnson tested these ideas and came to the conclusion that cancer patients "remembered their parents as more neglectful and cold" compared to the control group. This childhood trauma was, according to Bahnson, the reason for their inhibition of emotional expression.

Lerner (1994[283]) reported his observations of female patients with cancer of the reproductive system. He noticed that many patients with cancer had also experienced childhood sexual abuse. He suspected a correlation between these types of cancer and the abuse. Many of these women also attributed their cancer to the experience of being abused. He mentioned that certain psychological traumas could have a specific and direct link to the site of the cancer. This idea is supported by Hamer (1999[284]; 1999[285]), but is still highly controversial in the scientific community.

5.4.3   Depression

From a historical standpoint, Galen observed that breast cancer occurred most often in melancholic women as early as 130 AD (Lerner 1994[286]). Gendron (1759[287]) mentioned that depressed women with high anxiety levels had a higher chance of developing cancer.

Many researchers have indicated the influence of depression. However, the definition used varies greatly. Some studies have described it as similar to loneliness, while others place it closer to hopelessness. Depression is a combination of several emotions which have already been discussed separately.

In a Swedish study of 2500 participants, Thomas (1973[288]) noted that female cancer patients had a tendency towards depression before they became aware of the diagnosis. This tendency towards depression was absent in those participants not suffering from cancer. In another prospective study of more than 2000 Western Electric employees, Persky et al. (1987[289]) found a significant correlation between scores on the depression scale (Minnesota Multiphasic Personality Inventory) and the later development of cancer.

Section C

Current Psychological Cancer Treatment Programs

6

Current Treatment Programs

Many psychological therapies have been used with cancer patients. Several of these programs are outlined in books, articles or on websites. Most consist of a combination of different interventions associated with increased health. Research focusing on specific interventions, or the effects of complete programs, has yet to be conducted. Descriptions of complete treatment programs are very rare. Only Simonton and Spiegel describe their programs in more detail.

In this chapter, I will focus on the major therapeutic programs for cancer patients. I will describe two programs in detail, and will highlight other programs by describing their key elements. The actual interventions are discussed in the next chapter.

6.1   Simonton Program

The program developed by Carl Simonton and his wife, Stephanie Simonton-Matthews (1978[290]), is probably one of the most widely known psychologically-focused therapies for cancer patients. The couple started at the Cancer Counseling and Research Center in Dallas, and later established the Simonton Cancer Center in California.

Their "Whole Person Approach to Cancer Treatment" is geared towards enhancing the patient's immune system with psychological interventions and developing constructive beliefs. The enhanced immune system is more actively involved in fighting off the cancer, and constructive beliefs support the activity of the immune system. By imagining an active immune system, the patients themselves become more involved and active in their healing process.

The Simontons noticed that spontaneous remission was often associated with patients who had positive images of themselves, and imagined themselves as being healthy. Using imagination interventions, they noticed that patients' fear and stress were reduced, depression was reduced, and there was a noticeable decrease in feelings of hopelessness and helplessness.

Physiologically, they noticed an increase in the functioning of the immune system after the imagination interventions (Simonton 1978[291]).

6.1.1 Results

In their study, Simonton et al. (1980[292]) concluded that patients with advanced cancer lived twice as long as expected from statistics when they were also treated with psychological interventions. They studied 159 patients with medically incurable malignancies. The estimated survival time for these patients, based on national statistics, was 12 months after the diagnosis. With complementary psychological therapy, the average survival time increased to 24.4 months.

In a follow-up, conducted four years after the initial study, they noticed that 63 (of the original 159 patients) were still alive. These patients had outlived the statistics by at least four times! For 43 of those patients, the cancer was stable, decreasing, or had even disappeared completely.

Example:
The patients in our study who are alive have lived, on average, two times longer than patients who received medical treatment alone. Even those patients in the study who have died lived one a half times longer than the control group.

Adapted from Simonton (1978)

6.1.2 Goals

The goal of psychological treatment, as proposed by Simonton, is to improve the patient's overall quality of life, increase immune functioning, and assist patients in becoming active participants in their healing process.

The main focus is on increasing the quality of life, but suggestions that one can change the course of the disease to improve physical health are also given.

Therapists try to accomplish this through the use of imagery, belief change interventions, reduction of emotional distress (anger, fear, blame and guilt), reading assignments, and education sessions.

In addition to these interventions, they also ask patients to focus on activities that are important to them, which provide them with an experience of joy and fulfillment. Helping patients spend more time on fulfilling activities influences their quality of life, as well as the functioning of their immune system.

6.1.3 Interventions

The main intervention used is aggressive imagery. Patients are instructed to imagine their immune system combating the cancer cells three times a day.

Every imagery process starts with relaxation. During this time, imagery patients are asked to imagine the tumor as a weak, soft and confused organism.

Traditional treatment is imagined as being very potent, effective and capable of shrinking the tumor easily. The immune system is imagined as being strong, and working with traditional interventions to fight and destroy the tumor. White blood cells are imagined as a large army that overwhelms and destroys the tumor while easily disposing of dead cells. Finally, patients are instructed to imagine themselves as healthy and energetic.

Therapists also make use of cognitive restructuring. They focus primarily on recognizing unhealthy beliefs and turning them into healthy beliefs. The following areas are investigated for unhealthy beliefs: the nature of our universe; our nature; life; death; health; illness, pain and suffering; purpose and destiny. Patients are also taught to recognize and change limiting beliefs themselves, without the aid of the therapist. This gives patients more control over their own lives.

During this program, patients are also taught generic empowering beliefs about health and cancer. These beliefs include:
- People are healthy by nature.
- Disease is a blockage of the natural healing powers of the body.
- Cancer cells have been eliminated by our body since the time we were born. It is a natural process.

- People do the best they can with the resources they have at that moment.

Hope is addressed by having patients recognize the possibility of health while also accepting the possibility of death. Forced hope of health is avoided. Patients are taught to hope for better, and at the same time accept that things could become worse. Typical statements are: "I want to get better and it's acceptable to get worse," and "I want to live and I'm ready to die."

Over the course of treatment, therapists also make use of assignments which patients can do at home. Assignments increase patients' feeling of control.

6.1.4   Key Alements of the Approach

The program includes the following components:

Goals:
- Increase the patient's quality of life.

Elements:
- Mind-body education.
- Increase hope.
- Secondary gain.
- Resolve emotions (guilt, failure, fear, anger).
- Reduction of distress.
- Active patient.
- Patient participation.
- Pain management.
- Enhance joyful activities.
- Meaning of life.
- Communication skills.
- Accepting death.

Interventions:
- Imagery.
- Relaxation.
- Suggestions.
- Cognitive therapy: Rational Emotive Therapy (RET).
- Goal setting.
- Reading assignments.

6.1.5 Program

The Simontons designed a 6-week protocol to help patients increase their health and quality of life.

6.1.5.1 Week 1: Becoming Active

The first week is geared towards increasing patient participation through reading assignments and relaxation exercises.

Reading

Patients need to become active in their own process. They are given reading assignments which they can do at home. These books gradually increase hope and explain the mind-body connection. Patients learn the value of psychological work, gain insight into how their minds influence their health, and learn techniques that they can do by themselves.

Suggested books are:
- Simonton, O. Carl & Simonton-Matthews, Stephanie & Creighton, James L. (1978) Getting Well Again, New York: Bantam
- Hutschnecker, A.A. (1953) Will to Live, Thomas Y. Crowell Company
- Pelletier, Kenneth R. (1992) Mind as a Healer, Mind as a Slayer, New York: Delacorte
- Samuels, M. & Samuels, N. (1975) Seeing with the Mind's Eye, Random House

Relaxation and Imagery

Patients are taught relaxation techniques, and are instructed to practice these three times a day with the use of tapes or CDs. This teaches patients how these imagery techniques work, and how they can perform these types of imagery exercises on their own. They learn how they can relax.

Patients are motivated to continue to use these relaxation exercises throughout the program. During the program, patients need to reduce their use of tapes and CDs and rely more and more on their own forms of imagery. Every week, the use of audio is reduced by half. Occasionally, if their level of distress increases and imagery becomes difficult, patients can revert to using the tapes or CDs again.

Activities

During the first week, patients are motivated to find activities that they enjoy. They create a list of at least 5 things or activities that add significant value to their lives. They write down activities that give them joy and fulfillment. Over the next few weeks, this list should grow in size. Patients are instructed to pursue the activities on their lists.

6.1.5.2 Week 2: Learning from Stressors

During the second week, the daily relaxation exercises are continued. In addition, patients are asked to complete a questionnaire in which they list their major life stressors in the 6-18 months prior to the onset of the disease. This list of stressful events serves as a starting point for investigating patients' coping styles and participation. Patients are helped to recognize their participation in those stressful events.

One of the major interventions during this week is to aid patients in recognizing the secondary gains from their disease. Patients are helped to recognize the benefits they experience as a result of the disease, and how they can maintain those benefits when they are healthy.

6.1.5.3 Week 3: Psychotherapy

This week, psychotherapy starts to aid patients in expressing their emotions and discussing the issues they face. Patients are asked to discuss their issues with their friends and family. This continues to be the theme for the psychotherapy throughout the rest of the program.

6.1.5.4 Week 4: Death and Resentment

Existing imagery is expanded upon with dying and death imagery. Through the use of this imagery, patients start exploring their beliefs about death. This helps them to come to terms with death, and face their feelings about dying.

The other issue that is addressed during this week is overcoming resentment.

With the help of another imagery exercise, patients learn to forgive other people. This imagery reduces feelings of resentment, and assists patients in gaining insights into their own mental processes.

6.1.5.5 Week 5: Goal Setting

Patients are taught goal setting techniques, and are instructed to create 3, 6 and 12-month goals. These goals are then incorporated into their imagery exercises, so that they actually imagine themselves after overcoming obstacles and reaching their goals.

They are also assisted in composing a 2-year health plan. This plan includes joyful activities, continuation of the imagery exercises, and finding ways to keep the benefits of the disease that were discovered during week 2.

6.1.5.6 Week 6: Inner Guide

This final week of therapy is used to help the unconscious mind assist the patient in achieving health.

A new exercise is added to the list of imagery exercises: "the internal guide." This imagery is intended to aid patients in listening to their unconscious mind and to the messages from their body. During the imagery exercise, a communication is established between patients and their unconscious minds. The information and actions presented during this communication guides patients towards health.

6.1.5.7 After 6 Weeks

One of the goals of the program is to assist patients in becoming active participants in their healing processes. When the program is over, patients have learned all they need to know in order to continue on their own.

After these 6 weeks, many of the exercises are integrated into daily living, and it should be very easy for patients to continue performing them indefinitely.

6.1.6 Spiegel Program

Spiegel (1991[293]; 1993[294]) developed "Supportive-expressive group therapy," which is based on the expression of emotions towards others. This program is the only group therapy I will discuss because it has been described very well. The program focuses on current issues that arise in the group spontaneously. Planned and structured interventions do not take place.

The program is designed as group therapy, although most of the group issues are related to personal issues. They use the group as a "playground" for patients to express their emotions. Spiegel uses the group to decrease feelings of loneliness, to generate different options (during a discussion), and to express emotions. The manuals (1991[295]; 1993[296]) are created for breast cancer patients, but the techniques can be used for other cancer patients as well.

6.1.7   Results

Participation in group therapy was shown to prolong survival times by 17.7 months (Spiegel 1983[297]; 1991[298]; 1991[299]). The control group (36 participants) had a median survival time of 18.9 months, whereas the intervention group (50 participants) had a median survival time of 36.6 months. The survival time of the intervention group was almost doubled. The difference in survival times was only noticed after 20 months (Vries 1997[300]). This could indicate the time the body needs to recuperate.

They formed groups of 7 to 10 people, which lasted for one year. The groups were designed to be supportive, including self-disclosure and sharing mutual fears and concerns. Groups were formed with only breast cancer patients to increase the homogeneousness, and therefore the cohesion of the group. A cohesive group easily shares support, and suggestions from peers are more easily accepted. Homogeneous groups reduce feelings of isolation, and provide validation of patients' personal experiences. Patients were given the opportunity to stay as long as they wished, but for investigation purposes the therapy stopped after a year. After this year, an increase in survival time was noticed (Spiegel et al. 1989[301]).

6.1.8   Goals

The primary goal is to enhance the patient's quality of life. This is accomplished by also pursuing the following sub-goals:
- Increasing openness and emotional expressiveness both inside and outside the group.
- Improving social and family support.
- Accepting the changes in the body and in the patient's self-image.
- Improving coping skills.
- Improving the doctor-patient relationship.

- Detoxifying feelings about death and dying.
- Development of a life project.

Accomplishing these goals automatically increases the patient's perceived quality of life. When these goals are achieved, patients have a satisfying social network, where they can express their emotions, and have discovered more effective coping skills for handling situations. They also feel less isolated, and have an increased feeling of control over their health and obtaining their personal goals. Patients' fears (including existential fears) are reduced.

6.1.9   Therapeutic Overview

One of the major pillars on which Spiegel based his approach was the field of existential psychotherapy. This type of therapy deals with basic issues of existence that might be a source of problems. These are common for all people and include issues such as death, freedom, loneliness, and meaninglessness. Patients learn to reduce the tension associated with these issues.

Existential psychotherapy focuses on the here and now in order to increase self-knowledge and awareness, personal responsibility, choice, and learning to tolerate anxiety (Edgerton 1994). There is no search for truth, but the patients' views are accepted for whatever they are. Within existential psychotherapy, different emphases can be noticed. Deurzen (1990[302]) puts the emphasis on what it means to be alive, while Frankl (1959[303]) focuses on what is most meaningful in life for patients. Others focus on death.

This is the opposite of the "positive thinking" movement, where one should only express positive emotions. In existential psychotherapy, acknowledging and expressing negative emotions is valuable. As a matter of fact, the most important part is accepting and expressing one's true feelings. The utterance of hostility and feelings of depression are interpreted as signs of life. Based on the idea that emotional expression is the greatest difficulty with these emotions, the willingness and ability to express them is considered a good sign.

These fundamental issues of existential psychotherapy can be found throughout the Spiegel approach (1981[304]). The therapy program places the greatest emphasis on the present, sometimes taking a look at the past and future, but always focused on the here and now. Patients are supported in fully accepting the present situation, of mind and body, without repression or denial. Patients are motivated to live the life they want for themselves, and not what others expect their life to be. They are supported in accepting the negative sides of the present situation, while expressing their emotions and goals in life.

The therapy consists of a 1.5-hour group session once a week. During these sessions, group discussions take place and hypnotic procedures are taught to reduce anxiety and pain. Topics of discussion are: fears, reactions to bad news, family problems, limitations, communication with physicians, mortality, losses, life priorities, and relationships.

During the meetings, the therapist facilitates emotional expression by the members and discussion of issues they face at that moment. If certain issues do not arise spontaneously during the sessions, the therapist makes sure those issues are discussed. By virtue of fully accepting the current state of the group and their current issues, no planned structure is possible for the sessions.

This lack of structure does not leave the therapist without responsibilities. The task of the therapist is to:
- Increase openness to feelings and thoughts and encourage emotional expression, ensuring that everything can and will be discussed.
- Create an atmosphere of acceptance and a suspension of direct confrontation.
- Build a cohesive, respectful and mutually supportive group in which members can contribute to the extent they like.
- Place emphasis on the present, rather than past problems.
- Promote the development of relationships outside the group, and acceptance of relationships within the group.
- Deal with existential issues of death and dying when the group is ready to consider them.
- Address coping with the illness rather than attempting to correct long-standing problems or change personalities.
- Deal with personality issues only when they interfere with group processes.

6.1.10 Key Elements of the Approach

Goals:
- Increase quality of life.

Elements:
- Focus on the present.
- Emotional expression.
- Pain management.
- Reduction of distress (especially fear).
- Acceptance of the current state of mind and body.
- Acceptance and reduction of the fear of death.
- Meaning of life.
- Patient participation.
- Assertiveness.

Interventions:
- Group support.
- Cognitive therapy.
- Group discussions.
- "Testing" behavior within the group.

6.1.11 Program

This type of therapy cannot be structured the way other programs are. By fully accepting the current issues that the group faces and dealing with them as they arise, the program will be different for each group. The program is composed of elements which should be discussed. Only when a certain subject is structurally ignored by the group will the therapist address that issue.

The following elements are present throughout the program:
- Discussion of fears and anger about death and dying. Teaching patients that they can come to terms with their own mortality.
- Discussion of how patients can use the rest of their lives as fully as possible. Giving new meaning to life goals and reordering priorities.
- Reduction of isolation by making new friends and creating a sense of belonging. This is partly established through the use of coherent groups, in which the disease is the "belonging" factor. Groups are also stimulated to create meaningful relationships inside and outside the group.
- Discussing conflicting feelings towards patients' friends, families and medical teams.

6.2   Autonomy Training Program

Grossarth-Maticek (1982[305]; 1984[306]; 1991[307]) created a form of cognitive behavioral therapy that he initially named "Creative Novation Behaviour Therapy." He later renamed it "Autonomy Training" to reflect the main purpose of the program: to increase the autonomy of patients.

He studied the differences between healthy people and people with a disease. Cancer patients showed distinctive patterns. They tended to repress their emotions (especially anger and anxiety) and felt hopeless and helpless. This eventually led to indecisiveness towards their actions. He concluded that such patients tended to display a lack of autonomy and a high degree of emotional dependency. Cancer patients tend to depend on relationships with people, jobs, objects or situations (object relationships) and show a passive role for their own needs. They place others' needs above their own. Based on these notions, he created his program.

6.2.1   Results

Grossarth-Maticek (1985[308]; 1995[309]) developed a test to measure how much control people experience in getting maximum pleasure out of their lives. He selected a group of 1200 cancer patients who scored low on this test, indicating that they did not experience control over their lives. These patients were randomly divided into two groups, one of which received psychotherapy while the other served as a control group. The group who received psychotherapy survived 18.6 months on average, compared to 12.6 months for the control group.

These studies were later repeated by Grossarth-Maticek (in Simonton 1992[310]), who noticed that a six-hour psychotherapy program was already sufficient to produce noticeable effects on health outcomes. The program was later evaluated by Eysenck (1991[311]), who concluded that the program was effective in preventing the onset of illness and prolonging life.

6.2.2   Goals

The Autonomy Training Program is geared towards the reduction of dependent behavior, expression of emotions, decreasing feelings of hopelessness and reducing stress-inducing thoughts and negative self-interpretation.

"The aim of autonomy training is not to be a completely independent person, but someone who is able to create the possible conditions which lead to pleasure and contentment."
- Thomas R. Blakeslee - (1997)

6.2.3   Key Elements of the Approach

Goals:
- Reduction of dependence on relationships (object dependence).

Elements:
- Feeling of control.
- Emotional expression.
- Increasing hope.
- Decreasing stress cognitions.
- Reducing negative self-interpretation.
- Assertiveness, actively pursuing one's own needs.
- Active patients.
- Reduction of dependencies.
- Secondary gains.

Interventions:
- Relaxation.
- Imagery.
- Hypnosis.
- Goal setting.
- Suggestions.
- Cognitive therapy.
- Changing beliefs.

6.2.4   Program

During the program, patients are supported in making decisions independently and are stimulated to look towards the long-term positive effects of their new behavior. They learn to develop these new behaviors through self-observation.

Patients analyze their own behavior and are motivated to discover the consequences. They determine whether the results of their behavior are desirable or undesirable (for themselves). Patients also investigate the secondary gains from their current behavior.

After they have analyzed their current behavior, patients define their desired behavior. Desired behavior is defined as behavior which generates the most desirable outcomes in the long run, even if this means negative consequences in the short run. These desired behaviors are written down, including when and in what situations they should take place. This paper is read back on several occasions to commit the goals to memory.

Desired behaviors are practiced in a hypnotic trance with the help of suggestions and imagery. This imagery helps patients in discovering the positive results, and reinforces the belief that one can perform the new behavior.

During the program, psychotherapy is used to aid self-analysis and reduce anxiety about developing new behaviors. Special attention is devoted to patients who externalize the cause of their behavior. If they do not feel that they are in control of their behavior, this limits them in changing that behavior.

6.3   Cancer as a Turning Point Program

The research by LeShan focused mainly on personality factors, life events, and the onset and progression of cancer. He tried to distill a personality type that was prone to develop cancer.

He concluded that the combination of certain personality characteristics and experiencing certain distressing events suppresses the immune system. With a suppressed immune system, cancer had the chance to develop (LeShan 1977[312]; 1989[313]).

6.3.1   Results

LeShan claimed that during the 20 years he used this approach, half of his terminal patients went into remission and were still alive. Others seemed to live longer. Nearly all patients experienced a higher quality of life and found more enthusiasm in their lives.

6.3.2   Goals

The primary goal of the psychotherapeutic program developed by LeShan (1989[314]) was to free up the energy to live. The program is geared towards identifying patients' creative potential and tapping into their self-healing resources. In this way, LeShan intended to develop:

"The perception and the expression of the individual's special song
to sing in life."
- Lawrence LeShan - (1989) -

Patients are encouraged to take more time for themselves and put more effort into reaching their personal goals, regardless of others. To live life to its fullest, they increase their egocentrism and expand upon those things they like and reduce those things they dislike. The program focuses on increasing fun in life, and not on the causes of the lack of fun. At the same time, it focuses on health rather than no-cancer.

6.3.3 Key Elements of the Approach

Goals:
- Increase the quality of life.

Elements:
- Meaning of life.
- Emotional expression.
- Enhance fun.
- Assertiveness.
- Self worth.

Interventions:
- Goal setting.

6.3.4 Program

Throughout the program, patients are motivated to see the disease as being a "turning point" in their lives. This turning point should be the opportunity to reexamine their life and make new choices to fulfill their dreams.

LeShan initiated the focus on what is right with this person. Later, other programs would also use this approach. It is best illustrated by the following questions which are used.

Example:
- *What is right with this person?*
- *What are his special and unique ways of being, relating, creating, that are his own and natural ways to live?*
- *Etc.*

LeShan (1989[315])

6.4   Type C Transformation Program

Temoshok (1992[316]; 1993[317]) developed a program which she called "Type C Transformation." She was able to identify a cancer-prone behavior which she called "Type C." This behavioral pattern contains: emotional repression, anti-emotionality, unassertiveness, extremely compliant behavior, and excessive concern with the needs of others while repressing one's own needs.

Her program guides patients through the process of changing these patterns into healthier behaviors. The program is geared toward expressing emotions and becoming more assertive in relationships.

6.4.1   Results

I was not able to find the results of the actual application of this program. Temoshok attributes her results to the results of studies by Spiegel (1983[318]; 1989[319]; 1991[320]), Levy (1989[321]) and Fawzy (1990[322]).

6.4.2   Goals

The overall goal of the program is to increase the quality of life. The program places emphasis on patients being assertive and making self-directed decisions. Cancer patients seem to be extremely nice to other people, as if other people are more important than themselves. This was even noticeable after they heard the diagnosis of cancer. Transforming this behavior is one of the pillars of the Type C Transformation.

6.4.3   Key Elements of the Approach

Goals:
- Increase the quality of life.

Elements:
- Assertiveness.

- Emotional expression.
- Awareness of thoughts and emotions.
- Secondary gain.
- Feelings of control.
- Anger reduction.
- Patient participation.
- Hope.
- Communication skills.
- Laughter.

Interventions:
- Relaxation.
- Imagery.
- Cognitive therapy.

6.4.4 Program

During this program, patients are made aware of what their own needs are, and where their personal boundaries are. They might need the attention of friends or the absence of other friends at certain times. Other needs can be on a mental, emotional, spiritual, or physical level.

When patients become aware of their needs, the program moves on to having them assertively pursue those needs. This involves displaying assertive behavior towards friends, family and especially towards the medical or therapeutic team.

Example:
A clear example of this assertiveness was a client asking the nurse if the injection could take place in an hour, because the client was in a conversation and did not want to be disturbed. This was no problem for the nurse, and was a great relief to the patient.

To develop such assertiveness and aid patients in expressing their emotions, therapists make use of cognitive therapy.

Temoshok argues that in Type C behavior, emotions are repressed to such an extent that patients are not even aware of what emotions are present at a given time. The program teaches patients to become aware of emotions, recognize them, and be able to express their emotions.

6.5   Other Programs

The following programs are described in less detail, and less information is available. However, they seem important and offer many interesting possibilities. This chapter will briefly introduce these programs.

6.5.1   Wellness Community Program

The "Wellness Community" was founded by Harold Benjamin in 1982. It is a well-known center which offers psychosocial support to cancer patients and their families. The center encourages patients and their families to be active in their role against cancer. The goal is to improve the patients' quality of life and possibly prolong their lives.

The center makes use of support groups and teaches self-help techniques such as imagery. Central to the program is the idea that positive emotions and mental activities may improve patients' chances of recovering from cancer. Group activities focus on bringing laughter and smiles into the lives of patients (Melia 1987[323]).

One of the main issues is the "Patient Active Concept" created by Benjamin. He states that:

> *"People with cancer who participate in their fight for recovery*
> *from cancer will improve the quality of their life and may enhance*
> *the possibility of their recovery."*
> *- Harold Benjamin -*

Patients are encouraged to take small steps to increase their control of their lives and their decisions. They are actively involved in treatment decisions which promote an active stance and hope.

6.5.2   Exceptional Cancer Patients (ECaP) Program

The "Exceptional Cancer Patients Program" (ECaP[324]) was founded by Bernie Siegel (1989[325]) in 1978. This program is based on the notion of careful confrontation called "carefrontation." By giving patients therapeutic feedback in a loving and safe environment, they tend to aid patients in becoming an "exceptional cancer patient" (patients who get well unexpectedly). In addition to individual-oriented therapy, this program contains group support sessions.

The program is designed to help patients reduce stress, raise their level of control, and increase their personal value to life. Patients are assisted in discovering a new purpose and meaning in life and are actively involved in their treatment decisions.

Patients are taught to accept themselves and others as they are. One of the main goals is to remove psychological blockages.

6.5.3   Commonweal Cancer Help Program (CCHP)

The "Commonweal Cancer Help Program" (CCHP[326]) was founded in 1976 by Michael Lerner, in Bolinas, California. The overall goal is to increase the patients' quality of life. This is the only program that is promoted as an educational program, rather than a treatment, for people with cancer.

The program consists of groups of patients who meet for a week-long session. During separate sessions, patients are taught to reduce stress and resolve fears and anxieties (particularly about pain, illness and death). In addition to these teachings, patients work actively to explore the emotional and spiritual issues that they are facing. With the help of imagery, deep relaxation, meditation and creative means of personal expression, patients work on their issues.

> *"Our goal is to help participants live better and, where possible, longer lives"*
> *- Commonweal - (2005[327])*

6.5.4   Mind/Body Medical Institute (MBMI) Program

The "Mind/Body Medical Institute" was founded by Herbert Benson and colleagues in 1988 at the Harvard Medical School. Their research on the relaxation response formed the basis of their mind/body program.

The relaxation response is described by Benson (1975[328]) as:

> *"A series of coordinated physiologic changes elicited when a person engages in a repetitive word, sound, phrase or prayer, and passively disregards intrusive thoughts."*
> *- Herbert Benson -*

The goal of their 10-week Mind/Body program for cancer patients is to manage or reduce physical symptoms, cope with distress, teach patients to take better care of themselves, and maintain hope.

Interventions[329]:
- Stress management.
- Goal setting and meaning making.
- Cognitive restructuring.
- Journal writing.
- Relaxation and imagery training.
- Humor therapy.
- Support groups for patients and their families.

6.5.5   Fawzy Psychosocial Group Therapy Program

The Fawzy Psychosocial Group Therapy Program, as developed by Fawzy (1993[330]), resulted in psychological and immunological improvements. Fawzy (1990[331]; 1990[332]; 1993[333]) studied the effects of a short, structured intervention program. He worked with melanoma patients who had a good prognosis (whereas Spiegel studied patients with bad prognoses). The groups consisted of 7-10 people who met 90 minutes each week for 6 weeks.

6.5.5.1 Results

Unlike many other programs, this program's results have been published. In a follow-up study conducted 5 to 6 years later, Fawzy found a correlation between death rates and patients who had followed the psychotherapy program. Significant changes were observed in the therapeutic group after 6 months. The intervention group showed reduced psychological distress, greater use of active coping skills, and a significant increase in immune functioning. Only one-third of the patients in the control group showed similar results.

The therapeutic group also displayed a lower recurrence rate and a lower death rate compared to the control group. The difference in survival rates was shown 15 months after entry into the program (Vries 1997[334]). Even after a ten-year follow-up, participation in the intervention group remained predictive of survival (Fazwy 2003[335]).

6.5.5.2 Program

The therapy program included: enhancement of problem-solving skills, stress management through relaxation, psychological support, and education about the disease. To develop an active problem-focused coping style, cognitive therapy was used.

6.6 Summary and Overview

Key elements	Simonton ...	Spiegel ...	Autonomy Training ...	Cancer as a Turning Point ...	Type C Transformation ...	Wellness Community ...	Exceptional Cancer Patient ...	Commonweal Cancer Help ...	Mind/Body Medical Institute ...	Fawzy Psychosocial Group ...
Acceptance of current life		X			X					
Active Patient[1]	X		X				X	X		X
Anger	X				X					
Anxiety/fear	X	X							X	X
Assertiveness		X	X	X	X					
Communication skills	X				X					
Death	X	X						X		
Distress	X	X	X					X	X	X
Emotional/physical awareness					X			X		
Emotional expression		X	X	X	X					
Feeling of control			X		X	X	X		X	
Guilt	X									
Hope	X		X		X				X	
Humor/joy	X			X	X	X			X	
Meaning of life	X	X		X				X	X	
Mind-Body Education	X									X
Object dependence			X							
Pain management	X	X						X	X	
Patient participation[2]	X	X					X	X	X	
Quality of life	X	X		X		X	X		X	
Secondary gains	X		X		X					
Self-image/self-worth		X	X							

Therapeutic interventions	Simonton ...	Spiegel ...	Autonomy Training ...	Cancer as a Turning Point ...	Type C Transformation ...	Wellness Community ...	Exceptional Cancer Patient ...	Commonweal Cancer Help ...	Mind/Body Medical Institute ...	Fawzy Psychosocial Group ...
Cognitive therapy	X	X	X		X					
Creative expression								X		
Goal setting	X		X	X					X	
Group		X					X	X	X	X
Imagery	X		X		X	X		X		
Reading assignments	X									
Relaxation	X		X		X	X			X	X
Social support	X	X					X			
Suggestions (hypnotic)	X		X							
Writing									X	

Section D

Psychosomatic Model Applied To Cancer Treatment

7

Introduction

In Section B, the psychological elements associated with the development of cancer were discussed. Section C described some of the current psychological treatment programs. This section discusses the kinds of psychological interventions that can be used in cancer treatment based on the psychosomatic model. These interventions influence the clients' state of mind, which in turn influences their physiological well-being. The next section describes psychological interventions that directly affect physiology, without a mediating mental state.

Due to the nature of this section, there will be a slight overlap with regard to previous sections. The interventions discussed are not used exclusively with cancer clients, but can be used with a variety of people. In this work, I will focus on their use with cancer clients.

Previous chapters were more or less medically oriented. This chapter, as well as the succeeding chapters, will be more psychologically oriented. In this and forthcoming chapters, I will use "client" to reflect such a psychological orientation. This will be explained in detail in Section 8.1.2.2: Client, Patient or Student.

Unlike medical interventions, psychological interventions are primarily based on the relationship between the therapist and the clients. This relationship is of the utmost importance in any psychological therapy, especially when working with cancer clients. This relationship is partly defined by the personality of the therapist, which is why there is a separate chapter on the therapist, his beliefs, and his methods.

7.1   Psychological Therapy

Surgery, radiation therapy, chemotherapy, and other interventions are accepted treatments for cancer. They are based on scientific proof, including animal and human experimentation.

Other types of treatment often lack this scientific foundation. Every few years, the media is shocked by a new "miracle" therapy. The exact formula is usually kept a secret by the practitioner. Knowledge of the treatment usually spreads by word of mouth or through popular magazines sold at the supermarket. These "cures" are not backed up with extensive data or research, nor are they reported in the scientific literature. However, they do hold great appeal to people with cancer and their families. Particularly when mainstream medicine cannot heal them, people are willing to try unproven treatments, which could possibly be harmful.

There is a need to protect the public from such false claims. At the same time, there is a need to test and experiment with new paradigms. New (and unproven) methods should be investigated to determine their value. Without testing these claims, science is deprived of new insights. Many mainstream interventions grew out of ancient traditions. They used to be unproven and controversial, but somehow they produced the desired results. After careful scientific study, scientists were able to prove (or disprove) these interventions.

Unproven methods are not ineffective by definition; they might simply work in a way that we do not yet understand. In the case of radical new ideas, the paradigm could be so controversial that people cannot or will not believe it might be possible.

Example:
Copernicus said that the earth revolved around the sun. This was so controversial that Nicholas Copernicus published his paper anonymously. He was afraid of being prosecuted. His ideas were only ridiculous because they were not in accordance with current thinking.
In due time, he proved to be right. Eventually, his revolutionary thinking changed the way we view our world.

The fact that Copernicus' work was originally banned does not mean that the earth did not revolve around the sun. It means that people were not ready to understand the truth, and were unable to prove that his paradigm was false.

Several studies have shown that psychological intervention aids the immune system in overcoming diseases. Psychological therapy does not interfere with mainstream medicine. Although some *alternative* practitioners disagree, complementary approaches always work together with mainstream medicine. Medical interventions have proven to be successful in many cases. With the use of complementary psychological interventions, one can aid clients even more in their healing processes.

"A mind once stretched by a new idea never regains its original dimension."
- Oliver Wendell Holmes -

7.1.1 False Hope

In their quest for health, clients are willing to try anything, hoping for a miracle cure. They often reason that they might as well try it because "they have nothing to lose." Unfortunately, there *is* something to lose. Clients might gain a false sense of hope. They might lose interest in mainstream medicine or other complementary approaches. Finally, they might also be robbed of valuable time by pursuing an unsatisfactory therapy.

Complementary psychological therapy is often questioned on issues such as false hope. Some people are afraid that if cancer clients experience hope, they are fooling themselves, and will end up being disappointed. They think that as long as they are expecting the worst, they will not be disappointed. This is a form of false hopelessness. Such people like to call themselves realists, but are in fact pessimists.

Many people misinterpret the true value of an optimistic, pessimistic or realistic view of life. Pessimistic people view the world as a dark place, where there is only misery and everything is hopeless. They deny the positive side of things. Optimistic people view the world as one happy playground, where there is joy everywhere. They deny the negative side of life. Realistic people know that there are positive and negative aspects of everything in life. They fully accept both sides.

"No one really knows enough to be a pessimist."
- Norman Cousins -

Pessimist: "My glass is almost empty."
Optimist: "My glass is still full."
Realist: "I have half a glass."

When therapists work with the psychological issues that are described in this work, they are not providing false hope, but are assisting clients in being more realistic. Realistic hope is what is being communicated in this therapeutic approach.

Society and the medical team often issue some sort of death guarantee (although lesser every day) along with the diagnosis of cancer. Fortunately, this is not the case. There is no guarantee that one will die from cancer. On the other hand, there is also no guarantee that one will heal from cancer after the intervention. The issue of false hope only exists when the practitioner (medical or psychological) issues a guarantee that the client is healed after the intervention. False hope is thus only present as a false guarantee.

The presence of hope within clients is often associated with better health, and hopelessness is often a precursor for poor outcomes. Presenting hope, however, is no guarantee, but it assists the healing process.

Example:
When people marry, there is no guarantee that they will be happy. They hope they will be. This could be interpreted by a pessimist as false hope.
However, expecting the marriage to end in a few years is almost a guarantee that it will.
Hoping that one will be happy is no guarantee, but it surely helps.

Feelings of hope stimulate the placebo effect. The possible effects of a placebo cannot be denied, even in the context of cancer.

"Everybody knows that one dies of cancer, but I was not sure whether to apply this to myself. I considered this (belief) as nonsense."
Quote from a spontaneous remission patient
- Daan van Baalen - (1987[336])

False hope does exist, and can be seen as focusing solely on unrealistic and unachievable results, while denying the current truth. Such unrealistic expectations lead to disappointment and feelings of guilt. Hope of healing is a realistic hope. Realistic or mature hope is accepting the current feelings, thoughts, relationships, and possibilities of improvement. Focusing solely on hopelessness and self-pity is just as unrealistic as only seeing a positive and bright future.

False hope
- *"I only focus on the positive."*
- *"I can do whatever I want."*
- *"I can control everything."*

False hopelessness
- *"I am wallowing in despair."*
- *"I cannot control anything."*
- *"Everything scares me and the disease and emotions are controlling me."*

Realistic hope
- *"Sometimes I feel awful, and other times I feel more connected to life and others than ever before."*
- *"There are some things beyond my control. Yet, there are many things I can control."*
- *"I choose to live as fully as possible now. The quality of my life may be related to my physical health, but however long I may live, I plan to do it to the fullest of my ability."*

Hope triggers actions, and stimulates well-being. Without hope, people do not take action towards their well-being. Hope is a supporting emotion as well as a drive to trigger positive actions towards increased self-control.

Solano et al. (1993[337]) studied the relationship between psychosocial situations and the probability of symptom development. They concluded that "The best attitude with regard to prognosis appears to be full recognition of one's situation and a decisive will to do something about it." This conclusion is supported by many other authors. Hopelessness triggers inaction and letting things happen. Hope triggers the decisive will to take action.

"Trust in god and tie your camel to a tree."
- Muhammad -

7.1.2 Benefits of Psychological Therapy

Psychological therapy takes a lot of time; many techniques need extensive practice, and insurance companies most often do not reimburse clients for the costs. Clients must be actively involved and there are no guarantees. So, why should one consider therapy as a complementary intervention?

Karl Menninger, who founded the Menninger Clinic, noticed the reactions of cancer clients who were involved in complementary psychological interventions. Clients often reported that they felt far better and stronger than before the disease. They felt "weller than well." Similar comments have been made by clients who overcame cancer. They reported that after the therapeutic interventions, they had stronger psychological health, a positive self-concept, and a sense of control over their lives.

Example:
Like breaking a bone, the bone will increase in strength when it is healed. Exposure to environmental pollution will decrease the possibility of asthma.

In a review of studies on the effects of psychotherapy on physical functioning, Eells (2000[338]) concluded that "psychotherapeutic interventions are of great value in promoting physical health."

Research indicates that complementary psychological therapy is effective in improving the overall quality of life of clients. When clients are psychologically strong, the effects of traditional medicine are enhanced and often "catch on" better. Some people even attribute miraculous cures to psychological changes in clients.

Other benefits of psychological interventions are described below.

- The approaches are subtle and safe.
- The techniques can be practiced by clients without the presence of a practitioner. This allows them to be actively involved in their own healing processes.
- The techniques last a lifetime. They can be used independently by clients to alleviate other discomforts (psychologically and physiologically) as well.
- There are no contraindications when clients are complying with traditional medicine.

8

Therapy

This therapy has been designed for those clients who want to complement their traditional cancer treatments with psychological interventions. Cancer clients do not usually start with clear-cut goals, like other types of clients. "Regular" clients come in with a specific goal, or a specific issue to work on. When people come in for complementary cancer therapy, they have goals such as "getting well." Due to the wide-ranging nature of interventions to help such clients, complementary psychological therapy can be compared to "realigning life." Many changes to belief systems and behaviors are suggested during therapy. When clients have specific psychological or psychiatric issues, these should be worked through before the complementary cancer therapy can start. Although this model has been specifically designed for use with cancer clients, it can also be applied to many other therapeutic settings.

The overall goal of this therapy is to activate the client's internal healing resources, and remove blockages that could prevent healing. While working on these goals, physical, mental and emotional aspects are also balanced, and quality of life is improved.

Cancer treatment is multidimensional (Carter 1976[339]). One approach is to reduce the number of cancer cells by medical means. Another approach involves enhancing the immune system, which can be done with medical interventions, but also through other types of methods.

This work is about the psychological interventions that increase the natural healing powers of the body. Any intervention that elicits a "non-specific immunoenhancement" can be beneficial in the overall treatment of cancer.

It bears repeating that it is important to work with mainstream medicine, and not against it. From a psychological standpoint, this is also important. The therapist should accept the path that clients have chosen to follow. Both the therapist and the clients must believe in the healing power of current treatments, both medical and complementary (Simonton 1978[340]).

In previous sections, the basis for this therapeutic model was formed.

Based on the psychosomatic model, I will discuss all elements one by one, and describe how these elements can be used in psychological treatments for cancer clients. I will combine common techniques with new insights from different disciplines.

8.1   The Process

8.1.1   Timing

One important aspect of treatment is to determine at what point in time psychological therapy should be incorporated into the overall program towards health.

Just after hearing the diagnosis, or discovering that cancer has recurred after a long time, people are in a shock and often respond with denial and other defensive coping styles. During this period, the client might not be ready for any psychological help. Reassurance, acceptance, nurturing and simple relaxation might be more appropriate during this initial phase. According to Brody (in Simonton 1992[341]), the shock from the initial diagnosis lasts 3 to 6 months. The shock of a recurrence lasts about 2 to 4 weeks. When psychological treatment is forced upon the client during this time, Brody noticed that clients tended towards hopelessness. During this period of shock, clients are not ready for complementary psychological cancer treatment (CPCT). However, the therapist can still offer relaxation and pain management techniques. These interventions are easily accepted by clients. Slowly, the therapist can then introduce other items to start working on.

Although clients need to be ready, Peynovska (2005[342]) suggests that therapy should start as soon as possible after the diagnosis. Early on, clients are more energetic and can learn techniques for preventing further distress.

8.1.2   Therapeutic Goal

There have been many discussions about the goals of complementary psychological cancer treatment (CPCT). Some alternative practitioners promote the extension of life, while other, more conservative practitioners promote dealing with the cancer. The ultimate goal would be the extension of life; however, the therapist does not want to confront clients with possible failure or give them false hope. At the same time, one can question the value of life extension: What is the true value of a longer life, when quality of life is significantly reduced?

Newton et al. (1982[343]) started out with life extension as their major goal. During their research, their goal shifted towards increasing the quality of life. They noticed that unless the quality of life was improved, clients were not working fully with the therapist, almost as if they were holding back.

"The patient is in so much distress from symptoms and side effects of medical treatment that he has lost all or most of his desire to live and the energy to go on."
- Bernhauer W. Newton - (1982)

Although they continued to believe that they could reverse the course of the disease, they communicated only the goal of increasing the quality of life. Simonton et al. (1978[344]) already used this principle. While communicating the goal of increasing the quality of life, Simonton et al. and Newton et al. used interventions that suggested the extension of life (covert goal).

These overt and covert goals prevent the medical staff and most other people from objecting to the therapeutic approach, as it is "just" increasing the quality of life. At the same time, the covert goal allows the client's unconscious mind to be directed towards health.

The general consensus in scientifically-oriented research is that one should strive for improvement of the quality of life (LaBaw 1975[345]; Dempster 1976[346]; Simonton 1978[347]; Grosz 1979[348]). Quality of life can be increased by teaching clients healthy habits (eating, living, non-smoking, exercise, relaxation); developing forgotten interests (hobbies, music and other talents); redefining life goals and pursuing them; and improving relationships and completing unfinished business with friends and family (Grosz 1979[349]). When the therapist focuses on increasing the quality of life, this also gives clients more areas to work in. Research indicates that even the focus on increasing the quality of life as such is associated with increased survival times (Coates et al. 1992[350]).

> *"The unhappy person is the target for any and every type of illness."*
> *- B. Larson –*

8.1.2.1 Solution-oriented

In most psychological treatments, the focus is on clients' problems and alleviating their symptoms. This is based on the premise that finding and resolving the cause will also resolve the symptoms. Basic questions from this approach are: "What is wrong with this person?", "How did he get this way?", and "What can be done about this?" In his book, "Cancer as a Turning Point," LeShan (1989[351]) makes a strong argument about why this approach is not beneficial for cancer clients.

> *"Therapy based on these questions can be wonderful and effective*
> *for help with a wide variety of emotional or cognitive problems.*
> *It is, however, not effective with cancer patients. It simply does not*
> *mobilize the person's self-healing abilities and bring them to the aid*
> *of the medical program. We have now had enough experience in*
> *many different countries to state this as a fact."*
> *- Lawrence LeShan - (1989)*

He argues that these questions do not mobilize the healing resources within clients. He mentions that this is no longer a speculation, but an understanding based on hard experience.

LeShan proposes a different approach. His approach is geared towards what is *right* with the person, and how clients can increase their joy and fulfillment in life. This approach is also discussed in the section on treatment programs. Instead of focusing on problems and obstacles, he focuses on joy and fulfillment just by asking different questions.

Questions that he uses include:
- *What is right with this person?*
- *What are his special and unique ways of being, relating, creating; that are his own, natural ways to live?*
- *What is his special music to beat out in life, his unique song to sing, so that when he is singing it he is glad to get up in the morning and glad to go to bed at night?*
- *What life style would give him zest, enthusiasm, involvement?*
- *How can we work together to find these ways of being, relating, and creating?*
- *What kind of life would he have lived if he adjusted the world to himself instead of adjusting himself to the world?*
- *How can we work together so that he moves more and more in this direction, until he is living such a full and zestful life that he has no more time or energy for psychotherapy?*

Adapted from LeShan (1989[352])

The direction towards what is right is often new to clients, and the therapist needs to explain this clearly. Clients usually focus on what is wrong with them, and what should be fixed.

Working in this way does not exclude approaches that are geared towards the cause. The main goal is to create more fun and pleasure in the life of clients and resolve what is bothering them. This approach is adopted by many other therapists who are working with cancer clients, but also by therapists working with other clients (Berland 1995[353]).

When clients come in, they usually focus on their problems, and feel that they must explain everything that has happened to them in their lives. They believe that the cause must be found before any resolution can be felt.

By contemplating these questions, clients must shift their attention from problem-focused to solution-focused approaches. They start to feel that they are more in control of their life and their personal goals. This increases their fighting spirit and hope.

8.1.2.2 Client, Patient or Student?

As we have discussed, the primary focus is on increasing the quality of life, and questions are focused towards increased enjoyment. We may therefore require a different terminology for the person who is coming to therapy. Some researchers, particularly those who are medically-oriented, use the term "patient" for the person they are working with. "Patient" implies medical care and treatment, and should only be used by physicians.

> *"Patient: An individual awaiting or under medical care and treatment."*
> *- Merriam-Webster -*

Most psychologically-oriented researchers use the term "client." The word "client" implies a dependent relationship between the person and the therapist. The therapist steers the person in the most beneficial direction. It furthermore implies a fixed timeframe, in which the person is under the protection of the therapist. After the therapy, clients are on their own.

> *"Client: One that is under the protection of another, a person who engages the professional advice or services of another."*
> *- Merriam-Webster -*

The Huaxia Zhineng Chi Kung Center in China uses the term "student." They always address a person as a student, never as a client or patient, no matter how sick they are. They argue that the students are learning to influence their personal healing resources. They do not rely solely on doctors. They will learn how to heal instead of being treated. Although this is not made explicit, Simonton et al. (1992[354]) also make use of the student metaphor. They refer to the process as being a "Student of Life."

> *"Student: Learner, one who studies: an attentive and systematic observer."*
> *-- Merriam-Webster -*

Several mind-body clinics use the same metaphor. A student is more active and assumes more responsibility for his process than a client or patient does. At the same time, he takes more responsibility for the time when there is no interaction with the therapist, and continues to rely on his own judgment.

The term "student" is by far the best choice. However, the term currently used in psychotherapy is "client." For the sake of clarity and easy reading, I will continue to use "client."

8.1.3 Presuppositions

Anyone working with clients has certain therapeutic presuppositions, working hypotheses, or convenient or professional belief systems. Below, you will find the presuppositions which are most appropriate when working with cancer clients. These originate from different complementary cancer treatments and from the field of NLP and Hypnotherapy. These presuppositions will help the therapist in this direction, and discussing these with clients will aid them in their healing processes.

Presuppositions:
- *Healing is a natural bodily function, which has been performed for many years.*
- *Improved quality of life impacts one's state of health.*
- *Physiological processes, including immune system functioning and endocrine activity, can be influenced by clients themselves.*
- *Beliefs and emotions significantly influence health and recovery.*
- *Clients are in charge of their minds, their beliefs, and their emotions, and can change them.*
- *Changing beliefs and emotions can be learned easily.*
- *Health is the harmony between the physical, mental, emotional, social and spiritual/philosophical aspects of being.*
- *The current treatment program will help clients in their healing processes.*

8.1.4 Coping with Recurrence

When clients have recovered from their cancer, but the cancer later returns, many of these therapeutic elements have already been applied. There could still be a need for additional psychological therapy. Clients experience similar emotions as before, and similar themes apply. Some beliefs might have shifted back to their original state, and feelings of hopelessness might be even stronger than before. There is also a new theme that needs attention: the message of the recurrence.

Simonton (1978[355]) identified the psychological themes of recurrence:

1) Clients may be trying too hard, and making too many changes at once, by which they increase their stress level.
2) There might be emotional conflicts that still need to be resolved, or that were only pushed away by clients in earlier sessions.
3) The benefits of the illness may not have been met in a healthy way. There is a need to find new means of obtaining the same benefits as when the illness was present.
4) Clients may have stopped performing their tasks when they recovered, or might have slipped back into old behaviors.

Of course, there are many other possible messages. The therapist should assist clients in finding the meaning of the recurrence. Clients must actively explore their conscious and unconscious minds in search of meaning.

The therapist could focus on the time just prior to the recurrence. By examining that period for stressors, thoughts, behaviors, emotions and activities, a therapeutic direction could become apparent.

8.2   The Therapist

The therapeutic process is a highly individual process which takes places between the client and the therapist. In contrast to many other professions, the personality of the therapist greatly affects the quality of service. A therapeutic process cannot be seen as simply performing some interventions with clients. The therapeutic process is an intense relationship, whereby the therapist uses himself and his interventions to assist clients. If the therapist has a bad day, this influences the therapy, for good or for ill.

The personality and attitude of the therapist plays a very important role in complementary psychological cancer treatment (CPCT). The psychological processes of the therapist are usually an integral part of his professional education. Therapeutic education usually includes learning therapy to work though personal issues, and supervision to get feedback on the therapeutic process.

This chapter focuses on the therapist himself and his own mental processes, that could aid or prevent clients from reaping the greatest benefits from the therapy. Much has already been written about the interference of the therapist's personality issues with the therapeutic process. This chapter will only discuss additional issues specifically regarding work with life-threatening diseases, and specifically cancer.

8.2.1   The Therapist's Beliefs

Rosenthal (1966[356]; 1968[357]) conducted research on the effects of the experimenter's beliefs on the subject. He performed a test in which all children received a nonverbal intelligence test. This test was supposed to predict whether a child was about to "bloom" in their learning or not. The test was accordingly labeled "The Harvard Test of Inflected Acquisition."

Teachers were told that this test predicted surprising gains in competence by the children over the next 8 months. The group of children was randomly distributed between the teachers. The teacher of the experimental group was told that he was teaching the intelligent group, and the other teacher was informed that he was teaching the regular group.

After 8 months, at the end of the school year, the children were tested with the same test again. Rosenthal noticed differences in the competencies of the groups. The group where the teacher expected the children to bloom was indeed displaying a surprising increase in competence compared to the control groups. Based on this experiment, Rosenthal concluded that the Pygmalion theory was valid. The beliefs of the experimenter influence the results.

Rosenthal also discovered something peculiar: those children in the control group who displayed an increase in intellectual growth (were not displaying what the teacher expected) where judged unfavorably by the teachers.

This Pygmalion theory has been recognized by hypnotherapists for a long time. If therapists did not believe in certain hypnotic phenomena, clients could not perform them.

> *"The client will not actualize what the therapist does not believe to be true!"*
> *- Commonly expressed in hypnosis literature-*

LeShan (1989[358]) wrote of an experiment involving intentional covert communication by the experimenter. The participants were told that it was an experiment of free association.

The experimenter had a specific category of responses in mind (nature objects, plurals, movements or whatever). When the subject responded with a reaction that fell into the category the experimenter had in mind, he consciously confirmed it with a minimal reaction. The confirmation could be an "hmm," a small movement of the head or tap of the pencil on the notepad. These minimal reactions were very rarely noticed consciously by the subject. The subjects started to respond more and more in the category that the experimenter had in mind, without being aware of it.

> *"It is not possible –we know now- for a therapist to mask their assumptions and goals. They must behave or not behave, and both are communication."*
> *- Lawrence LeShan - (1989)*

When we apply the principles of Rosenthal, LeShan and what is commonly known in the field of hypnosis, it becomes clear that the beliefs and expectations of the therapist influence clients, even if these beliefs are not communicated consciously.

LeShan (1989[359]) also states that therapists cannot fake a belief or expectation. Clients will notice that the therapist is pretending, and will interpret the belief as not being true. When clients notice that the therapist pretends to believe that he likes a Chevrolet, clients interpret this as meaning that the therapist hates the Chevrolet. Pretending is therefore very counter-productive.

> *"Therapists cannot pretend belief or interest. It must be real or it damages the process...You can fake liking a Chevrolet and do as effective a job changing tires as you would if you really had a great deal of affection for the car. This is simply not true with people. You cannot, repeat not, fake it. You can only do damage."*
> *- Lawrence LeShan - (1989)*

Frank (1973[360]) published research indicating that young, inexperienced therapists seemed to produce results that more experienced therapists were unable to produce. He concluded that the inexperienced therapist had different beliefs about what was possible.

Realizing that the beliefs of the therapist influence clients becomes even more important when working with hypnosis. Hypnosis is a very intensive state in which clients pick up, and are influenced by, conscious and unconscious signals from the therapist. The hypnotic trance acts as an amplifier of these signals. Only therapists with constructive beliefs should work with clients, otherwise it obstructs the process and might even damage clients. This is actually true for all psychotherapeutic programs.

In the special cancer issue of the American Journal of Clinical Hypnotherapy, Newton (1982[361]) brought this to the attention of the readers.

> *"When we use hypnosis we need to recognize the intensification*
> *of the relationship between the people involved in the hypnotic*
> *experience .... The question of who does the study, what his motives*
> *are, what his beliefs are, what the structure of his personality is,*
> *what his expectations are, are to a very great extent as important*
> *as the concern over the experimental design, the selection of subjects,*
> *the hypnotizability of subjects and the statistical methods used in the*
> *analysis of the data."*
> *- Bernhauer W. Newton - (1982)*

During the therapeutic process, the therapist might notice that some of his own unresolved issues come up. These might be fears of his own mortality, guilt about his own past, doubts about the work he is doing, etc. When the therapist notices these issues, he should seek help to resolve them.

When a therapeutic program is described, attention is usually only devoted to the process and the interventions that took place. The beliefs of the therapist, as well as the definition of the relationship with clients, are usually left out of the description, even though these are vital ingredients. A well-described program includes the interventions and beliefs of the therapist to achieve success.

8.2.2   Relationship with Clients

Simonton (1978[362]) makes a clear statement about the relationship with clients. The relationship should be personal, passionate and non-attached. There is a difference between attachment, detachment and non-attachment. When the therapist is attached to the outcome, then it creates problems for both the therapist and the client. Clients will not feel free to discuss certain setbacks or express beliefs about giving up. The therapist could feel guilty about a cancer relapse, and might feel that he failed. The opposite of attachment is detachment, an impersonal approach. This also creates problems for clients, in such a way that they do not feel connected to the therapist, and might not feel cared for in the therapy.

Non-attachment involves caring about and loving clients, while at the same time respecting that the outcome is uncertain. By having a non-attached relationship with clients, the clients remain responsible for their own process. A belief that Simonton proposes in order to support this non-attachment is: "I want this person to get better; I accept that they might get worse or die."

8.2.3   Death

Dealing with death and dying is a special issue which is present when working with terminal diseases, such as cancer. Teaching clients to deal with death and dying is frequently found in psychological work (Simonton 1978[363]; LeShan 1989[364]; Spiegel 1991[365]).

Therapists have learned to listen and not to reassure. They must really listen to what the person is driving at, and what they have been experiencing. LeShan mentions that it is useless and counter-productive to tell a depressed client that they have a great deal to live for. This is commonly known; however, it seems to be forgotten when the person is dying. The anxieties of the therapist might increase in the face of their own mortality, so that they deny the death of a client by attempting to reassure them. It is important to accept death as an integral part of living, for both the therapist and the client.

In addition to teaching clients to deal with these issues, this also puts some constraints on the therapist. The subject of death will probably trigger the therapist's own emotions. This is very common; actually, not experiencing anything might be a source of concern. The therapist must be able to openly talk about death, and not reassure clients based on his own fears. This requires the therapist to be comfortable with his own mortality, perceptions, and emotions relating to death.

It is beneficial for the therapist to go through the processes described in the section on death before he begins working on these issues with clients. Just experiencing the exercises as if he were dying will reduce his own emotions about death.

9

Working With Events

Events that take place in clients' lives influence their psychology and may influence their health. Events are the triggers that fire the chain of psychological processes that eventually lead to health outcomes. Simply put, if there were no triggers, the stress response would be eliminated. Clients do not have control over the triggers that occur in their lives, so it is important to explore what the therapeutic process can do to reduce the effects of those triggers.

When working with clients, it is important to know their psychological makeup. In the case of cancer clients, this is even more important as the therapist tries to influence their state of health via the psyche.

The psyche is influenced by the triggers clients experience during their lifetimes. When the therapist knows the triggers (or events) that clients have experienced, he can determine what areas require interventions.

A list of triggers can be used to intervene with the trigger itself (this chapter), and/or as a tool for discussion in order to discover limiting beliefs or unresolved emotions (next chapters).

9.1   Diagnosis

Determining what issues clients have experienced is not actually a diagnostic tool, but operates more as a way-finder for the therapist.

Knowing what triggers have been present can aid the therapist in:
1)   Determining what issues can be explored further
       (i.e. by asking "How did you handle that situation?")

2)   Resolve possible emotions that clients were not aware of.
3)   Guess what future events will function as stressful triggers.

The diagnosis usually consists of a questionnaire on which clients indicate their triggers within a certain timeframe. There is some debate about the best timeframe to use. Some researchers use a timeframe of 3 months prior to the diagnosis of cancer, while others use up to 12 years prior to the diagnosis. Most researchers agree that a period of 6 to 24 months prior to the onset of the disease is most practical for resolving issues with cancer clients.

This list of triggers will be used as a tool for further discussion; I therefore propose the widest possible timeframe. When possible, ask clients to list all the triggers they can remember that have had an impact on their lives. This list will be used later for additional investigation into the client's beliefs, emotions, and coping styles.

As we have seen in previous sections, events of loss have a tremendous impact on the lives of clients. Statistically, they also have an impact on the prognosis of cancer. When interpreting the results of a stressor test, special attention should be devoted to such events (death, divorce, retirement, etc.)

Other issues that are very important to consider are primary relationships and work-related changes.

9.1.1   Questionnaire

Different questionnaires have been developed to gain insight into the triggers that clients have experienced. These questionnaires can be filled out by clients at their leisure, which also promotes an active role for the client.

The most widely used questionnaires are:
- Brown and Harris (1989[366]) "Life events and difficulties scales."
- Homes and Rahe (1967[367]) "Social readjustment rating scale."
- Cochrane and Robertson (1973[368]) "Life Events Inventory."

The above questionnaires can be used, or the therapist can ask clients to create their own lists. Having clients list events without using a questionnaire will generate a list of mostly conscious triggers.

The use of questionnaires will help clients to also include events they have forgotten about. The most detailed information can be obtained by asking clients to first make their own lists, and then use the questionnaire.

Intervention:
1.   *Have clients create a list of triggers they have experienced, including dates.*
2.   *Group these triggers into timeframes: 6 months prior to the onset of the disease, and 24 months prior to the onset.*

I have developed a website **(http://www.healingpsyche.com)** as a companion to this study[369]. This site contains several tools which are of help to therapists. One of these tools is the stressor inventory. To create this online stressor inventory, I have integrated the three questionnaires cited earlier. The questionnaire asks clients what triggers they have perceived, and on what dates. The dates are used to quantify the triggers during a certain timeframe.

After completing this questionnaire, clients can choose to print out several different pages, grouped by timeframe. These forms include the Homes and Rahe "Life Changing Units" and the Cochrane and Roberts "points."

The therapist can ask clients to fill out the online questionnaire and bring it in accompanied by three printed overviews: of all stressors, those experienced during the last 24 months, and those experienced during the last 6 months.

Intervention:
•   *Have the client create an account on the website: http://www. healingpsyche.com.*
•   *Have him fill in the stressor inventory.*
•   *He should print out 3 timeframes: all stressors, those experienced over the past 24 months, and those experienced during the 6 months prior to the onset of symptoms.*

From the different printouts, the therapist can determine what events or periods in the client's life have generated the most distress.

9.1.2   Creative Listing

Another way of having clients list their stressors is a more creative, unconscious method.

Intervention:
1.   Guide the client through his life using imagery.
2.   Have him make up a drawing using the colors of his life.
3.   Discuss the drawing and the metaphorical meanings of the triggers (or events).
4.   Ask the client what triggers he can identify.

Creative listing can also be used as a "warm-up" for the questionnaires. It will help clients recognize the triggers in their lives.

9.2   Therapy

Triggers "happen" to clients and can be perceived or not. The only real "intervention" is to evade all life situations. However, by forcefully trying to avoid all triggers, a new trigger is created, making avoidance impossible. The other intervention is to refuse to perceive events by closing your senses to all input, which is also unrealistic.

Real interventions cannot be performed upon triggers. The interventions discussed here are therefore semi-trigger interventions. Triggers occur, but clients can reduce the effects they have on their lives.

9.2.1   Evasion

Some people have more triggers in their lives than others. The list of triggers could indicate that clients have a tremendous number of them. In this case, an intervention could be to reduce the number of triggers by changing their lifestyles. Some people's lifestyles include a higher number of triggers than others.

The therapist can assist clients in determining the activities in their daily lives that trigger stress responses, and eliminate these to the greatest extent possible. One could think of the triggers that accompany a soccer competition, a demanding job, or visiting relatives. When these events elicit too much of a stress response, the client might consider giving up the events.

By reducing the actual number of triggers, clients experience less stress. This simple yet effective intervention seems obvious, but is often overlooked as a strategy for helping clients.

Intervention:

1. *Ask the client what activities elicit a stress response.*
2. *Work with the client to eliminate these activities from his life, or modify these activities in such a way that they no longer elicit the stress response.*

9.2.2 Desensitization

The level of uncertainty modulates the trigger and increases the stress response. Experience changes the uncertainty of the event. When someone has had prior experience with an event, uncertainty is reduced significantly. Richardson (1990[370]) studied the effects of an educational program on compliance with medical treatment. The educational program consisted of several hours of special instruction on medication and self-care. Those clients survived significantly longer than the control group, who did not receive the educational program. Education reduces uncertainty, which reduces the stress response.

Spiegel (1995[371]) noted the same phenomenon, that when clients are informed about the course of their illness, the prognosis, and possible treatments, their stress response is significantly reduced. In an educational study, Helgeson (1999[372]) demonstrated that those who received extra education showed less distress than the control group. Receiving timely information (not too soon and not too late) about an event also reduces the stress response (Fritz et al. 1954[373]; Elliott 1966[374]). By providing clients with information about their medical situation, treatment options and prognosis, uncertainty is reduced, as is the stress response.

Elliott (1966[375]) demonstrated that prior experience with shock reduced the stress response. The threat of the shock was perceived as less threatening after a similar previous experience. The surprising effects of the shock "wore off." This also applies to training programs for extreme situations, such as those experienced by military personnel or disaster workers. Such people go through such experiences as part of their training. The stress response will be reduced once they are actually working in the field. Such training or educational programs are highly recommended to reduce the stress response in cancer patients (Fritz at al. 1954[376]; Malmo 1956[377]; Rohrer 1959[378]; Vingerhoets et al.1994[379]; Rice 1999[380]). Through training or education, uncertainty is reduced and beliefs about the upcoming situation are changed. Beliefs such as "I can and will survive," and "I know how to handle the situation" could spontaneously form.

In addition to training and education, prior successful handling of the situation also reduces the stress response. Successful experience with the tasks will enhance levels of aspiration (Hill et al. 1962[381]; Feather 1965[382]). Another way of enhancing aspiration levels is by using communication patterns that imply that the task will be easy (Postman et al. 1952[383]; Feather 1966[384]).

Prior failure in dealing with the experience will increase the stress response. Failure in itself is a stressor because people want to perform. The higher the norm or group pressure, the higher the level of stress will be in the event of failure. Failure or potential failure leads to lower levels of aspiration, and to a decrease in performance effectiveness, such as learning, reasoning and psychomotor ability (Kalish et al. 1958[385]; Harleston 1962[386]; Feather 1965[387]). The therapist should avoid all situations in which clients could feel that they have failed.

A prior experience does not have to be a real one; an imagined experience works just as well (more on this in the section on imagery).

Imagery can be provided in which clients perform the task with ease, and complete the situation successfully. This increases clients' perceived level of competence and decreases their stress response.

Working With Perception

Perception as used in the psychosomatic model simply refers to registering an event with the senses. There is no intervention possible to work with perception as is. Therefore, I will not discuss it further.

Changing The Appraisal Process

In the previous chapter, I discussed triggers and possible interventions to reduce distress resulting from triggers. This chapter will discuss clients' thought processes and beliefs, as well as interventions to change limiting beliefs. Some of these beliefs stem from specific triggers, others are a product of the disease, and some were already present before the disease.

One of the most important things in working with appraisal is to move clients away from hopelessness and helplessness into a motivated healing state. Current thought patterns and beliefs about cancer could create feelings of hopelessness and helplessness. By changing these thought patterns and beliefs, clients will feel better.

> *"Suffering is produced and alleviated, primarily by the meaning that one attaches to one's experience."*
> *- Howard Brody MD -*

The belief that "Cancer cannot be cured" is one of those patterns that are detrimental for creating hope in the client. This belief creates hopelessness. The belief that "Cancer has been cured in many people, so it is possible for me to heal" is an example of a much more empowering belief that makes clients hopeful again. At the same time, this second belief is even more realistic than the first one.

Working with beliefs is a very powerful intervention. It is geared towards increasing the quality of life. Changing a client's beliefs changes his entire life - this is why clients often report that they feel better than before the disease. They not only recover from the disease, but gain a much stronger personality.

"Not infrequently we observe that a patient who is in a phase of
recovery from what may have been a rather long illness shows
continued improvement, past the point of his former "normal"
state of existence. He not only gets well, to use the vernacular; he
gets as well as he was, and then continues to improve still further.
He increases his productivity; he expands his life and its horizons.
He develops new talents, new powers, and new effectiveness. He
becomes, one might say, "weller than well."
- Karl Menninger - The Vital Balance 1963

The appraisal process is determined by what people believe about themselves and the world they live in. Beliefs are the driving force within the appraisal process. When referring to the entire appraisal process, I will start by using the word "beliefs."

Changing limiting beliefs is one of the core issues in complementary psychological cancer treatment (CPCT). In this chapter, I will discuss how these limiting beliefs can be discovered, and what interventions the therapist can use to change them. Besides generic interventions that can be used to change any limiting belief, I will discuss more specific interventions. These specific interventions are geared towards changing personality traits, the appraisal process, or clients' secondary gains. Finally, I will discuss some healthy and useful beliefs that can be installed to help clients in their healing process.

Interventions are discussed only in outlines. It goes beyond the scope of this work to discuss these interventions in detail. More detailed information can be found in the referred material.

11.1   Diagnosis

In order to know what areas to work on, we need to know what the client's true beliefs are. This is not always as easy as determining the triggers that someone has experienced. Some beliefs are conscious, and clients are aware of those thought patterns. Other beliefs are unconscious, and clients are unaware (or even deny) that they have such thought patterns.

In discovering the beliefs that are limiting him, the client becomes aware of them. This awareness helps him to change those beliefs. The therapist knows what beliefs he can intervene with.

Sometimes clients' true beliefs are so confronting that they are scared to utter them. Clients do not want to acknowledge that they have negative expectations, in which case the therapist cannot help them. This makes it clear that it is very important for the therapist to accept all expressions of beliefs that clients make. All expressions must be accepted in such a way that clients feel comfortable and supported in expressing their negative expectations and lack of hope.

Many people believe that positive beliefs help the healing process. Although this is true, there is more to it. When clients do not have these positive beliefs, the expression of negative beliefs is of vital importance. Working towards the resolution of one's negative beliefs is completely different from denying them and uttering positive statements.

Several diagnostic tools have been used to determine various kinds of beliefs. In this chapter, I will discuss some of the diagnostic tools that can be used by a therapist to determine possible conscious/unconscious beliefs.

11.1.1   Life Events

In the previous chapter, I discussed having clients create a list of the triggers they have experienced in their lives. This list can also be used to determine beliefs. The list contains events that could be interpreted as positive or negative.

Example:
Suppose I am getting married - this is mostly a positive event. If my dream is taking a trip around the world on my own, I might also associate getting married with never being able to realize that dream. This might then produce tension, which may be fully unconscious.

By discussing the list of events, the therapist is able to find out what the client's perceptions are, and what the underlying beliefs might be.

Diagnostic tool:
Ask the client to list the 5 major events that caused distress in his life during the 24 months prior to the onset of symptoms.

For each of these triggers, ask the following questions:
1.   What problems did you think might result?
2.   What did you worry about?

3.   *How did you feel about this event?*
4.   *How did you react; how did you handle the situation?*
5.   *What did you think about that?*
6.   *What did you believe at that time?*

After discussing all 5 stressors in this way, ask what the similarities are between these 5 stressors.

Adapted from Ellis (1977[388]); Simonton et al. (1978[389]); Arizona State University (1999[390]).

These questions give the therapist great insight into clients' beliefs.

11.1.2   Determined from Emotions

In Healing Journey, Simonton (1992[391]) teaches clients to become aware of their automatic emotional responses when they hear about the topic of cancer. These emotional responses are triggered by beliefs clients have about themselves, about cancer, or about themselves having cancer.

In order to find these beliefs, Ellis (1977[392]) suggests that clients write down the emotions they experience in a notebook. Emotions related to the topic of cancer are particularly important. They should also write down at least 5 beliefs or things they tell themselves at that time. Writing down at least 5 thoughts or beliefs helps to recognize both conscious and unconscious beliefs. If clients can easily write down 5 beliefs, the therapist might suggest writing down at least 10 beliefs. This will make clients think, and provide room for unconscious beliefs to surface. This notebook will be used at a later stage to investigate the beliefs.

Besides having a diagnostic value, this also increases clients' self-awareness and self-efficacy, and helps them take action and responsibility for their own healing processes.

11.1.3   List of Beliefs

In the group therapy sessions led by Spiegel, a list of topics is discussed to determine clients' beliefs. This list is discussed, and clients are asked to expand on these topics. While talking about these topics, beliefs arise which are noticed by the therapist. Using such a list of topics helps the therapist to address many subjects in a short time.

Examples of this topic list:
- *Thoughts about current or future treatments.*
- *Problems anticipated outside the group.*
- *Current stresses in relationships.*
- *Ability or inability to express feelings to family or friends.*

Adapted from Spiegel)1991[393]; 1993[394]).

Another way of listing beliefs is to work through the list[395] of beliefs commonly held by cancer patients. Clients can be asked if they recognize these beliefs. By having clients expand upon the beliefs on the list, their own core beliefs (both conscious and unconscious) can surface. The therapist goes through the list and asks clients to expand upon each belief listed. Through verbal and non-verbal communication, the therapist can make out whether the clients acknowledge having that belief or not. The therapist could also ask the clients to rank each sentence by how strongly they agree with that belief.

Example of the list:
- *Cancer is synonymous with death.*
- *Cancer is something that strikes from without, and there is no hope of controlling it.*
- *Cancer is a strong and powerful enemy, and is able to destroy the entire body.*

After having worked through the entire list, the therapist has some guidelines about what beliefs are limiting clients in their happiness.

The therapist can also ask clients to complete certain sentences to determine what their mindset is. McDermott et al. (1996[396]) asked clients to complete a set of sentences. Based on the answers, they could determine the clients' beliefs.

Example of Diagnostic Sentence Completion:
- *"When I am sick, it means that..."*
- *"I do not deserve to be healthy because..."*

11.1.4 Behavior

Another method for determining clients' belief systems is to discuss the way they are behaving. According to the Bandura (1977[397]) self-efficacy theory, one can determine clients' beliefs based on their behavior. Behavior reflects beliefs. When people believe that therapy will not be effective, they will behave as if this were true. This includes failure to do homework, canceling appointments, and not fully participating in exercises. In a study on patient adherence to chemotherapy treatment, researchers noticed that 23% of the clients (Itano et al. 1983[398]) did not keep their appointments for the administration of chemotherapy. In a follow-up study, 29% of the women did not return for treatment (Marcus et al. 1992[399]).

> *"If a person does not believe they can enact therapeutic behaviors that can bring about a positive outcome, they will not adhere to treatment regimens."*
> *- David Spiegel - (1997[400])*

When clients do not comply with treatment, they have assumed (consciously or unconsciously) that complying will not help them towards their desired result. This basic assumption can be further specified in that clients might believe that they cannot endure the (side) effects of treatment, cannot control their health, or consider their actions to be futile.

Ayres (1994[401]) studied 74 breast cancer clients, and noted that adherence to medical advice was associated with a fighting spirit. Those displaying better adherence also had a greater fighting spirit, and those with lower adherence received higher scores on guilt and hostility. This indicates that the beliefs distilled from behavior are more valid than those reported consciously by clients. By discussing clients' behavioral reactions, the therapist can determine the underlying beliefs. When these (unconscious) beliefs are changed, behavior will also change. Changing the behavior without changing the underlying beliefs will not yield results.

11.1.5 Imagery

The beliefs clients have can also be investigated through the creative expression of imagery. Clients go through an imagery process, and then express their experiences in some way. This can be done through painting, drawing, working with modeling clay, or any other form of creative expression. Following the expression, the therapist discusses the creation with the client. In this way, the therapist gathers information on the client's thought processes and beliefs.

This intervention usually takes place at the beginning of the therapeutic relationship. This allows the therapist to guide the rest of the therapy based on the beliefs he has discovered. The same process is sometimes used as an evaluative process where the therapist can determine the progresses made.

The use of imagery in the diagnostic process has been investigated by many people. Simmel (1967[402]) discovered that a phantom limb only develops when a limb is lost in a dramatic and rapid way. When his clients made a drawing of themselves at that time, they included the missing leg as part of themselves. He concluded that the clients' minds had not had time to readjust to the new situation. The drawings reflected the clients' true beliefs.

Moss (1978[403]) investigated people's self-perception in relation to weight loss. When clients drew a picture of themselves, they drew a picture of their old selves, before the weight loss. He noticed that very obese people who had lost substantial weight still walked the same way as when they were obese. Neither their behavior nor their self-image had changed to reflect their new weight. He concluded that the weight loss was not yet incorporated into the clients' mindsets. They believed that they were still obese. Moss concluded that the drawings clients made of themselves could be used as a diagnostic tool for determining their beliefs.

In his dissertation, Trestman (1981[404]) concluded that images are the reflections of beliefs. By investigating images, the therapist gains insights into clients' attitudes and beliefs. This can be used to determine clients' beliefs regarding disease, treatment, and their healing potential.

Simonton et al. (1978[405]) noticed during their imagery sessions that the actual symbols that clients used were important. They discovered that actual survival time could be predicted by analyzing the symbols clients used. They even concluded that images were more accurate than medical tests for predicting life expectancy.

Achterberg (1985[406]) continued Simonton's research on the diagnostic value of imagery. She had clients listen to a relaxation tape, followed by a short explanation. The therapist explained the treatment and how it would help them to heal. After this explanation, clients were asked to imagine their healing process and make a drawing of that process. During the following interview, clients explained the drawings they had made. The interview contained questions like "Describe how your cancer cells look in your mind's eye," and "How do you imagine your white blood cells fighting disease?"

The images and interviews were scored on several dimensions. All of these dimensions were rated on a scale of 1 to 5. The following dimensions were used:
- Vividness of the image.
- Activity and strength of the cancer cells.
- Relative comparison of size and number of cancer cells and white blood cells.
- Strength of the white blood cells.
- Choice of symbolism.
- Vividness and effectiveness of medical treatment.
- Regularity of a positive outcome.

Achterberg (1984[407]) came to the following conclusion: "The total scores were found to predict with 100% certainty who would die or show evidence of significant deterioration during the two-month period, and with 93% certainty who would be in remission." This supports Simonton's conclusion on the predictive value of diagnostic imagery.

She also noticed that the beliefs that surfaced using this methodology were often contrary to the beliefs that clients had previously expressed consciously. This stresses the importance of searching for unconscious beliefs.

In his Ph.D. dissertation, Trestman (1981[408]) added color and a metaphorical meaning to the dimensions used by Achterberg. His analysis showed that 13 out of 14 clients with a good prognosis imagined their cancers with primarily red or black colors. Of the clients with a poorer prognosis, 8 out of 11 imagined their cancers in lighter colors. This led to the preliminary conclusion that darker colors might indicate a healthier prognosis than lighter colors.

Shorr (1972[409]) noticed a strong link between the way people reacted during imagery and the way they reacted in real life. He asked clients to imagine a 100-foot well. Some of them experienced joy, while others experienced fear, just as they would in real life. They were instructed to imagine being at the bottom of that well and getting out. Some people imagined getting out on their own; others got out with help; and some were unable to imagine getting out. Shorr concluded that the way people react during imagery reflects what they would do in real life.

To determine clients' beliefs, Achterberg (1978[410]) asked clients to draw their immune system, which was then discussed. Simonton et al. (1978[411]) first guided clients through an imagery process in which they progressed through life until they were dead. After the imagery exercise, the therapist asked the clients to recall the images, which were then discussed. Sometimes they had clients draw the images.

Diagnostic Tool:

1. *Imagine a time 1 year prior to your death.*
2. *Notice what is going on in your life. Are you ready to die? What do you need to say or do to be ready? Are you alone? Who is there? What are they saying?*
3. *Imagine a time 6 months prior to your death.*
4. *Imagine a time 1 month, 1 week, 1 day, 1 hour prior to your death.*
5. *Imagine dying and the energy leaving your body. Relax and think happy thoughts.*
6. *Imagine your spirit flowing away, out of your head, and looking at your body.*
7. *Now imagine looking back over your life. What are you happy about? What do you regret?*
8. *Now, while looking back at your life, what will you make your top priorities?*
9. *Come back into your body and open your eyes.*

After this exercise, the therapist discusses the images and beliefs that the client has noticed during the process.

Adapted from Simonton (2003[412]).

A slightly different imagery was used by Gardner et al. (1983[413]). They had their clients imagine their lives each successive year after the diagnosis. During discussions of the images, expectations and beliefs were noted. Gardner used this imagery to determine clients' beliefs about their outcomes and lives after the diagnosis.

11.1.5.1 Symbols

The metaphorical meanings of the images clients used during their imagery sessions proved to be highly significant. One can imagine that an image of a group of big black rats creates different experiences than one of a single small ant. The metaphorical meanings of these images might be related to a fear of rats, or the ease of conquering the ant. Although interpretations of the images depend on the individual, some conclusions can be drawn based on research.

Simonton et al. (1978[414]) and Achterberg (1984[415]) discussed the importance of the interpretation of images for the healing process. In the case of images involving ants, Simonton noticed that they elicited an interpretation of small, disturbing creatures that one cannot get rid of because there are too many. Such imagery does not promote the conquest of cancer cells. When this imagery arises during a diagnostic imagery session, the therapist has a clear indication that the client might not believe that he can get rid of the disease. Although the interpretation is individual, research has indicated that certain images contain more healthy metaphorical elements than others.

When clients are able to engage in imagery, but cannot seem to imagine certain parts or processes, this might indicate certain underlying beliefs.

Example:
A client can imagine their body and different bodily functions, but cannot imagine the cancer itself. This might point to a strong fear that the cancer is stronger, and that he lacks the confidence to combat it.

A client can imagine the cancer, but cannot imagine the cancer cells as weak/fragile, or the treatment as strong/powerful. This might point to a belief that the disease is stronger than his immune system.

A client can imagine the white blood cells and the cancer cells, but he cannot imagine the white blood cells attacking and destroying the cancer cells. This could indicate that the client lacks the ability to express anger and hostility.

*A client uses some special (divine) intervention to flush away the
dead cancer cells. This might point to a belief that even when the
cancer cells are already dead, a very special intervention is required
to get them out of his body.*

Adapted from Simonton et al. (1978[416]; 1992[417]).

During the discussion of the imagery, the therapist should pay
close attention to the conscious and unconscious interpretations of the
imagery by questioning it.

Example:
*The client imagines the healing forces as a strong knight.
Questions that may be asked are:*
- *What does his armor look like?*
- *What is the armor made of?*
- *Does the knight like the armor?*

*It makes a difference whether the armor is rusty or strong and shiny.
If the knight wants to take it off, this might be because he thinks it is
useless, or because the fight has been won and all enemies have been
defeated.*

Example:
*When imagining the cancer as a big stone, the metaphorical meaning
might be something that is hard to break away. However, if the client
is an experienced stone sculptor the meaning might be that he can chip
away parts of it at his leisure.*

By questioning the imagery, the therapist receives detailed
information about the metaphorical meaning of the images, which
reflects the client's beliefs.

The discussion could include:
- How are the cancer cells imagined?
- How is the treatment imagined?
- How is the medication imagined?
- How are the immune system and white blood cells imagined?
- How are the normal cells imagined?

If the therapist tries on the image, he can get an idea of what the possible interpretations might be. By careful observation of his own experience when using that image, the therapist can determine the beliefs a client might have. This works very well as long as the therapist is aware that this reflects his own beliefs, and not the client's. The results can be used to guide the discussion with clients.

Achterberg et al. (1978[418]) created a structural interview to discuss the drawings made by clients. This allowed them to determine the appropriateness of the images used.

Intervention:
Ask the client the following questions:
- *What do you notice?*
- *What catches your eye?*
- *What do you miss on the picture?*
- *What is out of the ordinary, and what does it mean?*

Other items that can be discussed are:
- *Where on the page is the drawing located?*
- *Is it a large or small drawing?*
- *Did you press hard or softly with the crayon?*

Adapted from Achterberg et al. (1978[419])

11.1.6 Pitfalls

The therapist should be aware of some common pitfalls when working to identify clients' beliefs. Dilts et al. (1990[420]) identified these as: "Fish in the dreams," "Red Herring," and "Smokescreens."

The "Fish in the dreams" occurs when the therapist is determined to find a certain belief in the client. He will search for it until he finds the evidence, regardless of whether or not the belief was actually present.

Example:
The therapist is convinced that the client is afraid of the dark. The client does not recognize this fear. The therapist is so convinced, however, that he disregards the client's self-awareness and points out that this fear has yet to be recognized by the client. He argues that it is still unconscious to the client.

The second pitfall is the "Red Herring." This can become apparent when the therapist discusses behaviors in order to identify the client's underlying beliefs. Clients might create unrealistic excuses for their behavior, as if they were seeking a way out. They create such excuses because the discussion might be too confronting, or because they are not aware of (or do not want to be aware of) the real underlying belief.

Example:
One client was not showing up for his therapeutic sessions. He explained that it was impossible to come because someone had come over for coffee.

The "Smokescreen" provides (un)conscious protection from discovering real beliefs. When the therapist comes close to the underlying belief, clients might change the subject, draw blanks, or claim that they do not want to talk about that issue.

Example:
The therapist has just asked the client "What do you think about death?"
The client changes the subject to computers, or answers "I don't know," or "I'd rather not discuss that."

A "smokescreen" is also a good indicator that the therapist has touched upon a powerful issue that needs to be resolved. Farrelly (1974[421]) advises therapists to focus on the issue that caused the smokescreen to appear, no matter how irrelevant the client thinks it is. If the therapist does not discuss this issue, he allows clients to deny the core issue and run away from it. This is a disservice to clients.

11.1.7 Healthy and Unhealthy Beliefs

After having identified a client's main beliefs, the therapist needs to determine which of those beliefs limit the client. Some beliefs are healthy and support clients, while others are unhealthy and limit clients.

Based on Cognitive Behavioral Therapy, Maultsby (1974[422]) created a set of five simple rules for determining whether a belief is relatively healthy or not.

These rules can be applied to all beliefs. If the client answers "no" more than twice for a belief, that belief is not productive for health and well-being. Unhealthy beliefs should be changed during therapy. These rules can be applied to all beliefs to determine whether or not they support health.

Diagnosis Tool: "Rules for Healthy Thinking"
- *Is the belief based on facts?*
- *Does this belief help me feel the way I want to feel?*
- *Does this belief support my health?*
- *Does this belief help me protect my life?*
- *Based on this belief, do my actions support my health?*
- *Does it help me to achieve my long- and short-term goals?*
- *Does it help me to resolve or avoid my most undesirable conflicts (either within myself or with other people)?*

Based on Maultsby (1974[423]), and expanded by R.A.A. van Overbruggen (2006).

11.2   Therapy: Generic Appraisal Interventions

In this chapter, I will discuss some generic interventions that can be used while helping clients to change their limiting beliefs. The next chapter discusses interventions for specific beliefs. These interventions are not only intended for cancer clients, but can be applied to all clients with limiting beliefs.

When working with belief changes, the therapist needs to be aware of the client's changing behavior. A client's behavior is based upon what he believes. If clients behave the same way as before the intervention, the therapist can assume that the belief did not change. A truly effective belief change intervention will be visible in a client's (reported) behavior.

In some cases, the belief was actually changed, but changed back again. This is usually the result of a "metabelief," or belief about beliefs.

Example:
- *"My beliefs cannot be changed."*
- *"I am not worthy to become assertive."*

If the therapist encounters such metabeliefs, he should first work on changing these. For changing metabeliefs, the therapist can use the same generic interventions as for other beliefs.

11.2.1 Mapping Across Sub-modalities

An intervention that is often used to change beliefs is "mapping across sub-modalities." This method is based on changing the way clients make a representation of the belief at hand. Different image qualities representing the issue will render the belief as true or not true for clients.

This method is described in "Changing Belief Systems with NLP," by Dilts (1990[424]).

For example, a client might believe that he deserves to stay sick. The client is asked something that he definitely believes is not true - for example, whether he is 12 years old. The two beliefs are compared, and the differences in sub-modalities (such as color, size, location, etc.) are noted. The therapist asks the client to recall the original belief, and change the representation of that belief so that it reflects the same sub-modalities as the belief that is not true. This changes the perception of the old belief into the new belief. In this case, it goes from being true to not true. The result is that the client no longer believes that he deserves to be sick. Advanced additions to this are described in Dilts et al. (1990[425]) and James (1988[426]).

11.2.2 Rational Emotive Therapy (RET)

When Simonton started his work with beliefs, he used to rely only on relaxation and imagery as methods for changing belief systems (Simonton 1978[427]). Over the years, Simonton began relying more on Rational Emotive Therapy (Ellis 1977[428]; Simonton 1992[429]) to change clients' belief systems. He noticed that Rational Emotive Therapy (RET) was faster and more effective than using imagery.

> *"Cognitive approach (RET) is the best; I've used it the last 16 years to change beliefs and emotions."*
> *- Carl Simonton – (2003[430])*

The notion of Rational Emotive Therapy is that emotions are appropriate to the beliefs present. Clients are instructed to carry a notebook with them at all times, and to be aware of their emotions. When they notice strong emotions, they should write them down, including the situation and at least 5 beliefs they have at that moment. Unconscious beliefs surface easier when clients are forced to write at least 5 beliefs.

Later on in the therapeutic process, these beliefs are discussed, challenged (Ellis 1971[431]; 1977[432]), and replaced with healthier, more realistic beliefs. Finally, clients are instructed to perform imagery three times a day to reinforce the new beliefs.

More information on Rational Emotive Therapy (RET) and its applications can be found in Ellis (1961[433]; 1971[434]; 1977[435]).

11.2.3   Reframing

Many therapeutic programs make use of a technique from Neuro Linguistic Programming called "reframing." Although not explicitly mentioned, reframing is used throughout several programs. Simonton (1992[436]) makes extensive use of this type of intervention.

Reframing takes different forms, but they all focus on creating another frame around the same facts. Putting a different frame around a photograph changes the entire image. The same is true for placing a different frame around a belief. This changes the belief itself.

This intervention is fast, effective and can be applied throughout therapy (Watzlawick 1976[437]). An extensive description of this intervention can be found in Bandler et al. (1982[438]) and Erickson et al. (1985[439])

Dilts (1999[440]) extended and structured reframing with his "sleight of mouth patterns." He developed a specific set of questions for placing a belief within a new context that would change the client's entire perception.

Example:
When someone says "Cancer causes death," possible reactions could be:
- *That this belief causes depressive feelings...that belief is the real danger.*
- *Such a belief becomes a self-fulfilling prophecy because people stop exploring other options.*

- *It is not the cancer that influences life, but rather the workings of the immune system.*
- *Don't you think it is more important to focus on your purpose in life, rather than just on how long it will be?*

Adapted from the list created by Dilts.

11.2.4 Imagery

Imagery is often used to initiate or reinforce belief changes (Donovan 1980[441]). To facilitate belief changes, Simonton et al. (1978[442]), Achterberg (1985[443]), and Rossman (1987[444]; 2003[445]) made extensive use of imagery.

Dilts et al. (1990[446]) extended the traditional imagery process with a reality strategy. Clients have a mental strategy for determining whether something is real or not. When clients apply this reality strategy to the imagery process, the imagery becomes more real, and thus creates more effects.

Example:
The therapist elicits the sub-modalities of something that the client experiences as real (for example, the color, size and motion). These sub-modalities can be seen as reality criteria.

These sub-modalities are applied to the new imagery, thereby making this new imagery more real to the client.

11.2.5 Changing History

There are many techniques that are based on changing clients' perceptions of their own personal history. Somewhere in their personal histories, clients have experienced something that resulted in their limiting beliefs. If that situation had not taken place, the belief would not have developed either. Changing the client's perception of the experience from the past changes the belief in the present.

The following techniques all use some sort of time representations on which past events are located. Such a representation is called the timeline.

Example:
Clients can imagine their past, present and future as:

- *A line from behind them to in front of them.*
- *A line from left to right.*
- *Or in any other way.*

By representing their lives this way, this method helps clients to create emotional distance, and makes it easier to work with distressing situations. The actual form of representation differs.

11.2.5.1 Change Personal History

The goal of this intervention is to add resources to a problematic past event. By creating a physical representation of the past, the distressing situations are externalized. The therapist assists clients in locating personal resources that they would have needed in order to handle the problematic event. Clients are then regressed to that situation and instructed to apply the new resources. This leads to a better handling of the situation. When clients have handled the situation in a more appropriate way, other beliefs are formed. This intervention is described extensively in Cameron-Bandler (1978[447]), Bandler et al. (1979[448]), Dilts et al. (1980[449]; 1990[450]) and Dilts (1990[451]; 1994[452]).

11.2.5.2 Reimprinting

With the help of a physical representation of the past, clients are regressed, or taken back in time, to the event where the belief originated. When clients experience the situation again, they are instructed to identify the positive intentions of the other people present. Clients are instructed to identify the resources they need to better cope with the situation. Once they have found the resources on their timelines, these are copied over to the distressing situation. Finally, clients view the situation from all perceptual positions (3rd, 2nd and 1st position), with the others also present. This gives them a new perspective on the event, and changes the belief that was formed.

> *Example of perceptual positions:*
> - *1st position: This is associated with your own point of view, beliefs and assumptions. You experience the world using your senses. You talk about yourself using "I," "I am," "I think," and "I feel."*
> - *2nd position: This is associated with another person's point of view, beliefs and assumptions. You experience the world using their senses. You talk about yourself using "You," "You are," "You think," and "You feel."*

- *3rd position: This is associated with an outsider's point of view, beliefs and assumptions. You experience the world using their senses. You experience all people interacting with each other. This is also called the observer's position.*

This methodology of "perceptual positions" is described in Grinder et al. (1987[453]), Dilts et al. (1990[454]), Dilts (1990[455]; 1994[456]) and Dilts et al. (2000[457])

The main difference between this and Change Personal History is that reimprinting deals with the impressions other people have made, and the client's conclusions drawn from that situation. Another difference is the use of different positions, and the acknowledgement of positive intentions, which reinforce this technique.

11.2.5.3 Time Line Therapy

James et al. (1988[458]) redesigned the imprinting method and made more use of the concept of time. Time Line Therapy is based on the idea that emotions disappear when clients are regressed to a time before the disturbing event took place. With the disappearance of the emotions, the limiting belief disappears too. James does not represent the timeline physically, but has clients imagine that they "float" above the timeline. These and other timeline techniques are discussed in Andreas et al. (1987[459]), James et al. (1988[460]), Dilts et al. (1991[461]) and Bandler (1993[462]).

11.2.6 Installing Useful Beliefs

In addition to working on changing limiting beliefs, the therapist can also work on creating supporting beliefs. These beliefs are generic, and will support all clients in their healing processes. These healthy beliefs are not necessarily true, but support clients and keep their minds open to possibilities.

They have the choice of what to believe.

"Why should we think upon things that are lovely? Because thinking determines life. It is a common habit to blame life upon the environment. Environment modifies life but does not govern life. The soul is stronger than its surroundings."
– William James –

11.2.6.1 Creating Supporting Beliefs

Creating new beliefs can be seen as changing old beliefs into the belief to be installed. The following intervention, based on affirmative techniques, can also be used to install new beliefs:

Intervention:

1. *The client reads out the belief he wants to have, in the first person position, e.g. "I can heal."*

2. *Two assistants (one on the left and one on the right) repeat the belief aloud to the client in the second position, e.g. "You can heal."*

3. *Have the client notice the effects of these statements. Have them recognize any limiting beliefs or distressing emotions, and instruct them to write these down.*

4. *Rotate the clients so that the previous client becomes an assistant, and the assistant becomes the client.*

5. *Repeat this process with the same belief, e.g. "I can heal."*

Adapted from Dilts (1999[463]).

A list of useful beliefs to install can be found in the appendix[464].

11.3   Therapy: Specific Appraisal Interventions

This chapter discusses interventions for changing specific beliefs.

11.3.1   Personality Traits

In the section on the psychosomatic model I explained that some personality traits have been associated with a poor prognosis. A poor self-image, lack of assertiveness, and lack of autonomy are notorious for this association. This chapter discusses what interventions can be used to replace these personality traits with more constructive ones.

11.3.1.1 Self-Image

One's self-image is the view that one has of oneself and one's role, whether it be correct or not. A person's self-image is composed of many elements, including body image, psychological, and intellectual self-image. Our self-image is influenced by how we grew up, what work we do, who our friends are, were we live, how we look, how we dress, our economic status, etc.

The changes that occur during the cancer process, such as changes in appearance, health perception, and energy levels, can unfavorably influence clients' self-image. This could lead to the development or worsening of an already poor self-image. The first step is to accept the inevitable, after which a new, healthy self-image can be constructed.

Several interventions can be performed to improve a client's self-image.

11.3.1.1.1   *Accepting Self*

Cancer creates undeniable changes in the body and the mind. Sometimes these changes are very obvious. Sometimes they occur without others being able to notice them, or even outside the client's awareness. All of these changes, both physiological and psychological, have tremendous impact on clients. For example, the removal of a breast is a major physical change, and has a great impact on a woman's femininity. The same holds true for the amputation of the testicles, which has great influence on a man's feelings of masculinity. Certain changes might even leave clients with alienated or unfamiliar feelings toward their own bodies.

Many of these changes are irreversible, and must be accepted by the client. The client's view of himself as vital and healthy no longer agrees with reality. That view that he once held of himself might need to be abandoned.

If the current state is not accepted, a split is created between body and mind. The mind has a different view of the body than what actually is. The implications of this split can be found in research regarding "phantom pain." This is pain in a part of the body that has already been amputated, a pain in a leg that is not there anymore. The pain is still there after the limb is not, but the mind still thinks it is. The mind has a view of the body that differs from reality. This often happens when the change occurs so rapidly that the mind does not have time to adjust.

Accepting the current state of the body is one of the primary issues addressed by Spiegel. Clients begin by accepting the current situation, and then move towards the desired situation.

During the acceptance process, there might be a need to grieve for the lost elements (physiological or psychological). Grieving for what has been lost is a natural process. Clients grieve for the life they once had. There is no going back, but they can go forward. The fact that one can no longer do what one was used to doing can be shocking.

Intervention

- *Focus the client on the reality of the situation. Cancer can be deadly. This should not be denied. However, at the same time, people do heal from cancer.*
- *Communicate to the client that they are perfect, just as they are right now, and that the interventions will help them to enjoy life even more.*

Other interventions that promote acceptance are discussed in the sections on "Ideal Self Construction" and "Ego Strengthening."

11.3.1.1.2   Ideal Self Construction

Once the current situation has been accepted, a new ideal self-image can be constructed. This should be an enjoyable image (Olness 1981[465]). Brown et al. (1987[466]) suggest using the "Ideal Self" technique.

Intervention:

1. *Construct an image of your ideal self. This is your conception of the perfect self on a mental, physical and emotional level.*
2. *Make it a real, strong, and compelling image.*
3. *Imagine your current self while you gradually merge your current self with your constructed ideal self.*
4. *Imagine that you become a progressively stronger, healthier and more competent person.*
5. *Imagine yourself at various times in the future, feeling the way you want to feel and living the life you want to live.*

Adapted from Brown et al. (1987[467]).

11.3.1.1.3   Ego Strengthening

Another way to create a supportive self-image is by increasing the client's confidence and self-worth. Ego strengthening was first introduced by Hartland (1971[468]); its purpose is to increase clients' confidence, self-worth, self-acceptance, and belief in themselves. These techniques have been incorporated into many different therapeutic programs (not only cancer programs). This increase in confidence, self-acceptance, and self-worth is always beneficial to clients who come in need.

In her study of 25 children with cancer, Olness (1981[469]) concluded that hypnotic ego strengthening contributed to the well-being of the children by developing a sense of mastery.

Finkelstein et al. (1982[470]) had adults with cancer listen to a 10-minute hypnotic tape session. This tape session included hypnotic relaxation and ego strengthening suggestions. Listening to these tapes resulted in improvements in coping skills.

Association

Many clients with a poor self-image talk in a dissociated way about themselves. They tend to use the word "you" when they are actually talking about themselves.

Example:
If asked "Why did you do that?"
They answer "You have to do certain things. When people ask you, *you cannot simply decline."*

They actually mean "I have to do certain things. When people ask me, I *cannot simply decline."*

This kind of construction is a clear indication that they do not refer to themselves, and are dissociated from their sense of self. In these cases, the therapist should teach the clients to use "I" sentences when they refer to themselves. This will increase their self-concept, increase their awareness, and strengthen their ego.

Intervention
*   *I notice that you use "you" when you are talking about yourself. I want to make an agreement with you.*
*   *When you talk about yourself use "I" or "me." When you are talking about someone else, use "you."*

This very simplistic intervention should be repeated every time the client refers to himself as "you."

Many interventions to strengthen the ego are described by Hammond (1990[471]).

11.3.1.1.4   *Identification*

People often have a strong identification with their illness, especially in the case of cancer (Simonton et al. 1978[472]). When asked to describe what they are, they usually mention that they are "cancer clients." The roles they previously used to describe themselves may no longer seem to be present. Such people no longer view themselves as a father, manager, wife, friend of the family, or the funny woman at parties. This is not correct - they still have the same roles, and also happen to have cancer at that moment in time.

As soon as a client describes himself as a cancer client, he has made a shift in his perception of his identity. A client who describes himself as a person with cancer usually has a wider range of beliefs and behaviors than those who describe themselves as cancer clients. Language structures - the ways people think and talk about themselves - influence their self concept.

Spiegel (1993[473]) uses the "who am I" technique and the "Orpheus Experience" from Bugental (1973[474]) to loosen clients' identification with their illness. At the same time, these techniques reduce the fear of death and facilitate the acceptance of new roles. They help clients realize that they are much more than the roles they have used to describe themselves, and this creates room for new beliefs.

Intervention "Orpheus Experience":

1.   *The client is instructed to make a list of the roles he fulfills. Each is written down on a single index card. These roles could be something like: mother, father, piano tuner, cancer client, lover, technician, friend, brother.*

2.   *Next, he puts these in order, with the most important at the bottom and the least important at the top.*

3.   *He is instructed to take the top card (least important) and imagine the role that is written down on the card (e.g. Imagine your role as a father).*

4.   *Imagine giving up this role, and notice what remains. For extra impact, this card can even be torn up and thrown away.*

5.   *Continue with the next card until all roles have been thrown away.*

Adapted from Bugental (1973[475]).

James (1998[476]) developed the "Are you not more than that?" intervention, which can serve as a variation of the "Orpheus Experience."

Another intervention originally developed by Bateson (1972[477]), and later revised by Dilts (1990[478]), is called "Logical Levels." This intervention clarifies that the identity perception of a person influences their beliefs, and their beliefs influence their choices in life. Clients' identity perception can be seen as their core beliefs, which support all other beliefs. This "logical level" intervention is extensively described in Dilts (1990[479]) and O'Conner et al. (1996[480]).

11.3.1.2 Assertiveness

Assertiveness has proven to be an important area of concern when working with cancer clients. Many psychological therapies devote attention to increasing the assertiveness of cancer clients. Such clients often seem driven by a constant craving for love and the urge to please others, while avoiding all conflicts and complaints.

Changing this attitude is one of the core issues addressed in the treatments developed by Simonton (1979[481]) and Temoshok (1992[482]). Studies of spontaneously disappearing cancers often report that remission occurred after the clients' conscious decision to be more assertive in one way or another (Baalen et al. 1987[483]).

> *"Mice that spontaneously developed fighting behavior showed greater immune resistance to virus-induced tumors. It pays to get mad, even if you are a mouse!"*
> *- George F. Solomon MD -*

Assertive people know what they want and ask for it. This requires clients to actually know what feels good to them, and develop the ability to request it. When clients start expressing their needs, others will respond by expressing their own needs. This also enhances interpersonal communication.

Research on this subject is not as widespread as that in other areas. I will therefore devote some extra attention to it.

11.3.1.2.1 Awareness

The first step in developing assertiveness is for clients to know what they actually want and need. Temoshok et al. (1992[484]) helps clients decide for themselves what they need by constantly asking questions.

These questions include "When do you want me to come back?", "Who would you like to come visit?", and "Do you want our visit interrupted by the nurse?" These questions force clients to think about what they want and need.

To increase awareness, Temoshok teaches clients to ask themselves the following questions:

Intervention:
- *Do I want this now?*
- *Am I too tired for company?*
- *Am I satisfied with my doctor's explanations?*
- *Do I want more information from my doctor?*
- *What part of me hurts, and what can I do to alleviate the pain?*
- *Would I prefer a different meal than the one served?*
- *Which friends lift my spirits?*
- *Who can I confide in?*
- *Do I want to do that test now?*
- *Do I want more medication?*
- *Do I want less medication?*
- *Who do I want to help me?*

Adapted from Temoshok et al. (1992[485])

Another intervention used by Temoshok helps clients become aware of when they get tired.

Intervention:
When you feel tired in the upcoming week notice:
- *Who was present?*
- *What was going on at that time?*
- *Who was doing most of the talking: you or the visitor?*
- *What subjects were discussed?*

Adapted from Temoshok et al. (1992[486])

11.3.1.2.2 Taking Action

When clients become aware of what they want, they are only halfway there - they still need to express it. Expressing needs means saying "yes" to the things they want, and "no" to the things they do not want. Saying "no" is often harder than saying "yes."

*"Every habit and faculty is preserved and increased by
correspondent actions, as the habit of walking, by walking; of
running, by running."*
- Epictetus -

One of the first actions clients take could be asking for help, or saying no to a nurse. Clients should take small steps, and gradually move on to more difficult tasks.

"The journey of a thousand miles begins with one step."
- Lao Tzu -

Intervention:
Possible actions a client can take:
- *Have the client express his feelings, worries and questions to the staff.*
- *Speak up to the nurses and doctors if it is not the right time for him to receive his injections.*
- *Ask for help.*

Adapted from Temoshok et al. (1992[487])

Clients' failure to express their needs is often caused by a fear of losing their friends' love and support. Temoshok teaches clients communication skills to communicate their needs in such a way that they will not be rejected by their friends. At the same time, Temoshok helps clients to develop the confidence that they can express their needs and also keep their friends' love and support.

11.3.1.2.3   Assertiveness with Physicians

Assertiveness with the medical team often seems to be a different issue. Clients often feel (and are) dependent on their physicians and the medical team. They often feel that the physician is in charge of their lives. This misconception needs to be dealt with. The physician is a human being who is specialized in the human body; however, he does not know everything about all conditions. He does not know all there is to know about clients' physical, mental and emotional situations. Clients should therefore control their own lives. Their lives are their projects, and they have hired a consultant to provide help in dealing with the disease. This consultant does not run their lives, but merely gives advice and helps them with a specific situation.

The physician is not an authority with whom they cannot argue. Physicians provide clients with solid advice based on the knowledge they have. Taking charge of their lives means that clients actually form their own team of specialists to address the situation. If these do not perform well, they must be replaced. Furthermore, clients should learn all they can about their disease and ask questions. This helps to develop their autonomy.

In dealing with physicians' busy schedules, Temoshok advised clients to write down the questions they have. This allows them to ask their questions in the heat of the moment, without being overwhelmed. She also advises clients to continue asking further questions if the answers provided are not clear or specific enough. She provides clients with some standard questions that could help them to get more information.

Intervention:
- *What kind of treatment will I be getting?*
- *What kind of chemotherapy?*
- *How many times will it be administered? And for how long?*
- *What will the side effects be?*
- *Can I get assistance from a psychotherapist?*
- *How will I know when I no longer need the medication?*
- *Etc.*

Adapted from Temoshok et al. (1992[488])

For communication with physicians, Temoshok gives the following guidelines:

Guidelines:
- *State clearly and directly what you want and need from your doctor. Begin your requests with "I want..." or "I need..."*
- *Avoid criticizing your doctor. Like other human beings, he is more likely to respond to feelings than judgments.*
- *If your doctor has been unresponsive or insulting, do not accuse him of insensitivity. Instead, tell him how what he has done has made you feel. Statements of feeling are far more likely to be heard and understood than accusations.*
- *Listen carefully to your doctor and acknowledge his statements and feelings as well.*

- *Establish a partnership with him - the relationship is a two way street.*

Adapted from Temoshok et al. (1992[489])

In addition to these communication skills, the therapist can use another intervention which is quite powerful in changing the relationship with the physician. The "Social Panorama" intervention is designed to change the way clients perceive relationships with others. Clients are asked to represent the person in their mind. Then, the sub-modalities of the image are changed in such a way that clients find themselves equal grounds with the other person. Many people place their physicians on a pedestal. This intervention helps the client take the physician off of the pedestal, so that they can talk on the same level. This creates equality. The entire method is described by Derks (1996[490]; 1999[491]). Other widely used interventions are based on Transactional Analysis (Hellinga 1999[492]).

11.3.1.3 Autonomy

Van Baalen et al. (1987[493]), Schilder (1992[494]) tried to distill the psychological components of spontaneous cancer remission. What they discovered was that each of the people who spontaneously recovered experienced a "more or less radical existential shift" in their attitudes towards autonomy. Cunningham (2004[495]) noticed that those clients who showed a high degree of autonomy outlived their prognosis. Autonomy is defined by Merriam-Webster as "self-directing freedom and especially moral independence."

Grossarth-Maticek at al. (1985[496]; 1991[497]; 1991[498]; 1995[499]) came to similar conclusions, although they use the terminology of "Self-Regulation." This is defined as "the regulation of behavior to maximize long-term pleasure and well-being." This is essentially the same as autonomy.

Developing clients' autonomy is health-promoting. One way to accomplish this is through awareness, as with self-image and assertiveness.

Intervention:
Ask the client the following questions:
1.   *Do I try to perceive how this person wants me to behave, and then behave that way?*

2. *Am I often afraid of behaving in ways that this person will find unacceptable?*
3. *Do I suppress my real needs with this person?*
4. *Do I express needs with this person, but find myself constantly frustrated by him or her?*
5. *Am I frightened of expressing anger, fear, or sadness with this person?*
6. *Do I take care of this person to a large extent?*
7. *Is his or her love and approval dependent on my caretaking?*
8. *Is his or her love and approval dependent on my obedience?*
9. *Do I feel victimized by this person?*
10. *Is my sense of self-love and self-confidence dependent on the approval of this person or of my superior(s) at work?*

Adapted from Temoshok et al. (1992[500])

Explain to clients that just as they can be loyal without being obedient, they can be responsive to other peoples' needs without becoming a compulsive people-pleaser.

11.3.2   Primary Appraisal

In the section on the psychosomatic model, I explained that primary appraisal is the client's set of beliefs about how the situation influences his life goals.

11.3.2.1 Meaning of Life

Cancer clients have often lost their primary meaning of life prior to the diagnosis. The high incidence of people who have lost a primary relationship just prior to the diagnosis of cancer is remarkable. For them, that loss meant a loss of meaning in their lives. They ended up living a life that was unfulfilling, and not in accordance with what they consider the "real them." Such a loss of meaning could also be caused by the diagnosis of cancer itself, if they have lost their connection with their health and healthy self-image. Without meaning their lives, people are less motivated to do what is necessary to heal. Having meaning increases their general well-being, quality of life and immune functioning.

> *"Believe that life is worth living, and your belief will help create the fact."*
> *- William James -*

Borysenko (1984[501]) worked with clients to find renewed meaning in their lives. She attributed remarkable healings to such renewed meaning. Establishing a new connection with the true meaning of life is a very satisfying process that increases the quality of living. Dilts et al. (1990[502]) concluded that the main point in recovering is having a purpose in life. Bower at al. (2003[503]) studied the effects of finding meaning in life on the immune system. They studied 43 women who had lost a friend to breast cancer. They noticed that those who found a new meaning in life and emphasized goals, relationships and personal growth experienced increased immune functioning.

LeShan (1959[504]; 1977[505]; 1989[506]) pioneered his vision of the meaning of life and the mobilization of the immune system. He noticed that finding renewed meaning in life jolted clients' immune systems. They seemed to demonstrate that they were actively working to fulfill that new-found meaning, in order to achieve those goals.

Studies of clients whose cancer had spontaneously disappeared showed that an existential shift often took place prior to the remission (Hawley 1989[507]; Huebscher 1992[508]; Schilder 1992[509]). Roud (1985[510]) noted that two-thirds of the clients he interviewed associated the remission with "a new freedom to live a lifestyle congruent with their values."

Shanfield (1980[511]) noticed that those who survived reorganized their priorities and developed a renewed appreciation of life. Ikemi et al. (1975[512]; 1986[513]) reported that a "dramatic change of outlook on life" or a "dramatic existential shift" preceded spontaneous remission. Cunningham (2004[514]) noticed that those clients who outlived their prognoses were clearly aware of what was important in their lives.

A purpose in life is more than just the will to live or the will for the cancer to disappear. It is the reason why one needs to stay alive longer. What does it mean when the cancer goes away? What will health allow clients to do?

11.3.2.1.1 *Activities that Add Meaning*

Finding meaning in life can be obtained by creating peak experiences in life, or what Cskiszenthihalyi (1990[515]) calls "flow." These are moments of profound peace and harmony, both physical and emotional. Clients have often lost sight of what activities drive them towards personal satisfaction. Clients should recognize those activities and spend time and energy on them. Spending time on those activities actually increases the feeling of meaning in their lives. This creates joy and energy at the same time, and increases the quality of life.

> *"Ancient Egyptians believed that upon death they would be asked two questions, and their answers would determine whether they could continue their journey into the afterlife. The first question was: Did you bring joy? The second was: Did you find joy?"*
> *- Leo Buscaglia -*

One intervention is for the therapist to have the client make a list of meaningful activities:

Intervention:
Make a list of activities that:
- *You enjoy or have enjoyed in the past.*
- *Add meaning to your life.*
- *Give you more energy.*
- *Are valuable to you.*
- *Are worthwhile.*

Adapted from Simonton et al. (1978[516])

Periodically reviewing this list allows clients to change and add to their lists, and find new ways of seeking meaning.

11.3.2.1.2   *Living the Values*

In the face of terminal disease, there is a shift in what is important and what is not. Some activities or situations lose their importance, while others become the most important things in life. Being confronted with death puts a new perspective on the true values in life. Meaning in life is increased when clients spend more time on their true personal values. By investigating what these values are, clients are able to restructure their lives to meet those values. The values can be constant, or might shift throughout their lives.

One of the familiar techniques from Neuro Linguistic Programming is the value elicitation technique. This helps clients come into contact with their true values in life (James et al. 1988[517]). Another intervention that can be used is intended to help clients determine their purpose in life.

Intervention:
- *What makes your heart tick?*
- *What makes you feel most alive, vital or involved?*
- *What is your strongest connection to life?*
- *What is so important to you about ...?*
- *What is the true value of ... to you?*
- *What parts of ... are so valuable?*

Adapted from Simonton et al. (1992[518]).

11.3.2.1.3   Mission in Life

Developing a meaning in life often comes with a renewed major goal in life. This all-encompassing overall goal can also be called the client's life mission. It might sound enormous, but it does not have to be. A personal life mission is simply the direction in which the client wants to go. Other goals support this mission. The dramatic existential shift I discussed earlier often comes with a renewed sense of mission. This sheds new light on what clients think is important to them.

Example:
A personal mission of being the wealthiest person in the country creates different sub-goals than a personal mission of being the most loving father to one's children.

Writing a personal mission statement helps clients refocus their lives. This new focus also provides clients with an overall goal that holds and guides other goals. A mission could be defined as the role or purpose someone has in relation to the larger system of people, all other life and the planet.

A personal mission statement covers a very long timeframe. It actually guides the rest of the client's life (or until the mission is revised). It reflects his core values and the type of person he wants to be. What he wants to do is covered by his (sub)goals.

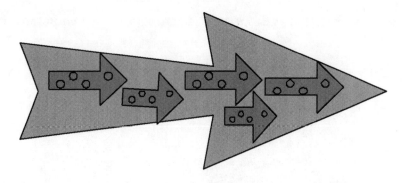

The mission serves as a compass for the client's direction in life, the goals that are important to him, and the choices he makes.

> *"If you don't set your goals based upon your Mission Statement, you may be climbing the "ladder of success" only to realize, when you get to the top, you're on the WRONG BUILDING."*
> - Stephen Covey -

The following process helps clients to discover their true meaning in life by writing their own personal mission statement.

Intervention:
The following questions can help the client in discovering his own personal mission in life:
- *Why do I exist?*
- *What is my life about?*
- *What do I stand for?*
- *Who do I admire, and what is my mission?*
- *What excites me in or about the world?*
- *What angers me in or about the world?*
- *What three things would I like to have changed in the world, as a result of my mission?*
- *What are my functions in life?*
- *What is the purpose of my life?*
- *What is the intention of god/the universe for me?*
- *What ignites my imagination?*
- *What would I love to pour myself into?*
- *What would I like to be remembered for?*
- *What moves me?*
- *What issue needs to be taken care of in this world?*

- *What would I love to learn or master?*
- *What are my favorite causes, and what interests do they reflect?*
- *With whom do I have my deepest conversations, and about what?*
- *On what cause, issue or problem that moves me would I spend a gift of a million dollars?*
- *On what need or problem that I strongly believe in would I love to work full-time, even if I am not getting paid for it?*

Adapted from Covey (1989[519]), Dilts (1994[520]; 1996[521]), Jones (1998[522]).

Covey refers to crafting a mission statement as "connecting with your own unique purpose and the profound satisfaction that comes in fulfilling it."

More on these types of personal mission statements can be found in Dilts (1994[523]; 1996[524]) and Covey (1989[525]).

11.3.2.1.4   Development of a Life Project

The diagnosis of cancer changes clients' perspective on life and the time they have left. Clients often focus on short-term problems, losing sight of their long-term goals. The development of a life project is a special long-term goal. It is a major goal to be pursued in life. A long-term project can be defined by using values as a starting point. Life projects increase clients' willingness to live because they want to fulfill that goal.

Example:
Life projects can be:
- *Taking up university studies.*
- *Setting up a community service.*
- *Guiding support groups.*
- *Writing a book.*
- *Taking a pet.*
- *Etc.*

Example:
BBC News, Friday, 6 August, 2004
"A 98-year-old woman who had never used a computer in her life has proved it is never too late to learn. Mary Robinson now uses her IT skills to do her shopping and other tasks after completing an

*adult learners' course. Ms. Robinson said: "It has been wonderful.
Computers are marvelous. There is so much you can do with them
and so much to learn." She really enjoyed the course and was always
one step ahead."*

Evaluation of life values and goals might indicate that clients are
putting off important goals for later. This time might never come.
Clients might discover that they need to live more in the present
(Spiegel 1978[526]).

> *"My breast cancer diagnosis gave me a new life. I would never have
> consciously asked for the disease, but I am grateful that it has helped
> me to fulfill my dreams."*
> *- Marilyn R. Moody -*

11.3.2.2 Detoxifying Death

Death is inevitable for every human being. Normally, we do not
pay attention to it. In fact, we actually ignore it most of the time. When
faced with a terminal disease, the possibility of death is forced into our
consciousness. Therapy is aimed at improving the quality of life up until
death. This means that when clients are about to die, therapy should be
geared towards a peaceful death.

> *"He who doesn't fear death dies only once."*
> *- Giovanni Falcone -*

Cancer is a terminal disease. Even though many people are healed,
the possibility of death is staring clients in the face. Upon hearing the
diagnosis, death might come closer than ever before. Fears and concerns
about death and the dying process could be present. Working through
these issues will help clients become more at ease with the inevitable.
Accepting death and being comfortable with it increases the quality of
life.

> *"Some people are so afraid to die that they never begin to live."*
> *- Henry Van Dyke -*

In many situations, the topic of death is denied. The possibility
of dying is usually not discussed in social, therapeutic, or even medical
settings. The topic almost seems to be off-limits. This leaves clients in a
conflicting situation, as they fear death, and yet cannot talk about it.

Clients are trapped in their own terrifying fantasies. Because there is almost no possibility of discussing these emotions, they are denied and repressed, which, as we have seen, is not beneficial to the healing process.

Fear undermines clients' well-being. By reducing their fear of death and dying, clients can more easily accept death as a part of life. By accepting death, clients can stop trying to avoid the inevitable (Spiegel 1990[527]). The energy that is freed when clients stop avoiding death can be used to enhance well-being.

Many psychotherapeutic programs for cancer clients incorporate working with issues relating to death. These issues are so existential that they should be an integral part of any therapy for clients with terminal diseases.

In the approach developed by Spiegel, death-related issues play an important role. "Detoxifying death," as he so eloquently calls it, is about coming to terms with death and reducing the toxic fears that can affect one's quality of life.

This topic is very delicate and confronting for clients. It should be handled carefully by the therapist. Clients should not be forced to work with these issues. Only when clients are able to confront these existential fears should the therapist continue. Simonton suggests that the therapist ask clients whether they are ready to face these issues. If they are not ready, this should be postponed for days, weeks, months, or even years (Simonton 1992[528]). Spiegel begins a discussion of death in the first week of sessions. This establishes a framework in which death and dying can be openly discussed. Only if it is not addressed by the group will Spiegel start the discussion again halfway through the program.

If clients indicate that they are not ready to face these issues, the therapist should remind them that the goal is to reduce those feelings.

Accepting death as a part of life is not the same as giving up on life. The main goals of working with death-related issues are to reduce the fears (detoxify death), and accept the possibility of death (while maintaining hope for life).

The issues relating to death can be divided into three groups (Simonton 1992[529]):

- Beliefs about death and dying in general: How are we going to die?
- Beliefs about life after death: What happens to our consciousness, awareness, body, and soul after death?
- Beliefs about what one's own dying process will be like.

The unhealthiest belief about what happens after death is the concept of a continuing consciousness that is undesirable. The concept of hell in certain religions is a clear example of this. If clients believe they will end up in hell, they suffer from a tremendous fear of death. If clients believe they will end up in "heaven," a good place to be, this fear is usually no problem.

Sometimes clients believe that there is nothing after death; death is the end of all things. In those cases, fear is usually not an issue.

11.3.2.2.1   Bringing Death Into the Open

The main goal in detoxifying death is to remove it from the realm of forbidden subjects. One way of accomplishing this is through discussion of the subject itself. It must be possible to discuss the topics of death and dying, just as one would any other topic. When clients experience a time and place where these emotions can be discussed, they will feel less alone in their feelings and their feared fantasies. These discussions should include emotional expression and utterance of their thoughts. This allows the therapist to work toward a reduction of those emotions, and the development of comforting beliefs.

During the discussion of fears about death, the therapist will break the topic down into manageable pieces. Clients will discover what part of death they actually have the most trouble with. This could be the dying process, the situation after death, or how other people might react upon their death. At the beginning of the discussion, fear and anxiety levels will be increased because the subject is brought into the clients' consciousness, but these will eventually diminish (Spiegel 1981[530]; 1983[531]). Clients have reported feeling relieved once they were able to discuss the subject of death openly.

> *"While it may seem initially that the talk of dying or death would be deeply anxiety-provoking and even destructive, in fact, the ability to face and deal with their worst fears is ultimately reassuring to patients."*
> *- David Spiegel –*

Starting this discussion is often difficult. Spiegel uses the following to start the discussion:

Intervention:
- *How do you feel about what is happening to you?*

Adapted from Spiegel (1990[532]).

11.3.2.2.2   Discussing Different Viewpoints

Every culture has viewpoints on death. In some cultures, people fear death, while other cultures celebrate reincarnation. There is no good or bad approach to death. It depends on the context, and the context here is to increase the quality of life. In that case, fearing death is less comforting than celebrating it.

> *"Death row is a state of mind."*
> *- Doris Ann Foster -*

In western cultures, death is often seen as something to be afraid of. To increase the quality of life, this belief could be changed, or the distressing impact could at least be reduced. Consider the "Rules for Healthy Thinking" based on Maultsby. (See 11.1.7 Healthy and Unhealthy Beliefs.) Western culture has an unhealthy view of death. It is not based on facts, and it limits clients in their well-being. By discussing viewpoints on death from other cultures and religions, clients discover that their view is not the only one. All views are equally true, but one supports an increased quality of life and others do not.

In many western cultures, death is thought to be the end of things, although some people present a different viewpoint. Kübler-Ross (1975[533]), one of the leading researchers on the topic of death, has clients contemplate the following sentences:

Intervention:
1. *You can influence your dying in much the same way that you can influence your living. If you want to die a certain way, then it is important to live that way.*
2. *Death is a brief transition period between physical life as we know it and an existence that comes afterward.*
3. *Death is the end of this physical existence, just as birth was the beginning.*

4.   *After death, your essence, or your soul, continues on in an existence that is desirable.*

Adapted from Kübler-Ross (1975[534]).

These beliefs support clients more in their well-being than traditional western beliefs. Incorporating these beliefs increases clients' quality of life by reducing their fear of death.

Eastern philosophy has a view of death that is quite the opposite of the traditional western "end of all things" view. It does not mean the "Inevitability of never returning" or the "absence of being." It means the concentration of life energy in the core of the being and moving that energy into a new state (Long in Kübler-Ross 1975[535]). Alaskan Indians celebrate a member of their tribe who died. That member progressed (Trelease in Kübler-Ross 1975[536]).

> *"Is death the last sleep? No, it is the last and final awakening."*
> *- Sir Walter Scott -*

The following is something which can be presented to clients as an alternative viewpoint.

Intervention:
"Death is not a permanent end, but a transition into a new state. Life is eternal in its essence, if not in its form. To grow, to move, to live - we must "die" to the old to give birth to the new.
Death represents an important ending that will initiate great change. It signals the end of an era; a moment when a door is closing. At such times, there may be sadness and reluctance, but also relief and a sense of completion."

Traditional Tarot Interpretation of Death.

By discussing different viewpoints on death from different cultures or peoples, clients' beliefs about death will change, sometimes even to a great extent.

> *"Death is not extinguishing the light; it is putting out the lamp because dawn has come."*
> *- Rabindranath Tagore –*

11.3.2.2.3   *Accepting Death*

Accepting death as an integral part of living is a hard process to undertake. People have problems coming to terms with death because they interpret it as giving up on life. This is not the same. Clients must learn to accept that they could die. They must accept that, and at the same time be fighting for their lives.

Intervention:
Simonton uses the following affirmations:
- *"Death is OK, life is better."*
- *"I am prepared to die, and want to live."*

Death is sometimes perceived as failure by clients. This perception creates more distress for clients than necessary. To reduce such distress, the therapist can point out that whether or not clients recover, they have succeeded in improving the quality of their lives, and have exercised great strength and courage.

To accept death, clients must be prepared to die. One of the interventions that aid in this process is having clients write up a will. At the same time, making the will increases their feeling of control over their lives (and over their deaths).

The therapist investigates what clients need to do in order to be prepared to die. This could be finishing some past business, forgiving, understanding death, or planning certain actions.

"Plan on living eternal, plan on dying today."
- Carl Simonton-

11.3.2.2.4   *Life Review*

The life review intervention helps clients gain a new and larger perspective on life. It changes their current views and makes them aware of goals that they want to accomplish. At the same time, it reduces their fear of the dying process.

The following intervention allows clients' unconscious beliefs to surface, regarding how they will die and what will happen to their consciousness afterwards. It helps them to investigate their beliefs about how others will react to their death, which helps them to deal with unfinished business while still alive. At the same time, newer, healthier, and more productive beliefs are formed through imagery.

The "Life Review" Intervention

1. *Sit back and relax.*
2. *Think of what you felt when you first heard the diagnosis. Who did you talk to?*
3. *Imagine moving towards death and experiencing physical and psychological deterioration. Experience the emotions and thoughts.*
4. *Imagine being on your deathbed. Who is present, and what are they saying and feeling?*
5. *Imagine being at your funeral. Who is present, and how are things organized?*
6. *Imagine that you merge with the universe, and review your entire life from there.*
7. *Create a new life just as you want it to be. Define your attitudes, beliefs and primary goals in life.*
8. *Appreciate the continuous flow of death and rebirth.*

Adapted from Simonton (1992[537]).

Clients frequently report that their fears and anxieties are reduced tremendously after performing this imagery exercise (Simonton 1992[538]). They are reassured that their friends will continue with their own lives, and they formulate ideas on how they want their funerals to be conducted.

Of course, this is not predictive imagery. It is a fantasy based on clients' current thinking, and what they think will happen when they die.

If their imagery is not satisfying, they can still change their lifestyles so that in the end, when they actually die, they do not have the resentments and distressing feelings they have just imagined.

To become aware of what clients need to do to create a fulfilling life, I designed an imagery exercise based on McDermott at al. (1996[539]). During this exercise, clients fantasize about the kind of person they want to be. They can design their life from scratch, with everything they need. This helps clients to clarify what they want to change in their lives.

"And when it is time to die, we need to understand what our life was about, to know and accept who we have become."
- Lawrence LeShan -

Another useful technique is to have clients write or tell about their biographies. The story should include everything that is relevant to them that they can remember, from childhood to major decisions, best and worst parts, things they never told anybody, etc. If this story is told to a loved one, it also enhances the relationship and might help resolve unfinished business.

11.3.2.2.5   Planning Death

Planning death consists of both the dying process and the organizational aspects of what happens afterwards. Most cancer clients fear the process of dying more than death itself. When clients take control of their dying process, arrangements can be made with physicians about medications and treatment decisions. In some countries, euthanasia can be planned if clients so choose.

Discussing and making arrangements for their funerals enhances clients' sense of control. At the same time, it is of value to clients because they can rest in peace knowing that their family members will respect their wishes. This reduces the distress of being a burden on the family, who would otherwise have to decide what must be done. It increases confidence because everything is arranged just as they want it to be. This also has an existential value, in that clients reflect on their lives and appreciate the people and events that were important to them. This adds to their quality of life.

As with all interventions dealing with death, other distressing beliefs and emotions might surface. Recognizing these beliefs and emotions motivates clients to change their lives while they still can.

One intervention that helps in the planning process is the following:

Intervention:
1. *Do you want to be treated at all times?*
2. *When do you want the medical staff to stop your treatment?*
3. *Do you want to be buried or cremated?*
4. *Who do you want invited to your funeral?*

5. *How do you want the ceremony to be conducted, and what do you want said?*
6. *Have you already created a will?*

Adapted from Spiegel (1993[540]) and LeShan (1989[541]).

11.3.2.2.6 Spiritual Growth

Death is often seen as a way of achieving spiritual growth, or reincarnation to another level.

> *"Death is for many of us the gate of hell; but we are inside on the way out, not outside on the way in."*
> *- George Bernard Shaw -*

This is all a matter of beliefs, as neither "death is the end" nor "reincarnation" can be proven. However, as discussed earlier, some beliefs support well-being more than others. LeShan suggests that clients view their "Dying Time" as an "exciting and interesting adventure in growth." LeShan shifts the perception of death toward a means for achieving spiritual growth. Believing this reduces fear and increases acceptance. In many cases, the deathbed is a sad and drugged time. By putting the emphasis on spiritual growth, this time can also be filled with joy, understanding, and peace with one's spiritual expectations.

Grosz (1979[542]) has clients hypnotically rehearse death, in such a way that they view it as a "journey and temporary separation," by which a belief is installed that everything will be better in a little while. Death is not the end, but part of the journey of life, and only a temporary separation from the people clients love.

LeShan (1989[543]) assists his clients in enhancing their explorations by asking a large number of questions. He composed a list of 33 thought-provoking questions that stimulate growth. Some of these questions are:

Intervention:
*   *What is the best thing that ever happened to you? What is the worst thing that ever happened to you?*
*   *What was the best thing you ever did? What was the worst thing you ever did?*

- *For the things you feel guilty about, what do you need to do now in order to be able to forgive yourself?*
- *For what do you most need the forgiveness of God?*
- *What do you need in order to finish your life, to complete it?*

Adapted from LeShan (1989[544]).

11.3.2.2.7   Ending Life Thoughts

When discussing death and accepting the possibility of death, it is not uncommon for people to start talking about their personal thoughts about ending their lives. People tend to avoid physical and psychological deterioration and pain; sometimes they are afraid of becoming a burden to their family. Many people with terminal illnesses have thoughts about ending their lives at one time or another. Ending one's own life is taboo in most conversations. It is therefore very important for clients to be able to discuss their thoughts on this subject during therapy.

Before I continue, there is an important distinction to make. People can, and do, recover from cancer and, in many cases, the chances of recovery are high. When working with clients who have a death wish, the therapist must differentiate between those clients with a high chance of recovery, and those with a very low chance. A client with a reasonable chance of recovery who expresses a death wish should be treated like any other suicidal client. Working with regular suicidal clients will not be discussed further in this study.

Clients with a very low chance of survival face different choices. For them, it is more a matter of timing. When such terminal clients express a wish to die, the therapist should still work to increase their well-being. The interventions described earlier could be used to ease the minds of such clients.

It is not always in the client's best interest to avoid death at all costs. The therapist's task is still to increase the client's well-being. Some clients are dedicated to their decision to end their lives. In those cases, the therapist should help them to think through their decision, and realize the implications for themselves and others. The therapist should focus on the psychological and social issues that clients might want to avoid by dying. Well-known examples are the fear of being a burden, and the avoidance of family conflicts.

Some countries allow clients to request euthanasia. The processes clients must go through are very well-designed to avoid allowing clients to make rash decisions.

The therapist should always allow clients to talk about their death wishes, and accept their decisions. The primary goal of the therapist is always to increase the client's quality of life, even when this is only for a short time.

11.3.3   Secondary Appraisal

The secondary appraisal filter, which was also discussed in the chapter on the psychosomatic model, is how people think they are able to handle a situation. It consists of what people think will happen, the outcome expectancy, and whether they believe they can control the situation.

11.3.3.1 Coping Potential

One of the issues that often arises with cancer clients is the belief that they are out of control. These self-efficacy or control issues are often overlooked, and are of great value in assisting clients. I will therefore devote some extra attention to them. Believing that one has control over the situation, or over one's life, is often associated with a better prognosis and a higher quality of life.

When clients go to a doctor, they usually reduce their own participation to a bare minimum. They go in with the belief and attitude that the doctor will cure them. Clients thereby place all responsibility for their health and well-being in the hands of the doctors, while they themselves "sit back" and wait to be cured. This lack of personal responsibility is often supported by the medical staff. They tend to take things out of the clients' hands, and decide what is best for them.

"Even if you are on the right track, you will get run over if you just sit there."
- Will Rogers -

The perception of being in control promotes well-being. In some cases, clients have been allowed to decide for themselves how much morphine they needed. Those clients who prescribed their own dosages generally used a lower dosage than traditionally prescribed, and perceived less pain (Ferrell 1992[545]; Owen 1997[546]; Ellis 1999[547]).

Those who administered their own dosages felt more in control of their lives than those who received the dosage from the medical staff. It could be that the feeling of control produces more natural morphine (endorphins). Sometimes client-directed medication has been shown to shorten hospital stays (Thomas 1993[548]). Vingerhoets (2000[549]) was puzzled that even though such client-directed pain medication is widely recognized as valuable, it is still barely used.

"Action may not bring happiness, but there is no happiness without action."
- William James -

Clients need to increase their level of control over their lives, and over their disease. They cannot control everything - some things are clearly out of their control - but sitting back and waiting to be cured is disease-provoking. Spiegel wrote that it is crucial for clients' recovery to take every opportunity they can to gain (some) control over their lives. Clients need to start participating in life and in their healing processes, rather than sit around waiting for it to happen. Making decisions and taking responsibility for their actions is one of the goals of therapy.

Even when everything seems out of their control, there are still issues that clients can exercise control over.

Example:
For Indians in Alaska, death has a different meaning. Most of the Indians who were dying were conscious of the process, and what they were going through. They were aware of their personal contribution to their deaths, and had arranged their own funerals. Many of them were already arranging their funerals days before they actually died. They were praying for those left behind, and told their life stories. Some even bought the food that was to be served at their funerals. Their actions in these matters show a high degree of control.

Clients should take full responsibility for their own healing, and form a close partnership with the medical team (Cousins 1979[550]). When clients experience a heightened level of control, they usually also experience an increase in their quality of life. Lerche (1999[551]) reported an increase in quality of life and reduced anxiety when breast cancer clients were allowed to co-decide on the time and types of checkups. De Vries (1987[552]) noted that spontaneous remission often occurred after a sudden change in clients' level of dependence: when they went from being in a helpless state to a state in which they felt in control of their lives.

Clients who had survived cancer against all odds were studied by Berland (1994[553]). Those clients recommended that one should take control of one's health, and take the time to choose the right physician and a treatment one truly believes in. Most of those clients attributed their remarkable recovery to the fact that they had taken responsibility for their healing. They played an active role in treatment decisions. They took full control of the emotional and spiritual issues involved in their healing. Cunningham (2000[554]) noticed a significant link between a high level of involvement in these processes and recovery from cancer.

One of the issues the therapist should point out when working on clients' level of control is that not everything can be controlled. Clients cannot fully control the course of the disease nor the outcome. What they can control is their behavior, and actions that influence their quality of life, and could influence the course of the disease.

> *"Grant me the serenity to accept the things I cannot change, the courage to change the things I can and the wisdom to know the difference."*
> *- A Saint Francis Prayer -*

Clients should take action to influence that which can be controlled, and let go of those issues that they cannot control. The following model illustrates this.

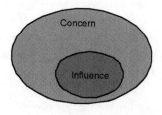

	Within Influence	No influence
Action	Autonomy Assertiveness Self-efficacy Control	Stress Worry Anxiety
No Action	Lack of control Helplessness Hopelessness Depressive feelings	Acceptance Ability to let go

Adapted from McDermott et al. (1996[555])

Certain issues can be controlled (Within influence), such as beliefs and emotions. If clients take action to control those issues, they will experience autonomy, assertiveness, self-efficacy, and control. However, if they fail to take action on those issues, they will experience helplessness, hopelessness, and feelings of depression.

> *"Don't let what you cannot do interfere with what you can do."*
> *- John Wooden -*

Other issues cannot be controlled (No influence), such as the weather. If clients forcefully try to take action to influence these, they will experience stress, worry and anxiety. If they do not take action, they will experience acceptance and the ability to let go.

The therapist should assist clients in taking action to influence those issues that can be controlled, and to resist taking action against those issues over which they have no influence.

> *"Influence is action, no influence is no action."*

11.3.3.1.1   *Assignments*

To increase clients' participation in their healing processes, the therapist can provide them with specific assignments to complete. When clients come in, they usually expect "to be healed." Assigning work that clients must take action to complete gets them participating. The actual assignment is more important than the content.

The actual level of performance shown through the assignments gives the therapist a wealth of information. If clients do not complete their assignments, they are somehow not participating in their own healing. This might indicate a belief that they will die soon, do not think they deserve to get well, or do not want to take responsibility for their own lives. In these cases, the therapist should also work with these beliefs. Such beliefs probably need to be changed before clients will participate in their own healing.

Example:
When people strongly believe that they cannot get well and will die in a week, what is the use of reading a book for the next session? In their minds, they will be dead by the next session.

The therapist can aid clients in finding ways in which they can exercise control. It does not actually matter how big or small these actions are, as long as clients feels that they can control (or partly control) them.

The most widely used assignments are:
- Reading supporting books.
- Performing relaxation exercises.
- Performing physical activities.
- Belief-supporting actions.

Taking the time and effort to perform such assignments not only increases participation, but also supports clients in their quest for assertiveness and self acceptance. These assignments force clients to take time for the assigned tasks and for themselves.

Reading Assignments

Reading assignments should focus on the psychological side of healing. The books suggested below are full of metaphors on healing and well-being. These books not only allow clients to participate more actively, but also shift their limiting beliefs toward more supporting ones.

Intervention:
Suggest that the client start reading the following books:
- *Getting Well Again, Simonton et al. (1978[556])*
- *Healing Journey, Simonton et al. (1992[557])*
- *Cancer as a Turning Point, LeShan (1989[558])*

- *You Can Fight for Your Life*, LeShan (1977[559])
- *Mind as a Healer, Mind as a Slayer*, Pelletier (1992[560])
- *Spontaneous Remission - An Annotated Bibliography*, O'Regan et al. (1993[561])
- *Will to Live*, Hutschnecker (1953[562])
- *Seeing with the Mind's Eye*, Samuels et al. (1975[563])

Relaxation Assignments

Suggesting that clients perform relaxation exercises (which are discussed in the section on Imagery and Pain Management) is very beneficial. It helps clients to achieve the benefits from those exercises: relaxation, stress reduction, etc. At the same time, clients feel more in control of their minds and bodies. Relaxation assignments are used in almost every therapeutic program.

Physical Activity

Physical activity assignments are used by Simonton et al. (1992[564]), who have clients determine their own level of physical activity. By noticing when they become tired, clients come to know to what extent they can exercise. By recognizing and acting upon these signals, clients gain control over their activities, deciding whether to stop or continue. This feeling of control also enhances their bodily awareness and autonomy. Physical activity has also been linked to a healthier prognosis.

Belief-Supporting Actions

Another type of task which can be assigned is based on cognitive behavioral therapy. Desired changes in personality traits should be backed up by behavior.

Examples of assignments that support assertiveness are:

Intervention:
- *Ask the nurse to come back in half an hour for your shot.*
- *Request a different meal.*
- *Ask visitors to get you a drink.*
- *Say "no" to a request.*

These actions increase not only the client's level of control, but also his expression of needs, which has also been associated with better health.

11.3.3.1.2   *Accepting Responsibility*

Helping clients to accept responsibility for their actions is another element of increasing their perception of control. Accepting responsibility for the healing process is an important step. It moves clients away from an external locus of control, towards an internal locus of control.

Usually, the mere act of asking a psychological professional for help, in addition to the client's current medical treatment, is already a big step towards accepting responsibility for the healing process.

One of the major tasks of any therapeutic program is to assist clients in taking responsibility for their healing process. This is not only the case for cancer therapy, but in any psychological setting. There are generally two pitfalls that the therapist must be aware of. One is allowing the therapist to decide what is best for clients. This must be avoided, as it is a disservice to the clients. It prevents them from taking control of their own lives. What they have to learn is how to regain control. Another pitfall is having the therapist check whether clients have done their homework. Performing the assignments is the clients' responsibility. If they do not complete their assignments, the therapist could take that as an indication that they are not fully participating yet.

The first step in taking responsibility for healing is to have clients identify their own participation in their sickness. This might sound a bit harsh, but if the therapist explains it carefully, clients will grasp it (see also 11.3.3.1.5 Pitfall of Guilt). The clients' participation in their sickness may have been creating, maintaining, or failing to solve certain distressing events. Examples of such participation could be:

> *Example:*
> *   *Allowing distressing events to enter your life.*
> *   *Denying your own limits.*
> *   *Creating distressing situations.*
> *   *Only taking care of others.*
> *   *Failing to say no.*

- *Ignoring emotions.*
- *Failing to accept help.*
- *Etc.*

These distressing events can be major life-changing events, traumata, minor events, or simply thoughts or feelings that have bothered them.

In the section on life events, clients listed the distressing events they had experienced. This list can be used to start a discussion with them concerning their participation. This discussion should lead to the recognition of their actions during the process. As clients control their actions, they control the level of distress. This recognition supports clients towards an internal locus of control.

Intervention: "Past stressors"
For each distressing event listed, ask:
- *How did you create that situation?*
- *What did you believe at that moment?*
- *What was your behavior?*
- *How did you react?*

When clients become aware that they did participate, the discussion moves on towards developing new coping mechanisms for these specific situations. By finding new behavioral coping styles, clients can reduce the level of distress in those situations.

Intervention: "Present stressors"
1. *Mark the five most distressing events in your life today.*
2. *Examine your participation in each of them.*
3. *Remove the situation from your life, if possible.*
4. *Think of alternative ways of reacting (beliefs and behaviors) to the situation.*
5. *Think of supportive elements in your life that help you to deal with the situation.*

Based on Simonton (1978[565]).

When clients fully accept responsibility, it will have a tremendous impact on the effect of every intervention, both medical and psychological.

The medical team provides clients with the information needed to make informed decisions, although the physician usually decides what is best for clients. If clients feel responsible, they will request much more information about treatment options, side effects, and prognosis. They will weigh the risks and benefits when they decide. These decisions include choices about what diets to follow, what exercises to perform, what medication to take, and what treatments to undergo.

The following is one simple piece of communication advice that can help clients persuade the medical team to provide them with the answers they need:

Intervention:
"I want to feel like I am part of this treatment. It will ease my mind to know the purpose of my medication. Can you tell me?"

Another element of taking responsibility is recognizing the benefits that come with the situation, as well as finding alternative ways of obtaining those benefits without the disease. This is an important and very extensive element; it will therefore be discussed in a separate chapter (11.3.4 Secondary Gain).

11.3.3.1.3   The Patient-Doctor Relationship

The relationship between the patient[566] and the physician is inherently associated with someone who is responsible (the physician) and someone who undergoes treatment (the patient). This is a dependent relationship; the patient is sick and depends on the physician in order to be cured. In the medical system, the physician is most often not to be questioned. This inherently produces passive clients.

Clients often feel dependent and powerless with regard to their physicians. They are often afraid to ask direct questions, or to continue asking when the answer is not satisfactory. Sometimes, clients even fear their physicians. Many clients treat their physicians as gurus or all-knowing-oracles, and feel that their physicians are controlling their lives. This reduces participation by clients.

Clients should perceive the relationship with their physicians as a consulting relationship. The physician is a messenger of good and bad news, a provider of healthcare and a source of knowledge. The most helpful metaphor for such a relationship is to imagine a decision maker and his consultant. The physician is an expert in medical issues, who advises clients in their decisions. This advice should be taken seriously, but clients will decide for themselves whether or not to follow the advice.

Example:
Take a plumber, for example, who is fixing your water system at home. You would usually ask questions about the situation and options, such as what rates he will charge and how he is going to fix the problem. If you do not trust his abilities or promises, you can change plumbers. He is only there to advise you, and perform the work you agree upon.

Although the physician is a medical expert, he should be viewed as an adviser, not the core decision maker. (See also the section "Assertiveness with physicians.") Clients need to develop a partnership with their physicians, and must be able to ask for the help they need. The following questions might help clients in their communication with their physicians.

Intervention:
- *Request anything that you need in order to feel involved in treatment decisions.*
- *Ask that the physician clarify any procedures that you do not fully understand.*
- *Continue to ask questions if you are not satisfied with the answers you have received.*
- *Ask for a second opinion if you want one.*
- *Ask to be involved in treatment choices.*
- *Discuss your concerns with the physician.*
- *Ask for information about side effects from the treatment.*
- *Make a new appointment if the physician is too busy.*

Adapted from Spiegel (1991[567]; 1993[568]) and Temoshok (1992[569]).

One thing that could help the client is to write down a list of questions he wants to ask. Additional questions can be added to this list. In situations of elevated distress, the list reminds the client of the important questions.

11.3.3.1.4   Imagery

Spiegel (1978[570]; 1991[571]; 1993[572]) makes extensive use of hypnosis to increase clients' feelings of control. By learning self-hypnosis, clients experience control of their minds and bodies.

Spiegel also uses the following intervention to increase feelings of control.

> **Intervention:**
> - *Imagine a large screen and split it down the middle.*
> - *Imagine a current problem in your life, which you feel you have no control over.*
> - *While remaining relaxed and comfortable, imagine something you cannot control on the left.*
> - *On the right side, imagine something that you feel you can control.*
> - *Look at both screens, and reflect on the meaning of those two sides.*
>
> *Adapted from Spiegel (1991[573]).*

This intervention helps clients realize that there is always something they can control.

11.3.3.1.5   Pitfall of Guilt

When working with gaining control and taking responsibility, there is one major issue to be aware of: the issue of guilt. Taking responsibility for healing and accepting one's participation in illness might be interpreted by clients as being guilty of their disease. In such cases, clients' thought patterns might include thoughts like "If I am responsible for my healing, I am also responsible for my disease," or "I am guilty of my own disease." This is counter-productive, and should be dealt with by the therapist. If the therapist does not handle this issue properly, clients' feelings of guilt will increase, and their quality of life will decrease. The focus of the therapist should be to increase participation in health without allowing clients to feel guilty for their disease.

Although an unhealthy lifestyle with unhealthy behaviors, thought processes, and emotions might increase the risk of cancer and result in a poor prognosis, clients are not to *blame* for it. Clients were not willing their cancer to develop. This issue is very important, and often does not receive the attention it deserves. I will therefore devote extra attention to it.

Example:
If you donate money to a charity, it does not mean that you made those people suffer earlier.

When a batter hits a home run, it does not mean that he made himself miss the previous times.

It is like having failed math at grade school, and then blaming yourself for failing that class (now that you have finished university) because you know the answers now.

Another way to view the perspective of guilt is to turn it around. It is not possible to create cancer, even if one wanted to. One can eat, drink, smoke, think, or feel unhealthy, but that is still no guarantee that a cancer will develop.

There is a huge difference between being "blamed" for a situation and accepting that one has "participated" in creating the current situation. This difference must be made clear to clients.

Blame suggests that someone consciously decided to create the situation, knowing very well what the outcome would be. Most people are not aware of any link between thought processes, emotions, and physical illness. Therefore they simply cannot be blamed; they were unaware of the influence of their mindset on their physical well-being.

> *"You are not creating your cancer, nor are you to blame for it. You learned a way to cope with stress in your young days, that was most appropriate to you at that time, but it ended up as less healthy than your body expected it to be."*
> *- Lawrence LeShan -*

The following is one intervention that can be used to reduce and eventually remove guilt, and keep the focus on participation:

Intervention:
Explain all the NLP presuppositions, and especially:
- *"There is no failure, only feedback."*

- *"All behavior is based on present resources and is the best choice available."*

Adapted from Alder (1996[574]) and Knight (1997[575]).

Temoshok (1992[576]) intervenes by explaining the difference between taking responsibility and feeling guilty. She spends much time explaining that clients are not to blame for their cancer, and that they do have influence over the course of the disease.

She uses the following statements to explain this to clients.

Intervention:
- *In the past, you were not aware of your behavior.*
- *Or, you were aware of your behavior, but did not recognize it as a psychological impediment.*
- *Or, you were aware of your behavior, but you did not know it would affect your health.*
- *Or, you were aware of your behavior, but you did not know you could change it.*
- *Or, you were aware of your behavior and its effects, but you were not able to change. Your inability to change was due either to lack of self-understanding; lack of social support; social pressures at work or in your family; or your own human limitations - not character flaws.*

Adapted from Temoshok (1992[577]).

The therapist must make sure that he communicates the message that clients can learn that their ability to control their health does not mean they were at fault for what happened before.

Example:
While growing from a child into an adult, people learn multiple ways of handling situations. Effective methods will be repeated, while ineffective methods will be discarded.

Some behaviors are effective only during the infant years, like crying to get attention. People learn how to think, express their emotions, and handle stress.

They form conclusions based on how they perceive their environment, and how their parents react.

Most of these decisions are made without consciously deciding. Some

*are made on the wrong premises, and some are false interpretations
of the truth.*

11.3.3.2 Expectations about Process and Outcome

*"A positive attitude towards treatment was a better predictor of
response to treatment than was the severity of the disease."*
- Carl Simonton -

Ikemi (1978[578]), Oliver (1982[579]) and Romo (1984[580]) noticed that
successful clients seemed to have very strong faith in the chosen
treatment program. These researchers noticed that clients' successes
did not reflect the objective effectiveness of the programs. They
attributed the success of the treatments to the clients' beliefs, and the
strong workings of the placebo response.

In the studies they conducted at Travis Air Force Base, Simonton at
al. (1979[581]) noticed the tremendous effect of expectations on outcomes.
When clients had positive expectations, their physical responses to
treatment were positive. When they had negative expectations, their
physical responses to treatment were negative. It seemed as if only their
expectations made the difference in their treatment.

Berland (1995[582]) studied cancer clients who had less than a 20%
chance of survival, but nevertheless survived. He noticed that clients
used methods that they personally strongly believed in. When Berland
asked them what they thought contributed most to their healing, they
mentioned their hopefulness (sometimes referred to as faith) for the
future. They also reported that this hope was present even when they
accepted the possibility of death.

Cousins (1979[583]) wrote that clients should have an "unshakable
confidence" in their bodies' ability to utilize its own wisdom to facilitate
healing. At the same time, they should maintain a partnership with their
physicians.

*"What the patient believes the treatment will do for him seems to be
more important than what the treatment actually is."*
- Daniel P. Brown - (1987[584])

This suggests, as does Newton (1982[585]), that the therapist should
assist clients in developing a strong belief system with positive

expectations. Taylor et al. (2000[586]) revealed in their investigations that optimistic beliefs about the future (even if they are unrealistic) may be beneficial to physical health.

A study by Cole et al. (2002[587]) explored the relationship between clients' subjective expectations and their objective recovery times. They studied 1566 injured workers. Their recovery times were estimated by a physician, and the workers were asked to fill in a questionnaire 3 weeks after the injury. The results of the study showed a strong relationship between expected and actual recovery times. Those who expected to recover actually recovered 30% faster than those without that expectation.

This is also nicely illustrated by a study conducted by Idler et al. (1991[588]). In a study of more than 2800 people, the researchers observed that one's opinion about one's health is a better predictor than objective factors.

A client who went into spontaneous remission attributed his remarkable recovery to his own belief, which he stated as:

> *"Everybody knows that one dies of cancer, but I was not sure whether to apply this to myself. I considered this (belief) to be nonsense."*
> *- Daan van Baalen and Marco J. de Vries - (1987[589])*

11.3.3.2.1   Common Expectations

The media and traditional medicine seem to overestimate the possibility of negative outcomes. Most of the stories that circulate are about the worst things that can happen, and people dying. Those cases with positive outcomes seem to be underestimated in the media, yet many cases are known. Research has demonstrated that positive expectations help the healing process. Because of what seems to be an emphasis on negative expectations, I will present only the positive side in this chapter.

A negative outcome is usually based on a belief similar to one of the following:
- Cancer is death.
- Treatment is drastic and negative, and has many undesirable results.

- Cancer is a strong and powerful enemy, and destroys the entire body.

Clients can be assisted in changing such beliefs for more positive (and realistic) ones by reading the proper literature (such as the introductory chapters of this work). Reading motivational stories about people who did heal, listening to biographies of former cancer clients, and reading scientific literature on spontaneous remission can also help to create positive expectations.

Reading such literature loosens the grip of the negative beliefs, and replaces them with more realistic and supporting beliefs.

Cancer is Death

One of the most common prevailing misconceptions concerns the deadliness of cancer in general. Cancer may be a terminal disease, but many people are healed. There is no guarantee whatsoever that death is approaching when cancer is diagnosed. One can die from breast cancer, but 96% percent of localized breast cancer clients now survive (5-year survival rate). A more realistic and accurate view is the belief that "Cancer is a disease that you may or may not overcome."

Intervention:
- *Have the client read the introduction to this study.*
- *Have the client read stories about cancer survival and spontaneous remission.*
- *Have the client read commonly suggested books. The titles that the client should read are listed in the section on assignments (11.3.3.1.1Assignments).*

By reading these books, a shift in beliefs will take place. The client will realize that people can be cured of cancer.

Another intervention which is very effective is the use of reframing, as discussed in the generic beliefs section (11.2.3 Reframing).

Treatment is Drastic

A belief that the treatment is drastic forces the mind to focus on the negative consequences. A more supportive belief is the fact that the treatment is an ally, one's friend while in need. The treatment supports the body in healing.

Cancer is Strong

Many people think that cancer is a very powerful disease. Scientifically, cancer consists of very weak and confused cells. According to current research, everyone has some cancer cells in their body, but only a few people develop cancer. In those rare cases of malignant tumors, the immune system was not powerful enough to recognize and destroy the tumor, or shield the body from it. It has even been shown that when cancer cells and normal cells are put together in a petri dish, the cancer cells are destroyed by the white blood cells (Simonton et al. 1992[590]). The truth is that the immune system is much more powerful than the weak cancer cells.

11.3.3.2.2   *Imagery*

A technique which is very often used to change outcome expectations is imagery. Clients construct a mental image of how they want the outcome to be. Then, through the use of several imagery techniques, clients are instructed to engage in a vivid imagery process with the desired outcome. A more detailed discussion of imagery techniques can be found in the chapter on imagery.

These techniques are also extensively described by Simonton et al. (1978[591]), Achterberg (1985[592]), and Rossman (1987[593]; 2003[594]).

11.3.4   Secondary Gain

Eliminating secondary gain is an issue that can be found in most therapeutic programs. In the case of complementary psychological cancer treatment (CPCT), the elimination of secondary gain is a very important subject. Early discoveries about the link between psychology and cancer suggest that secondary gain is involved. Accepting secondary gain can be viewed as an element of accepting responsibility (11.3.3.1.2 Accepting Responsibility). Because this is such an extensive and important issue, I have devoted a separate chapter to it.

> *"Disease can be a real opportunity, and it can be an opportunity without your having to lay a guilt trip on yourself. In other words, disease is not caused by a lesson you are giving yourself, but, if you choose, you can turn disease into something to learn from, or something to motivate you towards more balance or harmony in your life."*
> *- Ken Wilbur -*

As discussed earlier, a cancer diagnosis forces clients to make many changes in their lives. Their entire private lives, working lives, relationships, etc. will change. The diagnosis influences their whole lives. Clients start behaving differently, and feel different emotions than those they are used to. Their priorities in life change dramatically.

These changes do not have to be all bad. Some of the changes can actually be enjoyed. Cancer clients usually receive more attention and more love. People are willing to do anything for clients, and they accept more from them. People are less likely to get into a fight with cancer clients; conflicts with them are usually avoided. People do not strain clients as much as before, and try to release any pressure on them. People will accept most kinds of behavior from terminal clients. Many clients are confronted with more love and more attention than they were used to. Besides the fact that other people react differently, they might even allow themselves to act differently. They might allow themselves to skip certain tasks, request more attention, yell at people, cry endlessly, or be selfish. The illness gives clients permission to act out. It gives them permission to stop working, and run away from distressing situations.

"In the face of love and terminal illness, everything is allowed."
- Popular saying -

Although the disease is something negative, it almost seems like there are benefits that come with it. These benefits are also known as secondary gain. Clients are not aware of these benefits, but they do influence their behavior.

Almost any situation also conceals benefits. Only when clients are aware of these benefits can they find alternative ways of achieving them. When the benefits remain hidden, clients unconsciously move towards them and away from their overall goals.

Example:
- *A psychiatrist was blamed for his patient's suicide. The cancer diagnosis prevented him from receiving accusations.*
- *A man was under great pressure to achieve financial success. The diagnosis brought this man a generous disability allowance. When work became possible again, the man experienced serious flare-ups.*

Adapted from Simonton (1978[595]).

When they become aware, clients often report one of the following benefits:

- Permission to get away from a problem or situation.
- Receiving love, attention, and care.
- Taking time off to reflect on life and deal with current problems.
- Motivation to work on personal growth or change undesirable behaviors.
- Escape from high expectations of oneself or others.
- Expression of emotions.

"Many people tend to bottle up emotions and express only positive feelings. In the case of a life threatening disease, people allow themselves to express negative feelings and take more time for themselves."
- Carl Simonton -

This section is intended to help clients identify some of their own benefits, and find alternatives so that they can keep the benefits once they are healthy again. If these alternatives are not developed, there is a possibility that clients may wish to stay sick in order to keep the desired benefits.

Usually, these interventions are initially met with some rejection. This rejection is caused by people thinking that these benefits mean that they like their current situation. The therapist could explain that he understands that the illness is something they do not like, and that these interventions are about discovering the positive side effects that automatically come with the disease.

Example:
"I surely do not like it when I have a cold and must stay at home. I want to be cured and be able to do all my usual things. At the same time, I can enjoy sleeping in. Although the cold is something I do not want, the time off is welcome."

Research by Antoni et al. (2001[596]) concluded that efforts to find these benefits lead to a decrease in depressive feelings and increased optimism. Clients recognize the positive side effects of their traumatic experience, such as growth, appreciation of life, and the reordering of priorities and emotions.

Recognition of secondary gain also influences the immune system.

Cruess et al. (2001[597]) conducted a 10-week Cognitive Behavioral Stress Management program. Those women who recognized and acknowledged their secondary gain showed increased immune functioning. Cruess et al. concluded that the biological change was largely due to the effort devoted to finding benefits from the disease. They did not provide an explanation of how this effect was established.

Some cancer clients even reported that after having recognized the secondary benefits, they viewed their cancer as something that supported them in living a happier life.

The first step is accepting that there might be benefits. Next, these benefits need to be identified. Finally, alternative ways of achieving them must be developed.

"What does not destroy me strengthens me."
- Friedrich Nietzsche –

11.3.4.1 Accepting Secondary Gain

Accepting that there might be benefits associated with their current condition is the first step. Clients often find this very confronting. They most often interpret the existence of secondary gain as meaning that they do not want to heal. This misconception needs to be addressed by the therapist before clients will speak of what their benefits might be.

Discussing the above introduction with clients and explaining that secondary gain is always present changes this misconception. During the discussion, the therapist must stress that he acknowledges clients' wish to become healthy.

11.3.4.2 Listing Benefits

When clients accept that there might be benefits associated with having cancer, the therapist can help them to recognize their own benefits. Being consciously aware of their secondary gain increases clients' self-awareness and motivates them to change.

Example:
A client told Simonton: "At the time I became ill, I was having a lot of trouble finishing a job in which I had a great emotional and

financial stake. It was very important to me that it be completed in a splendid fashion, but the work was going slowly and I had doubts about the product I was producing. By getting sick, I was able to meet many needs at once:

- *I wanted my wife's help on the project but felt that, unless I literally could not do it myself, it would be wrong for me to distract her from her own activities to help me.*
- *I needed the excuse of "something beyond my control" for not finishing the project on time.*
- *I may also have been preparing an excuse for any imperfections that might appear in it.*
- *It gave me a reason to get seriously involved with my own health, which meant among other things resolving that when I got well I would find the time to play tennis, an activity that I enjoy but which I normally do not do because I am too busy.*
- *It was a simple rest from my daily labors, which were giving me a lot of stress."*

Case described in Simonton (1978[598]).

Realizing the benefits of the current situation could be embarrassing to clients. If the therapist stresses that he understands that they do not desire the illness, and that the benefits come automatically with the situation, their embarrassment may decrease.

Intervention:
Have the client write down all the possible benefits they can think of. The following questions can help the client in discovering these:
- *What positive side effects do you notice right now?*
- *What are the benefits of not getting healthy?*
- *What will happen (something you do not like) when you are healthy?*
- *What will not happen when you are healthy?*
- *What are you not doing because you have this disease?*
- *What will you lose when you become healthy?*
- *What are you doing that you like, which is not possible (or more difficult to do) when you are healthy?*

Another intervention was developed by Antoni et al. (2001). They developed a questionnaire on which clients can rate the kinds of benefits they experience.

Some of these benefits have underlying values. A benefit is only a benefit when it addresses something clients need or want. Usually, there are only a limited number of ways to achieve the benefit. However, there are many ways of satisfying the underlying need or want. When they discover the underlying need or want, clients have more ways to develop alternatives.

Example:
The benefit of vacuum cleaning the house could be removing dust from the room. The underlying "need" could be the desire to impress visitors with a clean house, or to breathe freely.

Another benefit of the disease could be that a major project has been blown off. The underlying "want" could be some time off for oneself.

The benefit from wasps were fresh organic plums. The "want" was healthy fruit.

Intervention:
Have the client investigate the true value of each of the benefits listed.
- *Write down the need or want that is satisfied next to each benefit you listed.*
- *What will it do for you?*
- *What does that benefit mean to you?*
- *What does it allow you to experience?*

11.3.4.3 Finding Alternatives

When the benefits and needs are clear, the therapist should assist clients in finding and developing alternative ways of satisfying that need. These new methods should be more attractive and healthier than the original.

The following metaphor could help clients discover those alternatives.

Example:
We used to have a plum tree. At the end of every summer, it was filled with delicious plums. Just before they were ready to eat, some fell on the ground and started to rot. Hundreds of wasps flocked to the tree every year to enjoy the fruit.

While we enjoyed the summer in our garden, we had to be very careful not to get stung by those wasps. Every year, we decided to get rid of the tree just after harvesting the delicious plums. But somehow, we postponed it every year, almost as if something prevented us from cutting down that tree.
This went on for years and years, only increasing our annoyance of the wasps.

One day, our mom decided to buy a pound of plums from the greengrocer right around the time when we could harvest our own. Insidious, we thought. However, now that we had delicious plums, we no longer needed the tree.
The next year, the tree was gone.

We were troubled by the wasps, but did not allow ourselves to cut down the tree because of the plums. Only after we got plums in a different way were we able to cut down the tree.

This metaphor explains that one must recognize the benefits and find alternative ways of obtaining them.

One intervention is to ask clients how they can satisfy the needs on their lists. Another possible intervention is the following:
Intervention:
Help the client to find as many alternative methods as possible for satisfying the needs on the list.
- *Write down each need on a separate form.*
- *Write down every method you can think of for satisfying that need.*

11.3.4.3.1   Listing Disadvantages

Some clients are not motivated enough to find alternatives for obtaining the benefit. Other clients show behavior which could lead the therapist to suspect that they do not want to heal. In those cases, the therapist could work to increase the clients' motivation to find alternatives.

Behavioral therapy suggests that one should motivate clients towards the desired situation and away from the current situation. In the case of secondary gain, the therapist can focus on the disadvantages of the current situation in order to increase clients' motivation.

Some disapprove of the use of this type of intervention because they believe it creates fear. In my opinion, such interventions are acceptable because the clients find themselves in a life-threatening situation. The therapist should nonetheless be aware that this could install fear, but increases the motivation to change at the same time.

Intervention:
- *What is the worst thing that can happen if nothing changes?*
- *How will your family and friends react?*
- *How much pain will you suffer?*
- *What will happen if you keep this disease?*
- *What are you not capable of if you keep this disease?*
- *What will it cost you if nothing changes.*

Adapted from Robbins (1987[599]; 1992[600]).

12

Emotion-Focused Coping

Many researchers have been discussing the different coping styles that are appropriate for cancer clients to use. As we have seen in previous chapters, there are basically three different styles of coping: problem-focused, meaning-focused, and emotion-focused.

1) **Problem-focused coping** involves taking action towards solving the problem. This has been discussed in the section on dealing with events.
2) **Meaning-focused coping** involves attributing a different meaning to the same event. This has been discussed in the section on changing the appraisal process.
3) **Emotion-focused coping** refers to handling the emotions that are present. This is the subject of this chapter.

A distinction must be made between the emotions that are present and how clients handle those emotions. The emotions themselves, such as anger, fear, or hopelessness, are the subject of the next chapter. This chapter deals with the way clients handle their emotions. Teaching clients how to handle emotions is a key element of many different treatment programs.

Many authors agree regarding the healing value of recognizing, listening, expressing, and acting upon emotions. Pert (1997[601]) even mentions in her research that clients must get in touch with their emotions for their healing to take place.

Research tends to focus only on coping with distressing emotions and their effects on health. There is no research available on the relationship between prognosis and coping with comforting emotions.

12.1   Diagnosis

The therapist can determine the client's dominant coping style during their conversations, or with the help of questionnaires.

During discussions with clients, the therapist receives information about their emotion-focused coping styles. If clients rationalize their emotions, or do not behave according to their emotions, a high rate of anti-emotionality could be suspected. If clients try to maintain a good, strong appearance, never seem to lose their temper, and fake a positive outlook on life, they probably have a high rate of emotional repression.

Questionnaires can also be used to determine a client's level of emotional expression. Spielberger (1988[602]) developed a questionnaire that measured emotional control of anger. Watson et al. (1993[603]) developed a questionnaire, based on the "Courtauld Emotional Control Scale (CECS)," to measure the extent to which clients withhold their emotions.

To determine clients' levels of anti-emotionality, Grossarth-Maticek (1979[604]; et al. 1985[605]) developed a questionnaire called the "Rationality and Anti-emotionality Scale (R/A Scale)." Other questionnaires to measure anti-emotionality were developed by Spielberger (1988[606]), Van der Ploeg et al. (1989[607]), Swan et al. (1991[608]), and Bleiker et al. (1993[609])

12.2   Therapy

12.2.1   Emotional Expression

Cancer clients have a tendency to feel that they need to be strong and able to handle every situation. To present such a strong and positive image, they have to mask their true emotions and thoughts. Cancer clients are not alone in this thinking. Many people share this false idea that they must think positive in order to increase health. They argue that expressing distressing thoughts and emotions is detrimental to the healing process. People who actually live according to this principle live a lie. Not only is the repression of such emotions bad for their health - it also turns their life into a façade. Their distressing emotions will not disappear; they are merely pushed into the unconscious, where they cannot be resolved.

These ideas are based on a false interpretation of research. Research did indicate that people who expressed happy emotions were healthier than those who expressed distressing emotions. The "Positive Thinking Movement" assumed that one only needs to express positive emotions to increase health. This is not the case. Research actually indicated that comforting emotions are healthier only for those who are really feeling happy consciously and unconsciously! Those people are happy from the inside out, and not just wearing a happy face.

When people only express comforting emotions, they deny the truth and repress their real emotions. Such repression is associated with poorer health outcomes.

Example:
Research has shown that nice red apples taste better than green apples. However, painting the green apple a nice red color will not improve its flavor.

When an apple has gone bad, just painting it a nice red color will not make it taste better. Quite the contrary is true. When an apple rots away, the paint covers it up and the rotting speeds up.

Positive thinking is definitely healthier than negative thinking, but distressing emotions should be expressed. Positive thinking should be based on a solid, realistic foundation, on which clients face their current situation. Only with a solid acceptance of the current situation can new, realistic goals be created.

Besides avoiding reality, forcing clients towards positive thinking also has other side effects that are detrimental to health. When clients are instructed by a therapist (or by society) to express only comforting emotions, they could develop feelings of guilt and failure when they experience distressing emotions. Forceful positive thinking also sets clients up for failure and self-blame in the event of a relapse. At the same time, it could induce them to think that they have created the disease themselves by still having those emotions. Not being able (or allowed) to express such distressing emotions increases clients' distress. This distress cannot be expressed, and a vicious cycle of ever-increasing distress is the result.

The huge potential of expressing dormant emotions is discussed by Pert (1997[610]). Clients who expressed their emotions often jump-started their healing processes. The expression of distressing emotions also seems to decrease the negative health effects of those specific emotions (which will be discussed in the next chapter. The expression of comforting emotions often increased the quality of life.

Most clients who generally do not express distressing emotions have a set of beliefs that support suppression:

Example:
- *I must exhibit courage at all times.*
- *The expression of depressive feelings, anxiety, and anger will make me sicker.*
- *I cannot allow myself any negative thoughts.*
- *I have to be strong for my family.*
- *If I express my distressing emotions, I will be rejected.*
- *If I express my distressing emotions, I cannot stop myself.*
- *It is useless to express my distressing emotions and needs.*
- *I should not burden my friends with my pain.*
- *Everyone's been so good to me. How dare I complain?*
- *If I express my pain and sadness, people will think I am a sentimental jerk.*

There could also be some repression of comforting emotions. When clients become aware of comforting emotions, they might not be able to express them either. If that is the case, they might have supporting beliefs that suppress those comforting emotions.

Example:
- *I cannot be happy in the face of this dreadful disease.*
- *Having fun is not appropriate at this time.*
- *There are so many people in misery, I just cannot have fun.*

All these beliefs are examples of limiting beliefs which should be changed. Such a change can be accomplished by using generic belief change interventions, which have been discussed earlier. This chapter discusses other (non-belief-based) interventions that can be applied to increase emotional expression.

12.2.1.1 Expressive Writing

Writing is a form of expression that is less confronting to clients than verbal expression. This makes writing an effective intervention to use, particularly when clients are not ready for verbal expression. Clients can be instructed to keep a personal journal in which they write down their experiences and emotions. Clients should write about distressing as well as comforting experiences, from the past and present. Writing about enjoyable experiences and comforting emotions increases their feeling of well-being. Being able to write about comforting emotions makes it easier for clients to write about other (distressing) emotions as well. Expressive writing helps clients deal with their memories and feelings from the past. Keeping a journal increases clients' participation and allows them to continue to work in between therapeutic sessions.

The therapeutic effects of writing have been extensively researched. Vingerhoets (1997[611]) reported studies by Pennebaker et al. (1988[612]) and Smyth (1998[613]). Pennebaker et al. had clients write for 20 minutes about their most stressful experiences for 3 to 4 days in a row. The results showed clearly that those who wrote about their most stressful experiences felt physically better than the control group. The writing group also reported fewer problems and showed an increase in health, measured by a reduced number of visits to their doctor. Even their immune systems showed higher efficiency (i.e. their T-cell activity). Some years later, Smyth (1999[614]) repeated the research and noted a reduction of symptoms in asthmatic and rheumatic clients.

Antoni (1991[615]) and Esterling et al. (1990[616]) concluded that writing about emotional traumas has a positive effect on psychological well-being. Such well-being has a positive effect on physical well-being. Their writing groups also displayed measurable changes in their immune functioning. Writing about emotionally disturbing topics measurably increases clients' immune functioning and reduces their distress.

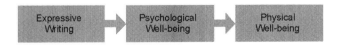

Intervention:
"For the next 3 (three) days, I would like for you to write about your very deepest thoughts and feeling about an extremely important emotional issue that has affected you and your life. In your writing, I

would like you to really let go and explore your very deepest emotions and thoughts. You might tie your topic to your relationships with others, including parents, lovers, friends, or relatives, to your past, your present, or your future, or to who you have been, who you would like to be, or who you are now.

You may write about the same general issues or experiences all three days, or cover different topics each day. All of your writing will be completely confidential. Do not worry about spelling, sentence structure, or grammar. The only rule is that once you begin writing, continue to do so until your time is up."

Adapted from Pennebaker (1997[617]).

Smyth noted that there is a stronger effect when the writing occurs over a longer period of time. It is more effective to write once a week for a month, than to write 4 times in a single week.

12.2.1.2 Expression

When clients learn to become aware and express their emotions, they could start with a single emotion in a setting they find the easiest. For example, they could start by expressing sadness to their best friend. In this way, they gain experience in expressing emotions. Through this experience, they gain confidence. When clients experience that there is a time and place for them to express their emotions, they are often better able to manage emotions in other situations as well (Spiegel 1995[618]).

They could express their emotions in a therapeutic group setting, by themselves, to family members, or to the therapist. The main issue is that they express their emotions, which prevents emotional build up. If they express their emotions to their loved ones, it will not only enhance their well-being, but also the intimacy of their relationships (Spiegel 1995[619]). Gradually, the therapist can move toward the expression of other emotions, as well as emotional expression in other situations.

"Openness and emotional expressiveness is a central goal in this treatment."
- David Spiegel -

An intervention used by Temoshok (1992[620]) is to discuss a time when clients were really angry. She has clients expand upon that incident, and asks them to become aware of their emotions at that time. Through the discussion, the clients express their emotions to the therapist.

12.2.1.3 Controlling Expression

When clients are confident with expressing their emotions, they must learn to control their emotional expression. This might seem to contradict earlier statements about expression and anti-emotionality, but it does not. The first step is to have clients recognize and express their emotions. The next step is to fine-tune their emotional expression. This consists of expressing emotions in an appropriate way.

The first thing that must be made clear to clients is that emotional expression is not the uncontrolled expression of emotions (emotional vomiting).

Research concluded that the expression of emotions is healthy. Some people took this to mean that every emotion should be expressed all the time. In their opinion, all distressing emotions and thoughts were harmful. Staps et al. (1991[621]) and Yang (1997[622]) made important distinctions regarding these issues. They concluded that it is not only the expression of emotions that should be of primary interest to the therapeutic work. The appropriate and effective expression of emotions to relevant other people is more important. This, of course, can only be learned when clients are already able to express their emotions.

Staps and Yang teach clients to be selective in their expression. Sometimes suppressing emotions is good, whereas at other times, or with other people, the emotions should be expressed. Their primary therapeutic goal is for clients to perceive a choice of whether to express or suppress their emotions. In the research that found suppression to be associated with poorer health, they discovered that clients did not experience such a choice. Those who did experience a choice ("flexible type C," according to Temoshok) did not display the negative health effects of suppression.

Somehow, when the concept of emotional expression is addressed, clients often fear that they are expected to start emotional-vomiting. When the concept of appropriate expression is explained, they often feel relieved. Based on the desired effects of their expression, clients choose either expression or suppression.

On the other hand, many people believe that extensive, prolonged emotional expression is healthy. This is also wrong. There is no evidence that prolonged crying facilitates catharsis. Crying might help to release some stress or request help from others. Labott (1987[623]) demonstrated that crying students more often reported high levels of mood disturbance, anxiety, depressive feelings, and anger. In a literature review, Vingerhoets (2001[624]) concluded that there is little evidence that tears improve health or well-being, in the short run or the long run. Both emotional suppression and prolonged crying seem to be unhealthy (Bolstad 2004[625].)

Some clients express their emotions and feel emotionally flooded all the time. They seem to cry almost constantly, and fully depend on others. This type of expression has become a habitual coping style for them. Experience has shown that these people tend to express only their surface emotions. By crying, they avoid expressing their true, deeper emotions. These clients need to develop the ability to stop their emotional vomiting and occasionally close the emotional valve. They also need to learn to express other emotions as well, particularly the emotions they avoid by crying. Within a group of 204 clients with mixed cancer types, Stavraky (1968[626]) noticed that those who expressed their emotions without losing control had longer survival times.

Clients need to learn that they can control their own emotional outlets like they would a valve. They are in control and can open or close it to express appropriate amounts of selected emotions.

Intervention:

1. *Explain what is expected with emotional expression, that controlled expression is important, and that endless crying is not a proper form of expression.*
2. *Assist the client in expressing some emotion.*
3. *Interrupt the client, have him stop his expression, and continue to another subject.*
4. *When he starts to express an emotion and then has to stop, he learns to control his own emotional valve.*
5. *Explain that by practicing this intervention, the client learns to control his emotional valve.*

Other clients seem to believe that if they truly express their emotions, other people will be overloaded. If these clients experiment with emotional expression on a small scale, they will notice that most people can handle it. They might even notice that many people are grateful when they finally express their true emotions. This changes their perception, and makes it easier for them to express their emotions freely.

These clients think they know what other people want, and how much they can handle. Such beliefs should be changed during therapy with belief interventions.

Sometimes it is not appropriate to express an emotion at a particular moment in time. If this is the case, clients can wait, write about it, and express it another time. The recognition of such situations and the ability to withhold the emotion is a huge step forward.

Intervention:
Assist the client:
1.   *In discovering what his purpose was when he expressed his emotions that time.*
2.   *In exploring when, and in what way, he can express his emotions and bring about the desired result.*

12.2.1.4 Communication Skills

To express emotions, clients need to communicate. Temoshok (1992[627]) teaches clients communication skills so they can effectively communicate their emotions and reduce the chances of rejection. She does this because, as she reasons, clients will otherwise be confronted with their fears that other people will not understand them.

While expressing an emotion, clients should not blame other people. Blaming increases the defensiveness of others. The same holds true for expectations of others. Clients should not expect others to miraculously behave differently just because they have expressed their emotions.

The following guidelines might be helpful while teaching clients effective communication skills.

Guidelines:

- *Express your emotion without blaming others.*
- *Formulate it in the "I" form without referring to the other.*
- *Expect nothing from the other. Do not try to change the other; simply express the emotion and mention your values and needs.*
- *Let the other decide for himself what to do with that information.*
- *If you feel this way because of a request someone has made of you, say no.*
- *Say yes to offerings of help.*

Adapted from Temoshok (1992[628]).

Friends, family, physicians, or others might interrupt clients' emotional expression. This could throw clients off-balance. Clients could ask them to be quiet until they are finished. The following introduction reduces the chances of such interruptions.

Example:

"When I am very upset, here is what I would like you to do. Just listen to me. Let me tell you my problem, and express my feelings, for however long it takes.
Please do not interrupt.
I know this will sound strange, but do not even say "right" or "uh-huh" or "I understand." Be as quiet as you can. Look at me, I need to see your response, but do not rush in to offer comfort or advice.
Wait until I am completely finished. It may take five minutes or twenty-five. I will let you know when I am done. After I am through, I would love to talk to you about the problem.
Until then, the most wonderful thing you can do for me is to listen."

Adapted from Temoshok (1992[629]).

This introduction prepares others to listen to the whole story. It reduces defensive reactions and frustration for both clients and any others present. Clients can fully express their emotions and thoughts. It often helps clients to achieve a deeper understanding of themselves.

Fiore (1986[630]) provides extra communication skills that can be useful for clients when communicating their emotions, especially when they fear that the other person does not understand them.

12.2.1.5 Social Support

Many researchers agree that the availability of a support system influences health in some way. The actual mediating variable has yet to be identified. This element might be the ability to express emotions in an accepting environment. During group sessions (Spiegel 1993[631]), clients express their emotions and are confident that others will listen and accept their emotional expression.

Simonton (1992[632]) asks the client to bring in a support person that follows the same therapeutic program. This support person should be someone the client trusts, usually their partner or a close friend. The support person goes through the same program as the client does. This ensures that the support person knows the goal of the therapy and the general issues the client needs to resolve. During the program, the therapist suggests that the client and the support person talk openly about many underlying thoughts and feelings. Those issues that were never discussed before, such as unspoken feelings or thoughts, are especially addressed. Such emotional expression by the client in the presence of the support person also enhances the bond between them.

Clients should also be encouraged to express their emotions with their family members. This increases their ability to express emotions, strengthens the bond between them and their family members, and reduces feelings of isolation (Cohen 1974[633]; Spiegel 1983[634]).

12.2.2 Anti-emotionality

The term "anti-emotionality" is used when clients do not react to their emotions, or do not trust them. These clients typically over-rationalize their emotions. Anti-emotionality is not the suppression of emotions, but the failure to act upon them. The opposite of suppression is expression, and the opposite of anti-emotionality is over-dramatizing.

Therapeutic interventions with cancer clients often include the recognition of physical and emotional signals. By becoming aware of the physiological signals, clients can more easily recognize the emotional signals. To reduce anti-emotionality, Temoshok (1992[635]) focuses on becoming aware of bodily and psychological sensations.

Intervention:

1.   *Sit back and relax.*
2.   *Breathe deeply and relax all the tensions in your body.*
3.   *Focus on the top of your head, inhale, and become aware of the sensations and feelings there.*
4.   *With that awareness, ask yourself: "What do I feel there? Tension? Hardness? Tingling? Softness? Pain? Flexibility? Warmth? Cold?*
     Become aware of all of the physical sensations.
5.   *Become aware of the emotions. Do you sense fear? Anxiety? Anger? Longing?*
     Become aware of all of the psychological sensations.
6.   *Exhale and relax that area.*
7.   *Focus on your eyes, inhale, and become aware of them.*
8.   *Become aware of all of the physical sensations.*
9.   *Become aware of all of the psychological sensations.*
10. *Exhale and relax that area.*
11. *Continue the same process with your jaw, throat, face, chest, arms, abdomen, pelvis, legs, and feet.*

Adapted from Temoshok (1992[636].)

To help clients to recognize their emotions, the therapist could suggest that they use a personal journal (Pennebaker 1988[637]; 1990[638]; 1997[639]). Writing about daily business, emotions, and hidden desires assists clients in becoming aware of sensations and distressing and comforting emotions. In addition to providing personal insights, writing is also a form of emotional expression (see also 12.2.1.1 Expressive Writing).

When the therapist asks clients to discuss and expand upon comforting emotions, clients also start recognizing them. Comforting emotions are often easier to recognize. The therapist gradually moves toward less comforting emotions until distressing emotions have been identified and recognized by clients.

The therapist can also assist clients in becoming aware of the true nature of their emotions. This helps clients to recognize their emotions and act upon the message inherent in the emotion.

Intervention:

Become aware of the emotion, and ask yourself the following questions:

1. *Why am I upset, or feeling this way?*
2. *What feels wrong, unfair, or cruel to me about what has happened?*
3. *What are my needs in this situation?*
4. *What can I do to make this right?*
5. *Is this emotion related to the current situation, or does it remind me of a time in the past?*

Adapted from Temoshok (1992[640]).

13

Emotions

Many clients repress their distressing emotions and focus only on other things. In the previous chapter, I discussed the healthy effects of expressing those distressing emotions. This chapter deals with actually resolving such emotions. When distressing emotions are resolved, they do not bother clients anymore, consciously or unconsciously.

> *"If you believe that feeling bad or worrying long enough will change*
> *a past or future event, then you are residing on another planet with*
> *a different reality system."*
> *- William James -*

The difference between denying and resolving distressing emotions is an important one. Denying or repressing emotions forces the emotions into the unconscious. Resolution means dissolving the distressing emotion.

Example:
Try to take an air-filled balloon and push it underwater. Maybe you do not see it anymore, and can focus on other things, but it still takes up a lot of energy. As soon as you stop pressing on it, the balloon will pop up and blow up in your face. This is the repression of emotions.

Resolution is like letting the air out the balloon. The energy previously used to keep the balloon underwater can now be used for other things.

In their study of spontaneous regression, Baalen et al. (1987[641]) noticed that those cancer clients who showed the most improvement accepted their desperation and resolved the issues relating to it. They suggested that the therapist should not try to force clients out of their depressive feelings or desperation, but should assist them in accepting and resolving those emotions.

When discussing the topic of emotions, people tend to make a distinction between "good" or "positive" emotions, and "bad" or "negative" emotions. People refer to "bad/negative" emotions to indicate emotions such as anger, fear, hurt and guilt, which they do not want to feel. Emotions that they do want to feel are generally termed "good/ positive" emotions, such as happiness, joy, courage, and excitement.

There is clearly a difference between such "positive" and "negative" emotions. Making such a distinction implies that one kind is better than the other. However, this is not the case. In her work, Pert (1997[642]) stated that all emotions are healthy by nature. Emotions are the union between mind and body. They are translated into neuropeptides, which help to run the body. Without neuropeptides, the body would not function well. All emotions therefore serve a healthy purpose. There are no "bad/negative" emotions, but neither are there "good/positive" ones.

Because a distinction can be made, and we cannot refer to "bad/ negative" emotions, I propose a different terminology. Emotions such as hope, joy, happiness, etc., bring clients peace of mind. Those emotions give comfort, so the descriptive term I propose is "comforting emotions." The other type of emotions, such as hopelessness, fear, and guilt, create pain and suffering. Those emotions increase distress, so a proper term would be "distressing emotions."

When distressing emotions are repressed, they start building up. They form a cluster which weakens the immune system. By expressing those distressing emotions, clients prevent the formation of such emotional clusters, and thus prevent the weakening of the immune system.

"The only bad emotion is a stuck emotion."
- Rachel Naomi Remen -

Emotional expression is discussed in the previous chapter. Distressing emotions can also be resolved; this reduces their distressing effects, so that build-up does not take place.

As in the section on beliefs, interventions to reduce emotional distress can be divided into generic and specific interventions. In addition to these interventions, this chapter also discusses specific interventions to increase emotional well-being.

Generic emotional interventions can be used to aid clients in their well-being. These tend to reduce all distressing emotions, and increase all comforting emotions. The most widely used generic emotional interventions are relaxation and physical exercise.

Specific emotional interventions are directed towards the resolution of a particular distressing emotion, or the enhancement of a specific comforting emotion. The reduction of hostility and anxiety, and the increase of pleasure, are most often used as specific interventions.

13.1   Diagnosis

Clients' primary distressing emotions usually become clear during the therapeutic discussions. Although many different distressing emotions might be present, the therapist should start with the resolution of the most troublesome ones.

The therapist could ask clients what their most troublesome emotions are. The most troublesome one could be the first to be resolved. If clients are unaware of their emotions, the therapist should start working on recognizing those emotions (see also the chapter on anti-emotionality), or begin with generic emotional interventions.

The application of generic emotional interventions is always beneficial to clients.

13.2   Therapy: Generic Emotional Interventions

Interventions that reduce general feelings of distress and increase general feelings of comfort can be called "generic" or "non-specific" emotional interventions. While distress depresses the immune system (Rossi 1986[643]), relaxation enhances immune functioning (Sachar 1966[644]; Katz 1969[645]). Distress is a general feeling. There are no interventions to directly reduce stress, although some have an effect on the level of perceived stress.

The topic of distress reduction can be found in most therapeutic settings, especially in programs geared toward cancer clients. The actual interventions used by different programs do not differ greatly. The most commonly used are different forms of relaxation and meditation. Spiegel (1993[646]) uses a more hypnotic type of relaxation, while Simonton (1978[647]) uses imagery and progressive muscle relaxation. Some programs also include physical exercise to create feelings of relaxation.

13.2.1 Relaxation, Meditation, Hypnotic Trance

Relaxation reduces distress and increases feelings of well-being. Clients can also be taught to perform it on their own, which increases their feelings of control. With relaxation, clients have a tool they can apply themselves to ease their minds and bodies. In addition to these positive effects, Kiecolt-Glaser et al. (1985[648]) showed that relaxation directly increases immune functioning.

To reduce feelings of distress, Fawzy (1990[649]; 1990[650]) used relaxation. Clients learned to relax beforehand, so that when they were in need of relaxation later, they could recall it themselves. Fawzy suggested also using relaxation as preparation for situations in which clients anticipated an increase in stress, such as operations, family meetings, or anything else that might be stressful.

Simonton et al. (1978[651]; 1980[652]) made extensive use of progressive muscle relaxation and breathing exercises. These exercises enhanced clients' quality of life, and in some cases even increased survival time. Relaxation techniques provided the foundation for all of their imagery exercises.

Learning relaxation takes practice. Clients must practice their exercises daily. Relaxation will not provide these benefits if only practiced in times of need. The more clients do the exercises, the easier they will achieve relaxation. Only when they truly master the techniques can they recall them when needed. Practicing on a regular basis also contributes to positive personality changes. Taking the time to practice requires changes in clients' schedules; they must make time for themselves in order to perform the exercises. This also enhances their assertiveness and feelings of control over their lives. A more detailed discussion of the techniques and benefits of relaxation can be found in Benson et al. (1975[653]).

Meditation can be seen as a deeper level of relaxation. Meditation adds another dimension: the awareness of the unconscious mind. Borysenko (1984[654]) defines meditation as "any activity that keeps the attention pleasantly anchored in the present moment." Different forms of meditation have in common a lack of rational thought and emotional experience (Meares 1982[655]). Regardless of the differences, they seem to produce similar physical and psychological results (Benson 1975[656]; Goleman 1978[657]; Chopra 1991[658]).

Most approaches focus on quieting the mind and concentrating on a single subject, such as breathing, a repeated word, or an image.

Meares (1979[659]; 1982[660]; 1983[661]) used a form that he called "intensive meditation." This method differs in essence from other types, and is typified by simplicity. The purpose is to keep the mind still, without any focus (not even on a sound or image). If there is a focus on breathing or a mantra, the mind is not completely still. The mind is supposed to be so still that clients are not even aware that their minds are still. Only afterwards do clients realize that their minds have been still. Meares claimed that such meditation enabled the immune and endocrine systems to work more effectively (Meares 1983[662]). He also attributed spontaneous remission to the effects of this type of meditation (Meares 1978[663]; 1979[664]; 1982[665]; 1982[666]).

Like relaxation, meditation must be practiced regularly to create the desired effects. According to Meares, meditating twice a day for 15 minutes already produces positive physical changes.

A very profound level of relaxation can be accomplished through hypnosis. In and of itself, the trance induced during a hypnotic session functions as relaxation. LeBaw et al. (1975[667]), Newton (1982[668]) and Kiecolt-Glaser et al. (1986[669]; 1992[670]) used hypnotic relaxation combined with imagery to relieve distress. Among a group of medical students, Kiecolt-Glaser et al. noticed a direct link between the number of times the students had practiced hypnotic relaxation and the effectiveness of their immune systems. The relaxation had directly influenced their immune systems.

13.2.2 Physical Exercise

Physical exercise has been shown to increase feelings of relaxation and well-being. Exercise not only reduces distress, but also enhances physical well-being. Many complementary therapies include physical exercise to enhance general feelings of well-being. Although this study is about psychological interventions, I would like to briefly discuss the value of physical exercise.

The value of physical exercise was studied by Silvertsen et al. (1921[671]). They analyzed 86,000 cancer-related deaths and noticed that mortality was the highest among people whose occupations required little muscular effort. Those people whose occupations required more muscular effort showed a lower incidence of cancer mortality.

Silvertsen et al. (1938[672]) supported these ideas with experiments on mice. Of a strain of mice that were bred to be cancer-prone, only 16% of those that exercised developed cancer. Those mice that did not exercise had an 88% chance of developing cancer. Other animal studies confirmed these findings. The positive health effects of exercise were also reported after animals received chemically induced and transplanted tumors (Rusch et al. 1944[673]; Hoffman et al. 1960[674]; 1962[675]; Thompson et al. 1995[676]; Westerlind et al. 2003[677]).

Studies showed that when animals were stressed and deprived of the ability to perform physical activity, their bodies would deteriorate. When stressed animals were allowed to be physically active, the damage to their bodies was minimized. Zielinski et al. (2004[678]) even showed that prolonged, intense exercise performed daily could decrease the growth rate and size of a tumor. The health effects of exercise were thought to be caused by the "channeling" of distress (Selye 1956[679]). It almost seems as if distress builds up something that can be released with exercise.

Example:
Imagine a rubber band. Twist and continue twisting towards one side. Eventually, the band will break.
However, when the band is allowed to release its tension occasionally, the band will not break.

Physical exercise can be used in psychotherapy. When clients become active and find ways in which they can release their physical distress, they increase their physical and psychological well-being.

Simonton et al. (1978[680]) instructed clients to become as physically active as their bodies would allow them to be. During physical activity, clients' levels of distress would decrease, simultaneously changing their state of mind. The researchers also reported that physical activity stimulated psychological flexibility. Clients on a regular program of physical activity tended to increase their sense of self-sufficiency and self-acceptance. They also showed less anger and fewer depressive feelings. Such an enhanced, stronger psychological profile, influenced by physical exercise, is often associated with a better prognosis.

Simonton et al. (1978[681]; 1992[682]) advised clients to exercise at least three times a week for a minimum of one hour, as shorter programs did not produce the same beneficial effects. The exercises they suggested could consist of different kinds of sports, walking, taking the stairs, walking to the restroom, or sitting and swinging their arms and legs. Essentially, the clients were instructed to create as much movement as possible with as many body parts as possible: arms, legs, head, neck, etc. In the event of physical or energetic limitations, clients can even vividly imagine that they are exercising or playing their favorite sports.

Physical exercise must be incorporated into the therapeutic program. The therapist should stress that clients must not overdo it. Physical exercises should be performed according to the clients' level of competence. Exercises must be done on a regular basis, at a slow pace, without causing pain or discomfort and progressively more strenuous as time goes on. The activities chosen should be those that clients enjoy.

In addition to reducing emotional distress and increasing physical well-being, exercise also gives clients the opportunity to actively participate in the process of regaining health.

13.2.3 Selective Support System

A technique which is often overlooked due to its simplicity is the selective use of family and friends. Some people bring clients positive energy and enjoyment, while others decrease clients' energy and reduce their hope. When clients are selective in their support system, they experience more situations accompanied by comforting emotions, and fewer situations that bring distressing emotions.

Simonton et al. (1978[683]) advises clients to be selective with regard to the people who surround them.

Intervention:
- *Identify those people and resources around you that influence your hope and energy* positively.
- *Identify those people and resources around you that influence your hope and energy* negatively.
- *Label each person as follows: "Listen to this one to gain more hope," or "Forget what this one says - health hazard!"*

Adapted from Simonton et al. (1978[684])

13.3   Therapy: Specific Emotional Interventions

13.3.1   Distressing Emotions

Holding on to distressing emotions, or denying them, is often associated with a poorer prognosis. In addition to expressing emotions, which has already been discussed in the previous chapter, clients should resolve their distressing emotions. Resolving such emotions, which have been accumulating over the years, dramatically reduces their distress.

Emotions such as anger, resentment, fear, anxiety, loneliness, isolation, and hopelessness have often been associated with the development of cancer, or cancer with a poor prognosis. Resolving these emotions is the subject of this chapter.

Unresolved distressing emotions are stored in the body (as neuropeptides). Every time the emotion is experienced, it is added to the store. Over the years, when emotions are not resolved, an "emotional cyst" develops.

Each time similar emotions are experienced and unresolved, the cyst gets larger. This continues until the cyst is so large that the person "explodes." They express all of their stored emotions at once.

Example:
This can be compared to blowing up a balloon. The first unresolved emotion creates a balloon. The next time the same emotion is

unresolved, a breath of air is blown into the balloon. The balloon grows (a growing emotional cyst).
This continues until the last blast of air causes the balloon to explode. This explosion includes all of the air that was put into the balloon over its lifetime.

Example:
Another concept is the "black bag" used in Hawaiian shamanism. There is a black bag for every emotion people can experience. Every time an emotion is experienced, it is either resolved or placed inside this black bag.

Some bags are almost empty, while others are almost full. Every time an emotion is placed inside the black bag, the person sees the emotional content and re-experiences the entire emotional content of that bag.

When clients place a new emotion in the "black bag," they re-experience the emotional content of the bag. This phenomenon can be easily recognized when clients react to a certain situation with much more emotion than could be expected from the situation. Clients experience a single emotion combined with the entire emotional content of their pasts. They then express the single emotion from that moment, as well as all the similar emotions they have ever experienced (which were stored). These "black bags," or emotional cysts, re-stress clients every time they experience that emotion.

Example:
Someone cuts into line at the supermarket. An appropriate reaction could be a slight feeling of anger.
When this person is beaten up for cutting into the line, the reaction is inappropriate.
In the second case, the load of anger was not related to the actual situation. The person who beat up the offender has experienced a slight feeling of anger in addition to re-experiencing all of the anger from their past.

When the emotions from a client's past are resolved, their "black bag" is emptied. Next time, the client will experience an appropriate emotional content, without the load of the past.

13.3.1.1 Resolution of Singular Emotions

13.3.1.1.1   *Anger and Resentment*

Many authors have noticed that cancer clients typically withhold anger and resentment. As discussed in the chapter on the psychosomatic model and emotions, there is a relationship between clients' levels of anger and the development of cancer. Some authors have noted typical anger or resentment issues that stem from abandonment and rejection. Resolving these emotions will also reduce much of the clients' distress. Simonton et al. (1978[685]) noticed that many clients with cancer harbor feelings of resentment towards themselves about having cancer. They need to resolve that resentment.

There is a difference between anger and resentment. Anger usually lasts for a short time, while resentment is more long-term, and is re-experienced over and over again. Some authors write about resentment, while others refer to built-up anger. One could say that resentment is the emotional cyst, or build-up, of anger.

Clients can suffer from distressing emotions that stem from their childhood. From time to time, these old emotions are triggered and re-experienced. Such resentment can be recognized when clients:
- Relive a distressing period over and over again.
- Seem to hold on to the emotion.
- Keep pondering how they should have handled it.
- Continue to recall others' behavior of which they disapproved.

When clients feel angry with many people, it might be useful to instruct them to make a list of all of those people, including why they feel that way. Each name on this list can then be used as a starting point for resolving resentment towards that person. This can continue until the list is empty and all resentment has been resolved.

To resolve emotions from the past, Simonton uses imagery:

Intervention:
1. *Guide the client into a state of relaxation.*
2. *Have him imagine the person he is angry with.*
3. *Have the client imagine all kinds of good and positive things*

happening to that person. See the other person receiving love, money, attention, or whatever the client genuinely believes is good and positive.

4. *Help the client to become aware of his own thoughts, feelings, and reactions, while imagining those good things happening to that person.*

5. *Examine the client's role in the stressful situation where the resentment originates.*

6. *Examine the other person's role in that situation.*

7. *Help the client to reinterpret the other person's behavior.*

8. *Imagine the situation from the other person's point of view.*

Adapted from Simonton et al. (1978[686]; 1992[687]), Fox (1938[688]).

This imagery exercise makes use of reframing ("reinterpreting the situation"), and a technique whereby clients look at the situation from different perspectives. These different perspectives are called "perceptual positions." The different uses of perceptual positions and their effects are described in more detail by Dilts et al. (1990[689]) and Dilts (1990[690]; 1994[691]).

Other techniques that are effective for overcoming anger and resentment are Ho'oponopono (James 1993[692]), Reframing (see the section on appraisal), and Time Line Therapy (James 1988[693]; 2000[694]).

In some cases, clients cannot imagine good things happening to those people. If this is the case, clients might be gleaning some hidden benefits from keeping their resentment. The therapist should first investigate these benefits before the emotions can be resolved.

13.3.1.1.2   Fear and Anxiety

Fear is often dominantly present in cancer clients. This is not only fear of the disease or the fear of death, but fear in general. It has been suggested that fear has been present throughout their entire lives. By reducing fear, clients experience a higher quality of life and can better handle all other therapeutic issues. The resolution of fear has often been associated with a healthier prognosis in the case of cancer.

Fear is imagining undesirable outcomes, possibly combined with an already present emotional cyst resulting from fear. Clients can be taught to set desirable goals. This helps clients to imagine desirable outcomes, which at the same time counters fear. When clients define goals and imagine them becoming reality, hope increases and fear is reduced.

The emotional cyst can be resolved by using Time Line Therapy (James 1988[695]; 2000[696]).

13.3.1.1.3   *Loneliness and Isolation*

Loneliness is a feeling that has been observed in many clients long before the onset of cancer. To resolve these emotions, clients could join a support group, in which each member shares similar feelings and issues. When all members face the same disease, the disease itself becomes a bonding agent that reduces loneliness. Clients feel that the group will support them when they are in need. Other members also understand what clients are going through, and this strengthens their feeling of belonging. Joining such a support group helps to reduce feelings of isolation (Spiegel 1981[697]).

Those support groups that follow Spiegel's guidelines are encouraged to keep in touch outside the therapeutic setting. Other therapists who guide support groups often discourage contact outside the therapeutic setting. When clients stay in contact with each other outside the therapeutic context, they create a kind of friendship and trust which is not associated with therapy. This leads to stronger relationships among group members, and decreases feelings of loneliness.

When clients are unable, or simply do not want to join such a group, the therapist could suggest alternatives. Clients could take up a hobby that helps them to meet people, or start taking care of a pet. Meeting other people decreases feeling of loneliness, especially when they share the same hobby or interest. A pet needs love and care, which stimulates clients to re-experience love and caring themselves.

13.3.1.1.4   *Hopelessness*

Hopelessness develops when clients believe that desirable outcomes are not obtainable, or that the outcome is undesirable. This makes it clear that attaining hope is closely related to reducing fear (see 11.3.1.1.2 Fear and Anxiety). Hope is also increased automatically when fear is reduced.

In addition to reducing fear, hope can be stimulated by having clients set attainable goals and imagine the desirable outcome. The therapist can also install beliefs that create hope, and eliminate beliefs that create hopelessness. (This has been discussed earlier.) The therapist must ensure that clients do not rely on hope alone; they have to take appropriate actions, too.

> *"Trust in God and tie your camel to a tree."*
> *- Arabic saying -*

13.3.1.2 Resolution of Emotional Cysts

Dealing with emotional cysts is important in order to reduce the intensity of a client's distress. Although many authors refer to such cysts, only a few discuss interventions that deal with emotional cysts directly. Most interventions, such as hypnotic regression and the different time line techniques from NLP, only deal with a specific emotion from the past, not with the actual emotional cyst. The only intervention that actually deals with the cyst itself is Time Line Therapy (James 1988[698]). It first resolves the cyst, and then all of the emotions that comprised the cyst.

Intervention:
1. *The therapist helps the client return to a time before the first event that caused the cyst to be formed.*
2. *With emotional resolution techniques, the emotions from this event (before the cyst was formed) are resolved. With those emotions resolved, the cyst itself disappears (the "black bag" is not present anymore).*
3. *The client reassesses his entire life based on those events that used to form the cyst. The therapist aids the client in resolving those emotions as well.*
4. *The client returns to the present. The emotional cyst itself is resolved, as well as all the emotions that comprised the cyst.*

Adapted from (James 1988[699]).

13.3.2 Comforting Emotions

> *"Life does not cease to be fun when people die any more than it ceases to be serious when people laugh."*
> *- George Bernard Shaw -*

Decreasing distressing emotions is only one way of increasing clients' quality of life. One can also work on increasing comforting emotions, such as pleasure and happiness, to develop well-being.

Example:
Norman Cousins was diagnosed as terminally ill with only a few months to live. His pain was so severe that he could not sleep through the night.
He decided to form an alliance with his doctor in which they both worked on his health. The doctor would take care of the mainstream medicine, and Norman believed that he could help his body to heal by using laughter. He rented all the movies he could find that would make him laugh. He read funny stories, and asked his friends to call him whenever they had a funny story or experienced something that could make him laugh. Every opportunity to laugh was seized with both hands.
While doing this, he noticed that a good 10-minute laugh would render him almost painless for a few hours, long enough to sleep through the night.
He eventually fully recovered, and lived another 20 healthy and productive years. He attributed his remarkable recovery to the combination of medical interventions, an active stance on his own part, and the use of laughter.
He wrote a book about his story to promote the use of laughter.

Based on Cousins (1979[700]).

Laughter is an expression of intense emotions of pleasure, happiness, and joy. Some researchers even suggest that faking laughter also creates feelings of pleasure. The emotion of pleasure, expressed by laughter, is the topic of this chapter.

Although researchers do not agree on whether pleasure influences the disease process itself, they do agree that pleasure dramatically influences clients' general physiological and psychological state. Pleasure reduces worrying, eliminates distress and, by so doing, increases the quality of life.

"The art of medicine consists of amusing the patient while nature cures the disease."
- Voltaire -

Dillon (1985[701]) demonstrated that watching a humorous videotape increased immune functioning, compared to watching a didactic videotape. Berk (2001[702]) noticed that the increase in immune functioning lasted 12 hours after watching only a one-hour humorous video. Levy (1988[703]) noticed that breast cancer clients who experienced joy at the beginning of her study had a higher survival rate than those who did not. Clients who performed joyful activities experienced longer disease-free intervals.

Futterman et al.(1994[704]) studied the effects of induced emotional states on the immune system. Actors who were trained in method acting (actually experiencing the emotion they are displaying) were able to create emotional states. Futterman et al. demonstrated that comforting emotions increased the actors' immune function, while distressing emotions decreased it. When the actors induced comforting emotions, an increase in their number of NK cells could be observed. The NK cells functioned more effectively than before. This increase in activity was established within 20 minutes of the start of the induced emotion. When the actor stopped inducing the emotion, the enhanced immune function lasted for 30 minutes.

Blakeslee (-year unknown- [705]) wrote an article together with Grossarth-Maticek, containing a follow-up of their previous research involving 3055 people. In the original study conducted in 1973, they had rated the well-being of those subjects.

Their follow-up study showed that of the group which initially scored high on well-being, 78% were still alive and 4% had developed cancer. Of those with low scores, only 5% were still alive, and 49% had developed cancer. This well-being score had a predictive value in determining who developed cancer. Feeling good reduces one's chances of cancer.

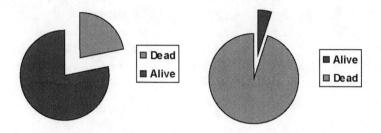

13.3.2.1 Finding and Creating Pleasure

Pleasure increases one's immune function and feelings of well-being. The therapist should help clients find ways to create as much pleasure in their lives as possible. By recognizing what gives them pleasure, clients can start pursuing and enjoying those activities.

Intervention:
Have the client find things that give him pleasure.
For example:
- *Movies.*
- *Sitcoms.*
- *Theater.*
- *Records, CDs, tapes.*
- *Stand-up comedy.*
- *Cartoons.*
- *Friends who share funny stories.*
- *Clowning workshops.*
- *Anything that creates pleasure.*

	Medical	Psychological	Psychosomatic
Considered cause	Body	Mind	Body-Mind interaction
Interventions	Biological	Psychological / Social	Biological and Psychological / Social
Patient's Involvement	None	Maximum	Maximum
Treatment	Fixing body	Fixing mind	Fixing the body and the mind

13.3.2.2 Playful Activities

Another way of increasing the amount of pleasure in clients' lives is by suggesting that they undertake playful activities. Simonton et al. (1992[706]) had clients create a list of at least 50 activities that are fun and free (or cost less than $5).

To ensure the fewest possible objections from clients, these items should preferably be cheap and take little time. Clients can engage in these activities when they need an energy injection, or simply a good laugh.

Clients should add new activities to this list on a regular basis. The same type of intervention was used by McDermott et al. (1996[707]). This list might look similar to the one discussed in the section on beliefs. The difference is that the list in the Beliefs section is about activities that add meaning to clients' lives, whereas the list discussed here includes only playful and fun activities.

This list of playful activities should only include pleasurable activities. If clients think of an activity that adds meaning to their lives, this should be added to the list in the Beliefs section. By keeping these lists separate, clients can actually focus on enjoying pleasure. The therapist should suggest that clients keep this list with them, so they can add new things that come to mind.

In addition to a list of pleasures, McDermott asked clients to keep a "Daily Pleasure Score." He instructed clients to keep a journal of every pleasurable event or occasion.

Intervention:
- *Keep your list of activities on hand.*
- *Score each event: 1 point if you experienced a little pleasure, 2 if you enjoyed it, and 3 if you really enjoyed it.*
- *A burst of laughter counts for 10 extra bonus points.*

Modified after McDermott et al. (1996[708]).

One caveat must be pointed out. Sometimes clients focus only on these playful activities in order to avoid the real psychological issues at hand. This must be avoided. These activities can be seen as rewards that they give themselves, or as energizers to help them start working on their psychological issues.

13.3.2.3 Imagery

Imagery can also be used to create or intensify feelings of pleasure and joy. With the help of imagery, clients can recall pleasurable activities and events, and experience the same pleasurable emotions. Margolis (1983[709]) used hypnosis to help clients develop happy and pleasant imagery. She also assisted clients in developing experiences which generated a strong sense of well-being.

Another usage of imagery is to create emotions of pleasure by mentally rehearsing fun activities. This could serve as a substitute when performing the real activity is not feasible. In that case, hypnotic experience is the next best thing.

Any intervention that helps clients to access pleasant memories or activities can be used to enhance their well-being.

Section E

Direct Psychological Influence On Physiology

14

Introduction

In previous chapters, I have discussed different psychological interventions based on the psychosomatic model that can be used to aid clients in regaining health and well-being. These interventions influence clients' mental and emotional state, and: (1) Through that state, influence their physiology. (2) Although this model covers most of the possible interventions used in complementary psychological cancer treatment (CPCT), it leaves two major issues untouched. These are the psychological interventions that directly influence physiology, (3) and psychological pain management.

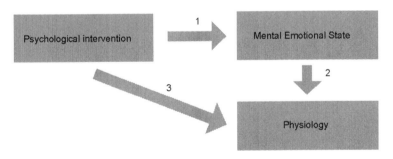

Studies of hypnosis, imagination, and suggestion have proven that physiology can also be influenced directly by the mind. Clearly imagining certain physiological processes actually influences those processes. When clients experience the ability to control their own physiology, their general feeling of control is increased, which produces healthy effects. Simonton et al. (1978[710]) discovered that the immune system could be influenced by having clients vividly imagine their white blood cells attacking the cancer cells. Based on this discovery, they began using imagery as a primary tool for influencing the body with the mind.

Another issue that is often overlooked is pain management. This issue alone could be the topic of an entire dissertation. When assisting clients with their well-being, pain management skills are of vital importance. I will discuss some of the most widely used interventions in the chapter on influencing pain directly.

In this section, I will discuss the psychological interventions that can be used to directly influence physiology, and those interventions that directly influence pain.

Influencing Physiological Symptoms

This chapter will discuss the four ways in which psychological interventions can influence physiology: conditioning, hypnotic suggestions, communication with symptoms, and imagery.

15.1   Conditioning

Conditioning is the association of a stimulus with an unrelated response.

> ### Example:
> *When dogs are fed, they respond by drooling. Pavlov rang a bell when the dogs were fed. Those dogs associated the sound of the bell with receiving food. After a while, the dogs began drooling when they heard the bell, regardless of whether there was food present.*
>
> *In this case, the bell (stimulus) produced the physical response of drooling.*

> *"When two things commonly occur together, the appearance of one will bring the other to mind."*
> *- Aristotle -*

Metalnikov et al. (1926[711]) continued Pavlov's research on conditioning, and observed that the immune system could be conditioned to respond to a stimulus. They combined the injection of bacteria with a scratch on the skin (stimulus). The bacteria triggered a reaction from the immune system (response).

They managed to associate a scratch with a reaction from the immune system without using the bacteria. By scratching the skin, they were able to induce the same immunological reactions that the bacteria had produced. Smith et al. (1983[712]) later conditioned subjects to experience the Mantoux reaction (red swelling of the skin). When they applied the stimulus, the Mantoux reaction would become apparent.

In their research on conditioning, Ader et al. (1990[713]) confirmed that the immune system can be conditioned to respond to a stimulus. They injected rats with an immunosuppressive agent, and gave them saccharine-flavored water at the same time. The taste (stimulus) and the suppressed immune system (response) were associated. When the rats drank the flavored water, their immune system was suppressed at the same time. The rats experienced the same immunological changes when they tasted the water and when they were given the real drug.

Buske-Kirschbaum et al. (1992[714]) exposed healthy subjects to a conditioning process. The subjects were given a sweet and, at the same time, an injection with medication that increased their natural killer cell activity. This procedure was repeated several times to solidify the conditioning. Both the sweet and the injection itself functioned as stimuli. Later, when the subjects were given a sweet and a neutral injection (a stimulus, but without medication), the same increase in natural killer cell activity was observed. Other researchers were able to use the sound of a horn as a stimulus to increase immune function (Pert 1997[715]).

There is sufficient evidence to show that the immune system can be conditioned to respond to a neutral stimulus, like a sound, taste, smell, touch or image. Although the existing psychological cancer treatment programs do not use this technique, it can be of great value. The therapist cannot accomplish this himself, as he does not administer the immuno-enhancing medication. Clients can learn how to perform the conditioning process. This allows them to start conditioning themselves when they receive immuno-enhancing medication in cooperation with their medical team. The therapist can aid clients by teaching them the conditioning process.

Sometimes conditioning takes place without people knowing it. Kornblith et al. (1998[716]) showed that clients became nauseous when confronted with a certain stimulus. The nausea was conditioned by a stimulus they had experienced many years earlier, during a stay in the hospital. The sight of the doctor or the smell of an antiseptic elicited the same symptoms they had displayed then. Those stimuli were still effective years after the actual conditioning. Bovbjerg et al. (1990[717]) noticed that a hospital setting could be conditioned to receiving immuno-suppressive medications. When those clients were later confronted with the same stimulus, their body reacted as if it had received the suppressive medication. When such prior conditioning exists, in which the stimulus elicits an unwanted response, the therapist should break the association.

These conditioning processes are known in the field of Neuro Linguistic Programming as "anchoring." Most books on NLP discuss the procedures for breaking such associations, as well as the conditioning processes.

15.2 Hypnotic Suggestions

Modulating physiological processes with hypnotic suggestions has been around for a long time, and is a well-known and effective technique.

> *"Suggestion is the process by which a physical or mental state is influenced by a thought or idea."*
> *- Merriam-Webster - Online Dictionary 2004*

When regular suggestion influences physiological processes, it is usually termed the placebo response. These suggestive interventions are rarely used with volition, but seem to occur.

Hypnotic suggestion is the use of a hypnotic trance to increase the effects of suggestion, and to use suggestion intentionally. Numerous studies are available that describe the effectiveness of hypnotic suggestion on physiology. One topic that has been intensively researched will be discussed in chapter 15.2.2, Treatment of Warts. The effectiveness of hypnotic suggestion has also been demonstrated through the creation of skin blisters, bruises, and warts by mere suggestion (Bellis 1966[718]; Johnson 1976[719]; Gravitz 1981[720]).

Hypnotic suggestion as an intervention is often associated with the formal induction of a hypnotic trance. However, for suggestions to take effect, a hypnotic trance is not required per se.

Bennett (1984[721]; 1985[722]; 1993[723]) discovered the tremendous influence of the discussions that occurred during surgery. He observed that clients picked up the conversations that they overheard while anesthetized. Clients reacted to such discussions as if they were hypnotic suggestions. Bennett played a three-minute tape containing suggestions during surgery. A week later, he interviewed the subjects. They were unable to remember having heard the tape, or to recall its the content. However, 82% of those clients had reacted according to the suggestions on the tape. Bennett concluded that clients will not remember what the surgeons say, but will react to their words as if they were post-hypnotic suggestions.

The effects of such suggestions can also be observed in the area of the placebo response. A placebo response can be explained as a suggestive effect. The physician explains (suggests) that a pill will help, and the client will experience relief, regardless of the contents of the pill.

In some cases, (hypnotic) suggestion is even more effective in relieving physiological ailments than traditional medicine.

15.2.1 "Towards" or "Away From"

The effects of suggestion have been proven many times. However, there is no conclusive evidence on the most powerful kinds of suggestion. One of the controversies about suggestion regards the use of "towards" or "away from" suggestions. These are the topic of this chapter.

"Towards" suggestions indicate a goal to move "towards," a desired situation to be obtained. "Away from" suggestions, as the name implies, indicate a suggestion that moves the subject "away from" an unwanted situation.

> **Example:**
> *You will keep your bed dry, and wake up in time to go to the bathroom.*
> (Towards *a dry bed.*)
>
> *You will not wet your bed, and will not be asleep when it is time to go to the bathroom.*
> (Away from *a wet bed.*)

Among therapeutic professionals, it seems to be common knowledge that positive suggestions are more effective than negative suggestions. Yapko (1990[724]) prefers "towards" suggestions because they are more supportive and motivating. Such suggestions call for something desirable. Yapko and many other clinicians recommend that therapists use "towards" suggestions. They argue that "away from" suggestions cannot be processed by the unconscious mind. Yapko argues that the mind cannot compute negations, and only reacts according to the "towards" side of the suggestion.

Example:
"Do not think about your favorite color."
The first thing that comes to mind is your favorite color. The mind tends to skip the negation.

If this is all true, then all "away from" suggestions would have the reverse effect.

Example:
The suggestion:
"You will not wet your bed, and will not be asleep when it is time to go to the bathroom."

This suggestion would be processed by the unconscious mind as:
"You will___wet your bed and will ___ asleep when it is time to go to the bathroom."

The effect of this suggestion would be a wet bed.

Such reverse effects have not been reported. While researching the literature and dissecting hypnotic scripts, I came across many accounts of the extensive use of "away from" suggestions. The reported results of those studies corresponded to the therapist's intentions, and not the reverse, as Yapko hypothesized.

Research on the use of "towards" and "away from" suggestion is very limited. The topic itself is barely discussed, and most research publications do not include the suggestion scripts used. This also makes retrospective studies impossible.

In his study of the influence of hypnosis on the immune system, Hall (1982[725]) described his experiment with five subjects.

Part I: The subjects were injected with P.P.D. (Purified Protein Derivative of tuberculin), and tested for the Mantoux reaction. The reaction was measured by the amount of swelling and erythema (abnormal redness of the skin). In the first test, four of the five subjects displayed the Mantoux reaction.

Part II: To investigate whether the immune system could be influenced by hypnosis, Hall conducted a 12-day hypnosis course.

Suggestions used during the course:
"...You will no longer react to the injection as you did before: there will be no redness, no swelling, no heat, no itching, no pain."

"The skin will remain perfectly normal on both sides of your left arm after the next injections..."
(Emphasis mine.)

Part III: After the course, the subjects were injected with P.P.D. again. The four subjects who had previously experienced the Mantoux reaction displayed no reaction at all after the course. The hypnotic course prevented the Mantoux reaction. Hall thereby demonstrated the influence of hypnotic suggestions on immune response.

The first part of the suggestions he used contained many "away from" language patterns. The second part contained "towards" suggestions.

If "away from" suggestions were truly ignored by the mind, the suggestions used by Hall would have increased the symptoms. This was not the case.

There are many effective hypnotic suggestion scripts that use "away from" suggestions. This is particularly true of the suggestions intended to influence physiology.

Hammond, etc. (1990[726]) indicated that there is no evidence from research to support the notion that "towards" suggestions work better than "away from" suggestions. However, based on his clinical experience, he still recommends the use of "towards" suggestions.

Older literature provides more evidence of "away from" suggestions. At the same time, older literature also contains more research using a deeper level of trance, compared to more recent studies. In a deep trance, the mind reacts more literally to the suggestions given, and seems able to compute negations very well.

The choice of "away from" or "towards" suggestions could be based on the depth of trance. The conscious mind seems to react better to "towards" suggestions. It might be that the unconscious mind reacts better to "away from" suggestions. This would suggest that one should opt for "towards" suggestions when working with a light trance, and "away from" suggestions when working with a deeper trance. Further investigation is required to reach a conclusive answer to this question.

15.2.2 Treatment of Warts

Warts constitute an interesting research area. They have been treated very successfully with hypnosis, and are pathologically very similar to tumors.

Warts have been successfully treated with suggestions for a long time. The use of hypnosis in such treatments is very common and well-known (Bonjour 1929[727]; Sulzberger et al. 1934[728]; McDowell 1949[729]; Obermayer et al. 1949[730]; Allington 1952[731]; Ahser 1956[732]; Schneck 1959[733]; Sinclair-Geiben et al. 1959[734]; Ullman et al.1960[735]; Surman et al. 1973[736]; Finkelstein et al. 1982[737]; Spanos et al. 1988[738]; 1990[739]).

Clawson et al. (1975[740]) was very successful in his suggestive treatment of warts. He even provided a "no cure no pay" guarantee for clients who came in for wart removal. After the hypnotic induction, he suggested that the blood flow to the warts should be cut off. After such a session, warts that had been present for months (or even years) disappeared over the following weeks.

Example:
"... Your unconscious mind has the ability to control the blood supply to any part of your body. Now I want you to stop the blood supply to each wart on your body."

Adapted from Clawson (1975[741]).

There are even reports about the creation of warts through suggestion. Baudouin suggested that by touching the subject's arm, a number of warts would appear on that spot. When this suggestion was given, the warts appeared. He was also able to remove the warts by suggestion (Gravitz 1981[742]).

15.3   Communication with Symptoms

In dealing directly with physiology, therapists often make use of a technique for communicating with symptoms. They have clients communicate with their symptoms, or with their organs, in order to investigate the meaning of the symptoms. Therapists view the symptom as a message from the body. By communicating with the symptoms, or with the organs where the symptoms reside, clients gain insight into those hidden messages. When clients listen, respect, and act upon the message, the symptom (which was needed to communicate the message) is no longer needed (LeShan 1977[743]; Rossi 1986[744]; Rossi 1986[745]; Brouwer 1996[746], McDermott 1996[747]). How clients act upon the message depends, of course, on the content and intention of the message. When clients ignore the message, the symptoms are often aggravated.

> *Example:*
> *Some years back, I was hiking in the Grand Canyon. After five days of hiking, I was on my way out when a tremendous pain developed in my left knee. Even after a short rest, I was still unable to walk up the steep trail.*
>
> *I decided to start communicating with my knee. Strange as it may sound, I was able to make a deal with my knee. I asked the pain to stop because I had to get out of the canyon, for my own health. I agreed that if the knee needed attention once I was out of the canyon, the pain could reappear.*
>
> *The pain stopped, and I was able to get out of the canyon. The next day, I had to go to a doctor because the pain had reappeared.*

Of course, clients are not really talking to the physical organ. They are communicating with their unconscious mind. The unconscious mind is then able to provide the conscious mind with the message it wants to communicate. When clients learn to accept and listen to these messages, they also accept their symptoms. Most clients despise their symptoms, and essentially ignore the message that might be present.

Symptoms of pain are famous for having a message that they want to communicate. When the message is understood and acted upon, the pain usually recedes.

A book by Edelstien (1981[748]) quotes LeCron, who explains the most common reasons why symptoms develop, and what clients should do to resolve them.

A symptom can be represented as:
- A symbolic representation of unexpressed feelings: Clients should express those emotions.
- A result of the unconscious acceptance of an idea or image of oneself from early life: Clients should let go of that image.
- A result of past traumatic experiences: Clients should resolve the trauma.
- A way of resolving current life problems: Clients should find other methods for dealing with the situation.
- A result of unconscious identification with an important person in one's life: Clients should let go of that person, and change their identification with them.
- A manifestation of an inner conflict: Clients should resolve the conflict.
- The result of an unconscious need for punishment: Clients should resolve the need for punishment.

By viewing symptoms in this way, the therapist has some guidelines on where to look psychologically in order to alleviate the symptoms. This can also be discovered using ideomotor signaling techniques.

Several techniques have been developed for communicating with symptoms. The symptom is represented by clients in some way during imagery exercises. They then learn to have a respectful discussion with the representation, as if it were a person. The therapist must ensure that clients accept and respect the answers. If clients blame or disrespect the symptoms, or try to explain that the answers are wrong, the established communication disappears.

Intervention:
1. *Relax and close your eyes.*
2. *Be curious and full of respect for what is about to come.*

3. *Ask the symptom to represent itself as a symbol, person, or object.*

4. *Notice the size, colors, sounds, motions etc., of the representation.*

5. *Acknowledge the willingness of the symptom to represent itself, and its willingness to communicate.*

6. *Give the symbol a voice.*

7. *Ask what the symptom is attempting to communicate. Ask its positive intention, and what should be done to help the symptom heal.*

8. *Watch and listen to the answers, and do not get into a discussion.*

9. *Communicate to the symbol how you feel about it, and your positive intention. Take as much time as you need.*

10. *Imagine floating above yourself, and watch the symptom for a moment.*

11. *Float down into the symptom, and look at yourself. How do you, as the symptom, feel about the client? Express what you (as a symptom) want, hope, and feel.*

12. *Float up and watch the client communicate with the symptom.*

13. *Listen carefully to their interaction, without involvement.*

14. *Float back into your body, and look at the symptom. Thank it for its cooperation.*

Adapted from Dilts (1999[749]).

Using a similar technique, Temoshok asks, "If the part of your body with melanoma could speak, what would it say?" This question is very effective, as it directly accesses the unconscious mind.

Another technique that is often used to assist in establishing communication with symptoms is "inner guide imagery." This is a kind of imagery in which clients imagine making contact with their unconscious minds. This inner guide could take the form of a wise person, or another metaphorical image. In this way, clients ask for advice from their own unconscious.

If the message contained in the symptom is clear to the client, he still needs to act upon it in an appropriate way. Interventions for helping clients to act upon such messages cannot be described here, as they depend on the content of the message.

Example:
In the case of my knee, the message was that my knee needed attention and rest.
At first, I acted upon the message by taking a short break. I established an agreement that when I was out of the canyon, the pain could reoccur to tell me that the knee needed medical attention, and I would immediately respond by seeking such help.

This was sufficient for the pain to disappear in this case.

15.4   Imagery

Imagery is a process by which clients vividly experience a situation that cannot be experienced through their senses at that moment in time. It is a mental process that can be applied to a wide variety of psychological procedures used in complementary cancer and other therapies. Therapeutic disciplines that use imagery are numerous and include: Biofeedback, Desensitization, Neuro Linguistic Programming, Gestalt Therapy, Rational Emotive Therapy, and Hypnotherapy.

Imagery has a variety of denominations. It can also be referred to as directed concentration, visualization, active imagery, guided fantasy, or meditation.

The literature tends to use "imagery" and "visualization" interchangeably. Both refer to a mental experience that includes all of the senses. Imagery defines the completeness of the senses in the image (i.e. sight, hearing, smell, taste, sense of movement, position, and touch), whereas visualization focuses more on mentally seeing. The completeness of the experience is vital for the effect to influence psychology and physiology. I have therefore opted for imagery.

Imagery procedures are geared towards changing beliefs, changing behavior, increasing coping skills, reducing distress, setting goals, or changing physiological reactions. Most complementary psychological cancer treatment programs use some sort of imagery.

> *"Imagination is more important than knowledge."*
> *- Albert Einstein -*

This chapter discusses the general concept, the different types, and the physiological applications of imagery for cancer clients. The techniques and principles they describe can also be used for psychological change, but those interventions have already been discussed in previous chapters.

Merriam-Webster defines imagery as "The product of the act or power of forming a mental image of something not present to the senses or never before wholly perceived in reality."[750] Imagery is often defined as a thought representing a sensory quality, such as a sight, sound, feeling, smell or taste (Horowitz 1970[751]). In her book, Achterberg (1985[752]) describes it as mental scenery in which a thought process invokes and uses all of the senses.

Example:
Imagining the sea means that:
- *One sees the color, shape, etc., of the sea.*
- *One feels the structure, temperature, etc., of the sea.*
- *One hears the volume, sounds, etc.*
- *One tastes the saltiness of the sea.*
- *One smells the scents of the sea.*

Another interesting concept was developed by Paivio (1971[753]) and McGuigan (1966[754]; 1978[755]), who viewed imagery as the creation (or re-creation) of perception. This view includes the notion that the mind cannot make distinctions between what happened in real life and what is vividly imagined (Shannon et al. 1963[756]; Birnbaum 1964[757]; Epstein 1967[758]; Nomikos et al. 1968[759]).

Example:
When someone feels frightened while walking through a dark and dangerous alley, their physiology reflects their emotions.

When this person vividly imagines walking through such an alley, he will demonstrate the same emotional and physiological reactions, as if it were real.

His mind does not distinguish between reality and vividly imagined images.

The interactions between imagery and physiological reactions can be compared to the workings of a "desktop" on a computer (Rossman 2003[760]).

When one drags an item to the "trash," that item is deleted. There is no wastebasket inside the computer. The pictures on the screen are not the actual processes that occur; only a representation of intention. The screen visualizes the intention, which is removing the item, and the computer takes care of the deletion process.

Just as the body consists of cells, the computer consists only of the numbers 1 and 0. The desktop is designed to allow a person to interpret and instruct the computer; to instruct the 1's and 0's to do something. Imagery is designed to interpret and instruct the body; to instruct the cells to do something. Or, as Achterberg defines it: "Imagery is the communication mechanism between perception, emotion, and bodily changes."

"The spirit is the master, the imagination the tool, and the body the plastic material."
- Paracelsus -

The effects of imagery on clients is highly individual, even when the therapist uses the same script for all clients. Clients interpret the imagery symbols in their own personal ways. Although there are some archetypical images that the therapist can use, clients will still create their own experiences from these archetypes.

15.4.1 Types of Imagery

There are several different types of imagery. Distinctions can be made to describe the ways in which the image comes to mind, and the nature of the structure of the image itself. Based on Achterberg (1994[761]) and research on the complementary cancer therapies available today, I have distilled the following categories, each consisting of two types and excluding other items. All imagery contains one item from each category.

Creation of imagery:
• Receptive or Guided.

Structure of imagery:
• Realistic or Symbolic.
• Process or Goal.
• Fighting or Cooperative.

In this chapter, I will discuss these different types. The actual application of these types is discussed in another chapter (15.4.3, Applications).

15.4.1.1 Creation of Imagery

The creation of the image is based on the source of the imagery. Did the imagery come spontaneously from the client's mind, or was the symbology instructed? Receptive imagery (also referred to as autogenic or spontaneous imagery) stems from the client's mind without instruction. Guided imagery is when the therapist guides clients with his instructions while they create or recall certain images.

Receptive Imagery

Receptive imagery means that the images stem from the client's unconscious mind. The therapist does not provide any guidance or suggestions towards the content of the imagery or the symbols, but helps clients to access their own unconscious images. The most common forms of receptive imagery are those that appear in dreams. This type can also be used for diagnostic purposes.

By focusing on feelings, thoughts or symptoms, the image spontaneous arises. The therapist asks questions about the images that appear. Such images are frequently used for diagnostic purposes (Simonton et al. 1978[762]; Achterberg 1985[763]; Rossman 2000[764]).

Intervention:
The therapist could give the following instructions:
1. *Be curious about what is going to happen.*
2. *Become relaxed.*
3. *Focus on the symptoms, body parts, beliefs or whatever else your goal is.*
4. *Accept every image that comes to mind. The first image is particularly important.*
5. *Thank your unconscious mind for bringing up that particular image.*
6. *Accept and observe the image in detail.*
7. *Ask yourself, "What could the message of this image be?"*

Based on Achterberg (1985[765]).

Guided Imagery

If the content of the images is instructed by the therapist, this is referred to as guided imagery. Based on the desired results, the imagery is constructed and appropriate symbols are included.

For creating a numb hand prior to an operation, the image of the "hand in a bucket of ice" is often used. The therapist helps clients to vividly imagine the hand in the bucket in order to create the desired numbness. Due to its instructed nature, this form is not suitable for diagnostic purposes. This type of imagery is very effective for creating specific physiological results.

15.4.1.2 Structure of Imagery`

15.4.1.2.1   Realistic or Symbolic Imagery

Realistic or symbolic imagery can be found only in physiological imagery. This category is based on the extent to which the imagery corresponds to scientific knowledge. Realistic imagery is an actual scientific representation of what is to be imagined. Symbolic imagery uses metaphorical representations.

Realistic Imagery

Realistic imagery corresponds to scientific knowledge. Clients make a mental image, as if the procedure were being viewed under a microscope. This method is most often used in direct physical imagery. To use realistic imagery, the therapist must possess realistic, detailed knowledge of the workings of the human body.

Example:
"The mast cells lining the airways are hyperactive. When the cells react to release histamine, this causes a constriction in the airway. Imagine the mast cells holding the histamine inside."
Symbolic Imagery

Symbolic imagery uses a metaphorical representation of the desired result. It does not correspond to scientific models of the human body. The metaphors used can be devised by clients or by the therapist. If the therapist composes the metaphorical images, he must be aware that interpretations are personal. The same symbolic image has different meanings for different people. The metaphor must correspond to the client's interpretation.

Example:
Symbolic imagery for the immune system, in order to eliminate all cancer cells:
- *You can imagine Pac-Man eating all the blobs it can find.*
- *The toilet is clogged. However, with careful attention and the proper tools, you can unclog it.*

15.4.1.2.2   Process-Oriented or Goal-Oriented Imagery

Depending on the timeframe and the desired effect, one can choose process- or goal-oriented imagery. Experiencing the process step-by-step, creating many sequential images in order to reach the desired result, is called process-oriented imagery.

Example:
- *Imagine your immune system eating all of the cancer cells.*
- *Then, imagine it transporting them.*
- *Finally, imagine it escorting the cells out of your body.*
- *Imagine a restored, healthy body.*

During goal-oriented imagery, the end goal is imagined directly. For example, the body is imagined as restored and healthy.

15.4.1.2.3   Fighting or Cooperative Imagery

This distinction is made almost exclusively for physiological imagery applications. It is based on how one views disease in general: as something to beat, or as a message that must be listened to. Fighting imagery is based on the notion that clients need to overcome the situation by being stronger than the cancer. Cooperative imagery is when clients work together with the cancer to obtain health.

The imagery scripts in the appendix contain an example of fighting imagery and one of cooperative imagery.

Fighting

A fighting metaphor interprets the disease as a foreign body that must be destroyed.

Intervention:
- *Imagine the immune system as a very strong army that joins*

forces with another large, strong army in the form of the medical intervention (chemotherapy/radiation).

- *The small, weak and confused opponent cannot handle the enormous fighting power of the immune system army.*
- *Bullets fly through the body, killing all cancer cells in the area.*
- *Finally, the army calls in the garbage disposal teams, who collect all of the dead cancer cells, and kill the one or two cells that have survived.*
- *The garbage collectors carry the dead cells out of the body.*

There are different degrees of aggressiveness for the fighting. The above is an aggressive example. Dilts et al. (1990[766]) describe an imagery script in which they used a fighting metaphor, but one that was less aggressive. They used an imagery of sheep (the medical treatment) grazing and dissolving the grass (tumor).

Cooperative

This type of imagery interprets the disease as something that belongs to the body, that seeks to communicate a message. Working together with the disease will therefore achieve the desired health effect.

Example:
Imagine that the disease is helping you. What does it want you to know?

Barely any research on the application of cooperative imagery in complementary psychological cancer treatment (CPCT) is available.

15.4.2 Elements of Imagery

There are many different forms and ways in which imagery can be used. This chapter focuses on the elements of imagery that produce the greatest effects with clients.

When teaching clients imagery techniques, not all of these guidelines are incorporated the first time. Imagery is a developmental process, in which each successive imagery session should use more of the proposed guidelines in order to increase the effect.

15.4.2.1 Preparation

For clients to benefit the most from imagery, they should prepare and really take the time for it. The following guidelines can help clients in their preparation.

Preparation tips:
- *Schedule regular times to relax and do the imagery exercises.*
- *Create a special seat, place or room where the imagery can be done.*
- *Before you begin, take the phone off the hook and make sure you will not be interrupted.*
- *Take a piece of paper and write down everything you want to remember. Now you do not have to think about it anymore.*
- *Take enough time to sit back and relax.*
- *Expect and believe you will benefit from the imagery exercises.*
- *Believe you deserve to get well.*

15.4.2.2 Relaxation

Before the actual imagery exercise begins, clients must enter a relaxed state of mind, and find a physically relaxed position.

This relaxed state of mind is a precursor to imagery and, at the same time, produces many positive effects (see relaxation). The most widely used relaxation method is the "progressive relaxation" technique developed by Jacobson (1964[767]). This technique is relatively simple to use, and allows clients to relax easily even if they are in a very stressed state. The actual method chosen must be one that clients can perform on their own, when they need or want to do so.

15.4.2.3 Using All Senses

The effects of imagery increase when the images are perceived as more real. This means that imagery should include as many sensory systems as possible. The sensory systems, which are often referred to as modalities, are: sight, hearing, emotions, touch, smell, and taste.

If one or more modalities are not present, the therapist should help clients to include them. This can be done by asking clients about the missing modality. For example, the therapist could inquire "What do you smell?" This will help clients to incorporate the missing modalities into the image.

The more modalities are present, the stronger the effects of the imagery.

15.4.2.4   Optimizing Sub-modalities

Each modality consists of smaller elements called sub-modalities. The modality of sight consists, among others, of the elements color, movement, and size. The modality of tactile sensations consists, among others, of the elements weight, temperature, and vibration.

Sub-modalities influence the effects of a single image. By changing the sub-modalities, the effects of the image increase or decrease. Changing the distance from "nearby" to "far away on the horizon" alters the effects of the imagery dramatically. If this is done with the image of a problem, the usual perceived magnitude of the problem is reduced. Trestman (1981[768]) and Achterberg et al. (1978[769]) wrote that changing sub-modalities influences the immune system immediately.

Depending on the situation, different sub-modalities should be used. In some cases, a colorful image is more effective, while other times a black and white image produces a greater impact. Images are personal, and so are the effects of different modalities and sub-modalities. There is no preferred set of modalities or sub-modalities.

By experimenting with different modalities and sub-modalities, the therapist can determine which are most effective for a specific client and result. Clients can change colors, sounds, and feelings to the extent that they feel will be most effective for them (Rossman 2000[770]). By carefully observing what sub-modalities produce the greatest effects, clients learn to use their own most effective sub-modalities.

Research by Trestman (1981[771]) concerning the effects of colors suggests that lighter colors used in imagery have different effects than darker colors. His observations are not conclusive with regard to which colors should be used.

To increase the effectiveness of imagery, McDermott at al. (1996[772]) used a technique called "mapping across sub-modalities." They noticed that many clients created images in a set of sub-modalities that corresponded to feelings of doubt or hope. McDermott et al. suggested that clients use sub-modalities corresponding to expectation.

Intervention:
1. *Define the sub-modalities of something the client expects to happen.*
   (Example: My expectation contains the sub-modalities "close by" and "in color.")

2.   *Map across these sub-modalities to define this new constructed image.*
    (Example: My new constructed image should include the sub-modalities of "close by" and "in color.")
3.   *This new image is now encoded in the sub-modalities of expectation.*

Adapted from McDermott at al. (1996[773])

15.4.2.5 Vividness

Some therapists strive for vivid imagery, while others prefer more vague images. After years of experimenting, Newton (1982[774]) stopped pursuing vivid images. He noticed that not all vivid images produced the desired effects, and that vague images also produced very good results. He concluded that pressuring clients for vivid imagery creates extra distress for them, and increases clients' chances of failure. For this same reason, Meares (1983[775]) simply instructed clients to let their natural images appear. Whether clients' imagery is vivid or vague is based on their preferences.

Although stressing vivid images increases the tension on the client, and weaker images also produce good results, vivid images are generally stronger. The therapist should motivate clients to make the images as vivid as possible without pressuring them if they are unable to do so.

15.4.2.6   Frequency of Imagery

"Practice makes perfect" is also applicable to imagery. The effects of imagery become stronger when the exercises are repeated. Clients who practice imagery most frequently and most enthusiastically will reap the greatest benefits.

Richardson et al. (1997[776]) concluded that performing imagery exercises with greater frequency increased the effects. They used immune-enhancing imagery, and observed a clear link between the frequency of the imagery exercises and enhanced immune function. Some therapists ask clients to do imagery exercises every day (Shapiro 1982[777]), while others suggest doing it 3 times a day for at least 15 minutes (Simonton et al. 1978[778]; Rossman 1987[779]).

Imagery exercises do not always have to be performed in a quiet place. When clients have practiced the exercises a couple of times, the process is familiar to them. They can practice while waiting for a bus, or during their daily routines. The more they practice, the stronger the effects will be.

15.4.3 Applications

Imagery is most widely known for its ability to produce physiological changes. Although this application is very old, Simonton et al. (1978[780]) were the first to publish the tremendous results they obtained using physiological imagery with cancer clients. They introduced imagery as a means of enhancing the immune system. Clients were instructed to imagine their immune systems attacking and destroying cancer cells, while joining forces with their medical treatments. They reported that repeated imagery sessions were associated with increased survival times, and sometimes remission among the target group. Based on their results, others later adopted and modified their approaches (Siegel, 1986[781]; Borysenko 1987[782]).

Gruber et al. (1988[783]) studied the effects of relaxation and imagery training on clients who suffered from metastatic cancer. They were instructed to imagine their immune systems becoming more actively involved with their medical treatments to aid in their healing processes. The instruction also included having them imagine becoming healthier each day. After six months of practice, their immune systems were functioning measurably better than before. In another study, Batt (1996[784]) noticed that the immune system destroyed cancer cells more actively after being instructed by such imagery.

Rossi (1986[785]) quoted a study by Schneider et al. (1984[786]), who reported their findings on the effects of imagery on the immune system. Students were shown a video on the biological workings of the immune system, and then listened to a tape-recorded imagery session. After six sessions, the students were able to increase or decrease the circulation of neutrophils in their bloodstreams. In a review of 22 studies, Hall (1993[787]) concluded that 18 studies had shown that clients could alter their immune systems with the help of voluntary imagery.

The possible physiological effects of imagery are extensive. Effects include pain reduction, reduced nausea and vomiting associated with chemotherapy (Frank 1985[788]; Scott et al. 1986[789]), reduced side effects, recovery from burns (Kenner 1983[790]), and preparation for spinal surgery

(Lawlis 1985[791]). Imagery has been used for diabetes in order to change glucose levels (Stevens 1983[792]), oxygen supply (Olness et al. 1985[793]), cardiovascular patterns (Barber 1969[794]), blood flow and temperature (Green 1977[795]), heart rate and galvanic skin response (Jordan et al. 1979[796]), and gastrointestinal activity (Barber 1978[797]). It is also used as a cardiac recovery approach (Ornish et al. 1983[798]; Ornish, 1990[799]).

The effects of imagery on physiological processes were also well demonstrated by Green et al. (1977[800]) in their biofeedback studies. They concluded that there is no mental image without an appropriate physical counterpart. This means that all mental images (desired or undesired) influence physiology. It has been demonstrated that when people watch a soccer game, tiny muscles in their legs become active, almost as if the body thinks it is playing soccer itself.

The effects of imagery can also be very specific. Hall et al. (1992[801]) describe a study in which students practiced imagery techniques. The students were instructed to imagine a specific way to enhance their immune system. Certain cells of their immune system were instructed by imagery to increase their adherence to other cells. Saliva and blood samples were taken some weeks later to investigate the subjects' immune function. The only significant change noticeable was the adherence between the cells, as instructed by the imagery. Other specific immunological changes were reported by Achterberg (1978[802]), Peavey et al. (1985[803]), and (Kiecolt-Glaser et al. 1985[804]).

When working with imagery to achieve physical effects, there are some choices to make regarding the structure of the images and the supporting language patterns. In this chapter, I will describe some of the most common structures and how to use them.

15.4.3.1 Receptive or Guided Imagery

Guided imagery is used in most applications for physiological and psychological change. Receptive imagery is mostly used for diagnostic purposes. Clients can communicate with their symptoms through receptive imagery.

Another application is to use receptive imagery as a starting point for guided imagery. The therapist helps clients to access their starting image for the current situation, and guided imagery is then used to change the current situation and move towards the desired situation.

Example:
- *Therapist: "How do you see your cancer and your current treatment?" (Receptive Imagery)*
- *Client: "My cancer is like white mushrooms on the lawn, while the lawnmower mows the grass."*
- *Therapist: "Imagine that at night, when the lawn is resting, a small group of squirrels eats all the mushrooms. They enjoy their dinner." (Guided Imagery)*

This type of intervention is increasing in popularity (Lawley et al. 2000[805]), and works with current thinking to facilitate change.

15.4.3.2 Realistic or Symbolic Imagery

Some therapists prefer realistic imagery, while others prefer symbolic imagery.

When using realistic imagery, which must be realistic in accordance with current medical thinking, clients become more informed about their condition. They can easily translate what they hear from their medical teams and apply it directly to their imagery.

Example
Current thinking is that there are always cancer cells in the body. This can be used in imagery by imagining that the immune system continuously fights the cancer cells, and is getting stronger with every battle.
Today, when a client hears something about cancer cells always being present, the belief described above is still in place, and their visualization is already adapted to this situation.

Realistic imagery does not necessarily elicit the response the therapist wants.
Try the following:
- Imagine increasing your saliva.
- Imagine increasing the blood flow to your face.

Realistic imagery also has a caveat. Clients could receive information that contradicts the imagery they are practicing. If they truly believe that new information, their imagery could be rendered useless, or even negatively influence their physiology. Furthermore, the therapist does not always know all of the specific processes that must take place in order to create a certain biological effect.

> **Example:**
> *A client has imagined the chemicals of his treatment adhering to the receptors of the cancer cells, depriving the cancer cells of nutrients.*
> *He has now heard, from the media or a physician, that this concept is outdated, and that the treatment works in a completely different way.*
> *This new information makes all of his previous practice useless.*
>
> *Or worse, science has come to the conclusion that adherence by the chemicals actually increases the size of the tumor. The client's previous imagery might have a negative effect on his physiological well-being.*

According to Barrios (1961[806]), physiological change occurs through unconscious association. To influence specific physiological reactions, one must find physiologically corresponding experiences. If there is a need for an increase in saliva, the therapist could use a corresponding experience such as eating a lemon. If there is a need for the client's hands to become sweaty, the therapist could use the corresponding experience of giving a presentation. Corresponding experiences are examples of symbolic imagery.
Try the following:
- Imagine slicing and eating a lemon, and your saliva will probably increase.
- Imagine that someone has caught you in the act, and you will probably blush.
- Imagine that you must give a very important presentation. It is likely that your hands will sweat a bit.

Achterberg et al. (1978[807]; 1994[808]) and Battino (2001[809]) believe that symbolic imagery is more powerful than realistic imagery. Symbolic images communicate the effects to the unconscious mind, rather than the physical procedure. It is easier for clients to think of their hand becoming numb in a bucket of ice, than to physically imagine all of the processes that must take place for the hand to become numb.

Pelletier (-year unknown-[810]) mentioned that it is not actually the kind of imagery that makes a difference, but the level of detail. Rossman (2003[811]) uses the imagery that has the most personal meaning and positive emotional response for clients.

Margolis (1983[812]) indicated that the therapist should draw on the clients' own experiences. This implies that clients choose whether to use a realistic or symbolic representation of the healing process. Although Rossman (2000[813]) concluded that there was no difference in the effects, whether the imagery was done realistically or symbolically, most imagery scripts are still based on symbolic imagery.

15.4.3.3 Process-Oriented or Goal-Oriented Imagery

To achieve the greatest effects, one could use both process- and goal-oriented imagery. Process imagery is used for the healing process, followed by the goal imagery of being healthy (Achterberg 1985[814]).

15.4.3.4   Fighting or Cooperative Imagery

As discussed earlier, Simonton et al. (1978[815]), who initiated the use of imagery in complementary cancer therapy, used a fighting style of imagery to combat the disease. In this style, the immune system allies with the chemotherapy or radiation to fight off the cancer cells. This fighting approach perceives the cancer as a foreign intruder that must be killed. It supports the medical paradigm of fighting the disease.

Fighting imagery disagrees with the holistic approach, in which everything in the body is interconnected. It also sets the stage for denying the message cancer could convey. Dilts et al. (1990[816]) proposed the use of cooperative imagery. They concluded that when clients use fighting imagery, they will be involved in a fight, which always includes a winner and a loser. It sets clients up for failure if the battle is not won in time, or if a temporary setback occurs. The fight could also trigger past conflicts and distressing emotions. Although they suggested using cooperative imagery, they actually used examples of fighting imagery in their book. They used examples of "sheep who graze the cancer away," which is less aggressive, but still a fighting style of imagery.

When using fighting imagery, the therapist should ensure that the image includes the following elements.

Guidelines for Imagery:
- *The disease is curable.*
- *Treatment is strong, powerful, and effective.*
- *The body is able to heal itself.*
- *Cancer cells are soft, weak, confused, and fragile.*
- *Cancer cells can be broken down and penetrated easily by the immune system.*
- *White blood cells outnumber cancer cells significantly.*
- *Healthy cells can easily repair themselves if they have been damaged by the treatment.*
- *The immune system is powerful and omnipresent.*
- *White blood cells are strong, clever, and eager for battle.*
- *Dead cancer cells are washed away from the body in a natural way.*
- *One feels good during the entire process of healing.*
- *One's goals in life are reached, and one enjoys being vital, energetic and healthy.*
- *There is action and movement towards health.*

Adapted from Simonton et al. (1978[817]), Temoshok (1992[818]), and Rossman (2000[819]; 2003[820]).

In addition to adhering to the above guidelines, the imagery should be powerful and active. Increasing the power and action in the image enhances the effects on the immune system (Achterberg et al. 1978[821]).

Margolis (1983[822]), Newton (1983[823]), and Shapiro (1983[824]) also used fighting imagery. The immune system was viewed as working together with the medical treatment to attack the cancer cells. Rosch (1984[825]) suggested that in combating an illness, people should use fighting imagery. Derogatis et al. (1979[826]) and Achterberg (1985[827]) suggested that fighting imagery produces more effects than cooperative imagery. Temoshok (1992[828]) took another approach. She believed that the imagery should not be imposed on the client. The imagery should spring from the client's unconscious mind, whether it be fighting or cooperative. The therapist aids the client in accessing those images.

15.4.4 Common Problems in Imagery

When clients begin practicing imagery, they might encounter some problems. They might find that images do not appear as quickly or clearly as expected. They might fear that they are fooling themselves, or notice that their minds wander. As with any other kind of learning, practice makes perfect when learning imagery. In this chapter, I will discuss these common problems.

15.4.4.1 Inability to Imagine

Some people believe that they must clearly see vivid mental pictures in order to imagine (Rossman 2000[829]). They think they are unable to imagine because they assume that they must see pictures. Imagery can take place through all of the senses. Some people notice primarily their feelings, while others notice mostly sounds or their predominant emotions. The five senses may all be present, or there may be an emphasis on one or two. This does not matter.

A mental image is not as clear as experiencing something through the senses. There is a difference between experiencing things in real life and through imagery. Imagery need not be clear or vivid (see also 15.4.2.5 Vividness). Many people have reported obtaining the desired effects with only vague images.

15.4.4.2   Denial of Images

Sometimes clients try to find the most appropriate images. Clients cannot always come up with a satisfying image, so another image appears. The original images are denied and repressed because they did not satisfy the client.

The therapist should explain that every image that comes to mind is a good image to begin with. Every image that appears is appropriate. When clients deny certain images, they are denying their unconscious, who is presenting the images.

15.4.4.3   Failure to Allow Healing

Interpretation of the imagery could suggest that clients are not allowing themselves to heal. If this is the case, the therapist should first focus on this (conscious or unconscious) belief. The interventions that the therapist could use to change such beliefs have already been discussed in the chapter on changing the appraisal process in therapy.

Example:
The imagery could show the cancer cells spreading and overruling the immune system, or a very potent and strong opponent.

15.4.4.4   Clients' Fear of Fooling Themselves

Clients could claim that the imagery is not real, and that by imagining themselves as healthy, they are fooling themselves. In this case, the therapist should explain that imagery is not about reality, but about focus and direction. Focusing on your goal will increase the likeliness of attaining it (Rossman 2003[830]). The following metaphor might be helpful for explaining this.

Example:
Imagine a person who is playing darts. The player focuses on the bull's eye. They imagine the dart going into the bull's eye.
This is not reality, but if they focus on their hands or on the wall, they will not throw as well as when they focus on the bull's eye.

15.4.4.5   Becoming Distracted

When clients begin practicing imagery, they sometimes notice that their minds wander. This is very natural. Many things can cause the mind to wander. It might be that they have things to remember, which can be solved by asking clients to write down everything they want to remember while preparing for the session.

Other issues might be beliefs such as "I don't have time for this." In that case, the therapist should work with such clients on the issue of taking time for themselves and their healing processes. There could be a belief present which resembles a lack of self-worth, or the idea that other people are more important.

Another way of handling a wandering mind is by having clients become aware of the locations that their minds wander off to. The therapist could ask clients to observe what their minds are trying to tell them by wandering off, or by going to that specific location.

16

Influencing Pain

Pain management is an important issue when working with cancer clients. Pain influences their psychological well-being and increases distress. Distress in turn increases pain. In this chapter, I will present some ways in which the therapist could work with pain.

"Change and pain are part of life, but suffering is optional."
- Anonymous -

The most obvious benefit of teaching clients pain management skills is the reduction of pain itself, but this is not the only issue. Clients could take medication to reduce the pain itself. The core issue in learning pain reduction is to increase the client's feeling of control. This feeling of control increases their well-being, and eventually reduces their pain perception.

Clients who experience control over their pain also experience control over their bodies. This increased control usually decreases the effects of stressors on clients' lives. Often, the ability to reduce pain also results in a decrease of fear. Pain and emotions of distress intensify each other. The reduction of pain reduces distress, and the reduction of distress reduces pain.

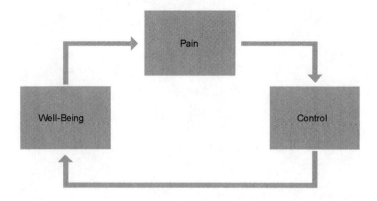

Most healthy people will not even notice small pains, but most cancer clients are well attuned to every pain. These pains are often interpreted as being signs of recurrence or other bad omens. Such interpretations intensify the clients' emotions of distress. This is a vicious cycle, and learning to control the pain breaks the cycle.

When clients begin learning pain management skills, they often report an increase in pain before it actually decreases. According to Spiegel, this is caused by the fact that clients start noticing and communicating with their pain. Before, the pain was suppressed and denied as much as possible, but now it is being stared at in the face. By explaining this to clients, their motivation to work on pain management remains high, even if the pain increases in the beginning.

In this chapter, I will discuss some interventions that can be used to increase the control and influence clients have on their pain.

16.1   Imagery

Imagery is also used as a pain management intervention. For acute pain, Simonton et al. (1978[831]) used a technique for helping clients to imagine themselves engaged in a healthful activity. This changes the client's focus and reduces his pain at that moment. In addition to this acute technique, Simonton et al. used imagery to decrease pain in general with techniques called "imagine your body's healing resources" and "imagine the pain."

"Imagine your body's healing resources" is an imagery process in which clients imagine making a journey through their bodies. When they arrive at the location of the pain, they are instructed to imagine those muscles and ligaments relaxing. At the same time, clients imagine healing that location.

The imagery process "Imagine the pain" involves having clients imagine the pain and describe all features of it. They describe all of the sub-modalities, such as color, size, shape, texture, weight, sounds, etc.

Clients are then instructed to change some sub-modalities. The representation of the pain could be changed by reducing its size, pushing it farther away, shifting it to the left, or changing the colors. By changing the sub-modalities, clients feel that they gain control over their pain.

The imagery session ends with a representation of the pain, and therefore a changed perception of the pain. This changed perception usually includes a reduction of the intensity.

Intervention:
1. *Sit back and relax.*
2. *Focus on the pain. Observe its color, shape, size, sound, etc. Did you notice what it looks like?*
3. *Imagine that you are pushing the representation of the pain slowly until it is one hundred feet away from you.*
4. *Notice how your body reacts.*
5. *Imagine bringing the pain closer and changing its size, making it as small as a pinhead.*
6. *Notice how your body reacts.*
7. *Imagine changing its shape and color.*
8. *Notice how your body reacts.*
9. *Open your eyes.*

Based on Simonton et al. (1978)

16.2   Communication with Pain

Pain itself is often viewed as communication between the body and the mind. The pain might convey a message about the activities, thoughts, or emotions that are present at that time. Receiving this message allows clients to act upon it. Once they have acted on the meaning of the message, the pain no longer needs to communicate the message itself. This usually leads to a reduction of the pain. If the message is ignored, or clients do not take action, the pain still needs to convey its message. If clients are not listening, the pain might need to "shout" (increase its intensity) in order to communicate its message.

Example:
A patient might tell us that on awakening he is free of pain. However, when he begins to think about getting out of bed, the pain begins.

After examining his own thoughts, he might notice that the pain increases when he remembers that he is ill and does not feel like "his old self."

During the day, he may experience low-intensity pain until the phone rings, at which time there is a sudden, dramatic increase.

Adapted from Simonton et al. (1978[832]; 1992[833])

This example could indicate that the client has negative expectations regarding the day, and particularly the meaning of the ringing phone.

Once the message conveyed by the pain is known, clients can do something about it. The following intervention helps clients to understand the message.

Intervention:
1.   *Sit back and relax.*
2.   *Imagine the pain as a friendly person or creature that is there to help you.*
3.   *Enhance the imagery by experiencing it with all your senses.*
4.   *Establish communication with the person or creature.*
5.   *Thank the representation for its cooperation.*
6.   *Ask what it is there for, what message it is trying to get across to you.*
7.   *Respectfully listen to the answers.*
8.   *Ask it what you can do so that the pain is no longer necessary.*
9.   *Ask it to replace the signal of pain with another signal, which you agree to listen to.*
10. *Open your eyes and act on the information you just received.*

Based on Simonton et al. (1978[834], 1992[835])

16.3   Secondary Gains from Pain

Every situation has a positive and a negative side. This also holds true for pain. In the section on therapy for changing the appraisal process, I discussed the secondary gains from the current situation. Pain often has specific secondary gains. This applies not only to cancer clients, but to any area in which pain is an issue. When clients become aware of their secondary gains, and take action to obtain them through different means, this often results in a decrease of their pain.

When clients experience pain, other people are more inclined to help and to relieve them of certain tasks. As in the case of cancer itself, clients must become aware of the benefits associated with pain. Recognition and acceptance of these benefits is the first step.

The therapist can begin investigating the possible benefits of pain by asking clients the following probing questions:

Intervention:
- *Why do I need this pain?*
- *What purpose is it serving?*
- *What does it allow me to do, or not do?*
- *What am I getting from it?*
- *When do I get it?*
- *What makes it worse?*
- *What reduces the pain?*

Adapted from Simonton et al. (1978[836])

These questions, like all questions regarding secondary gains, are often difficult and very confronting to answer. Sometimes clients do not want to discuss the possibility of the pain bringing any benefits at all. Sometimes clients know the answers, and have a hard time accepting them. Usually, the first thing they say is that there are no benefits, and that they just want to get rid of the pain. The therapist needs to continuously acknowledge the client's desire to get rid of the pain, while also pointing out that there are benefits to the situation, however small they may be.

Other interventions that can be used for challenging secondary gains are already discussed in the chapter on working with beliefs.

16.4   Creating Pleasure

One of the best-known methods of pain management is having clients do something they enjoy. However, this is barely used in therapy. By engaging in pleasurable activities, one is likely to forget both physical and mental pain for the moment.

Simonton et al. (1978) actively promoted seeking pleasure to reduce pain, especially after they observed that people in pain tended to engage in fewer enjoyable activities. They also noticed that when clients actually did participate in gratifying activities, they reported less pain.

Interventions that can be used to create pleasure are described in the chapter on meaningful activities, and in the section on creating comforting emotions.

16.5   Changing Focus

The experience of pain changes over time, and differs depending on the situation. Sometimes the pain might be excruciating, while at other times it might be very slight. Clients have a tendency to describe their pain as being constant and present all the time. Motivating clients to examine when they are in pain, and when the pain is reduced, allows them to make distinctions in their perception. Their minds become open to more moments of reduced pain. When clients are fixed in their thinking that the pain is always present, they will increase their own discomfort. Clients need to realize that there are moments of pain and moments of comfort.

Intervention:
- *Help the client keep a "comfort diary."*
- *Have the client write down how comfortable he feels each day (on a scale of 1 to 10).*
- *Have the client notice what increases his comfort, and what decreases his comfort.*

If the pain is overwhelming, avoidance techniques can be applied. This can be accomplished by helping clients focus on other parts of their bodies, for example the pressure of their feet on the ground, the feeling of their backs pressing against the chair, their buttocks on the chair, the temperature in the room, or the wind on their ears. Any sensation experienced by other parts of their bodies will do.

16.6   Hypnotic Pain Management

Spiegel (1978[837]) taught cancer clients self-hypnosis for pain management, and to control the side effects of medical treatments. These techniques can also be used when clients experience psychological pain.

Hypnotic pain interventions are well-known and effective. Esdaile (1846[838]) already applied hypnotic anesthesia to perform surgery. Other well-known sources for hypnotic pain interventions are: Hilgard et al. (1975[839]), Zeig (1982[840]), Hilgard et al. (1984[841]), Zilbergeld et al. (1986[842]), and Rossi et al. (1988[843]).

Many reports have been written on hypnotic anesthesia. Glove-anesthesia is particularly well-known and effective. There is extensive research available on hypnotic pain management, which is beyond the scope of this chapter.

Section F

Conclusions And Recommendations

17

Recommendations For Further Research

While reviewing the literature and gathering knowledge elsewhere, I came across many subjects meriting further investigation. These could provide valuable information for enhancing current therapeutic programs for complementary psychological cancer treatment (CPCT).

In this chapter, I will discuss some of these subjects and formulate questions that might be of interest for further study.

17.1   Mind-Body Connection

Much has already been written on how the mind and body interact (see chapter), yet there is still much to uncover. Many possible research areas could be pursued to further unravel the mysteries of the mind-body connection. One area of investigation that could provide interesting insights is Dissociative Identity Disorder (DID), formerly known as Multiple Personality Disorder (MPD). Although much research is available in this area, there is a lack of research on its implications for mind-body therapy.

Dissociative Identity Disorder provides interesting insights into how, and how quickly, psychological changes affect physiology. Clients who display the symptoms of DID seem to have multiple "personalities" (or "alters") inside their bodies. Each alter has its own mental and physical makeup and history. Each has its own age, attitude, IQ, memories, behavioral patterns, etc. For all practical purposes, several different people seem to be living in the same body. At a given time, only one personality (alter) is "actual," and the environment experiences only that personality. When another alter becomes actual, other people perceive this as a radical change in personality. When such a change takes place, the client also dramatically alters his attitudes, behavior, and even his talents and affections. In addition to these tremendous changes in psychology, the client's physiology also changes dramatically.

There have been reports of allergic reactions and scars disappearing when a change of alter occurred. The reports also described the later reappearance of the scars and allergic reactions when the original alter became actual again.

Although there is still much controversy about the causes, most people agree that the symptoms of radically changing psychology and physiology are real.

Daniel Goleman (1993[844]) wrote about some interesting cases that showed the physiological effects produced when another alter became actual. Remember, these involved the same person - only a different state of mind!

- Dr. Bennett Braun reported having sedated a person with only 5 milligrams of a tranquilizer (diazepam). When that person switched alters, even 100 milligrams was not enough to sedate him. This report is supplemented by others describing people waking up on the operating table after switching alters. The newly actual alters required higher doses of the anesthetic.
- A person who was drunk became instantly sober after changing alters.
- Another one of Braun's cases was the famous citrus juice case. All alters (except one) were allergic to citrus juices. When the client drank citrus juice, a terrible rash would appear. When the non-allergic alter became actual, the rash would immediately begin to fade, and the client would be able to enjoy drinking citrus juice. When another alter became actual, the rash would reappear.

These cases (and many others) clearly show the tremendous physiological effects caused by the actual alter. These changes all took place within the same physical body, with the same DNA, organs, and chemicals. The only difference was the psychology. The speed of such physiological change almost seems miraculous.

Several other cases are known that document such physiological changes. These include the appearance or disappearance of scars, epilepsy, burn marks, rashes, cysts, blisters, color blindness, sensory acuity, body posture, right-handedness, and many others (Braun 1986[845]). Phillips claimed (in Chase, 1987[846]) that he even saw tumors disappear.

Many authors have recognized that people who display symptoms of Dissociative Identity Disorder are also very good hypnotic subjects. DID phenomena (even the bizarre) can be induced in other clients by using hypnosis. It has been suggested that DID might actually be a pathological hypnotic state, or a form of spontaneous self-hypnosis. Dissociative Identity Disorder is also often viewed as a kind of hypnotic regression (see also 17.4.3.2 Symbolic Modeling). If these views are correct, the physiological effects of alter changes can be induced by hypnotic suggestion in non-DID clients.

Some hypnotically induced physiological changes were so severe (deadly allergies, cardiac changes) that they endangered the lives of the clients. Those clients also had severe repressed traumas. People often reason that such severe changes stem from repressed traumata (or emotional cysts). Research and reasoning in this area underlines the possibility of dramatic physiological effects being caused by emotional cysts.

Questions for further study:
a) *How is immune system activity influenced by the actual alter?*
b) *What happens to the tumor, its speed of growth, and the immune system when a non-cancer alter is in control? What happens when the non-cancer alter is in control for a prolonged period of time (multiple weeks/months)?*
c) *Do any positive physiological changes occur when another alter takes control? How can hypnosis be used to achieve those same benefits in non-DID clients?*

17.2   Psychological Markers of Cancer Clients

Many researchers have tried to find the psychological markers that characterize cancer clients. These psychological issues have been described in this study. Further research on discovering specific psychological markers is necessary in at least three areas: Metaprograms, Organ Language, and combined psychological markers.

17.2.1   Metaprograms

Metaprograms are psychological patterns that guide beliefs

and behavior. Current literature has identified over 20 different metaprograms (James 1988[847]; Charvet 1995[848]; Hall 2002[849]). These categories of patterns can be found in everyone.

One of these metaprograms is "proactive vs. reactive." A proactive client takes action and then thinks over his actions. A reactive client thinks first and then acts. This metaprogram corresponds to taking action and responsibility for one's healing process.

Another metaprogram is "self vs. others." This indicates whether a client is focused on himself or on others. Does the client listen first to himself, or first to others? This corresponds to assertiveness and self-worth.

Much evidence is present to suggest that the above metaprograms (proactive vs. reactive and self vs. others) influence the healing process. This evidence has been discussed in the Appraisal section, under the Psychosomatic Model. Only the two metaprograms described above have been studied and identified as having an influence on healing. A possible research area could be the influence of other (currently at least 18) metaprograms on the healing process.

Questions for further study:
a) *What metaprograms are typically found in cancer clients?*
b) *Are there metaprograms that are distinctive between cancer and non-cancer clients?*
c) *Are there any metaprograms typically found in clients who have experienced spontaneous cancer remission?*

17.2.2   Organ Language

Hamer (1999[850]; 1999[851]) presented a model of cancer development that was quite extreme. He claimed that a direct relationship existed between a specific psychological problem and the development of a specific kind of tumor.

His evidence suggested that the metaphorical meaning of a psychological problem was not just metaphorical, but literal, as if the metaphor itself created the corresponding type of cancer.

Example:
• *An indigestible anger is manifested as a tumor in the colon.*

- *The loss of physical contact is manifested as a skin tumor.*
- *Fear of suffocation leads to tumors related to respiratory functions.*

Besides Hamer's own research, there is barely any other evidence to support these bold statements.

The fields of Neuro Linguistic Programming and Hypnotherapy contain an element that comes close to Hamer's ideas, called "organ language." Organ language is normal language that metaphorically refers to a specific part of the body. There is a difference between organ language and the communication with organs discussed earlier. Organ language is specific language uttered by clients, which refers to different parts of their bodies. Organ communication is a therapeutic technique that allows clients to hold conversations with particular parts of their bodies.

Examples of Organ Language:
- *I made a rash decision.*
- *He gets under my skin.*
- *That really eats me up.*
- *I cannot crop that.*
- *I do not want to look at that.*
- *I hold in my problems.*
- *That is breaking my heart.*
- *He is a pain in the neck.*
- *It's eating away at me.*

The above statements are everyday language for many people. It seems that those people who use such language excessively have a higher chance of actually experiencing those symptoms. The resemblance between the metaphors clients use and their physical symptoms is often stunning.

Apparently, these metaphors (and organ language) are not merely a representation, but actually a guiding principle in the development of the symptoms. Hamer (1999[852]; 1999[853]), Dilts (1999[854]; 2000[855]), and Lawley (2000[856]) have suggested that the mind interprets these metaphors and statements as instructions, and creates the symptoms "on request." Perhaps these metaphors are not just figurative, but actually create reality.

Hamer has developed an extensive list of metaphorical descriptions that are thought to be associated with the development of cancer. Others have also identified possible cancer-creating metaphors. Dilts (1999[857]; 2000[858]) associated metaphors such as "I cannot maintain my boundaries," "I am dying to do that," and "That is out of my control" with the development of cancer. "Something is eating at me" was identified as a possible cancer-creating metaphor by Lawley (2000[859]).

Example:
- *The client feels badly treated by someone.*
- *Metaphorically, he creates an image representing the idea "I cannot digest what he has done to me."*
- *The mind creates symptoms related to the concept "cannot digest." This results in symptoms of the digestive organs.*

The process by which all of this takes place might be the following:

1) The client experiences something and attributes meaning to it.

2) The client creates a metaphorical image of that meaning.

3) Based on the image, the client unconsciously constructs his language.

4) The image influences his health.

Questions for further study:
a)   *What is the influence of organ language on the development of cancer?*

b)   *What evidence can be found that proves or disproves the theory developed by Hamer?*

c)   *What happens to the tumor and immune system if the client starts using different language patterns than before?*

17.2.3   Combined Psychological Markers

Research into psychological markers generally focuses on one or more specific psychological elements. Instead of concentrating on one isolated element, one could also study the effects of interactions between multiple elements. For example, Goodkin et al. (1986[860]) found a weak connection between stressors and cancer progression, and between hopelessness and cancer progression. When they combined stressors with pessimism and hopelessness, they found a much stronger connection to cancer progression.

Garssen (2000[861]) warns about the premature exclusion of certain factors from research, and suggests that psychological factors should also be studied in interaction with one another. A combination of multiple psychological factors might have more profound effects on physiology than single psychological factors.

Questions for further study:
a) *What relationship to cancer progression can be found when multiple psychological markers are combined?*

b) *If a specific set of markers is related to cancer progression, what happens physiologically if a change occurs in only one psychological marker from that set?*

17.3   Specific Cancers

In studies of the psychological markers found in cancer clients, most research is focused on cancer in general. Very few distinctions have been made between the different kinds of cancer when assessing the client's personality.

Martikainen (1996[862]) observed that bereaved men had a higher mortality rate from accidents, violent encounters, heart disease, and lung cancer. No increase in mortality was observed in relation to other types of cancer. He suggested that bereavement has more of an effect on mortality from lung cancer than from other types of cancer.

Levav (2000[863]) studied over 6000 people who had lost sons in wars or accidents. Bereaved parents showed an increased incidence of lymphatic cancers, melanomas, respiratory cancers, and hematopoietic malignancies, but not other types of cancers.

On this subject, I agree with LeShan (1961[864]) and Greer (1982[865]), who suggested that there is a need for further research regarding the links between specific psychological markers and the types or locations of cancers. Specific psychological factors might actually lead to specific cancer growths (Hamer 1999[866]; 1999[867]; Garssen 2002[868]).

Questions for further study:
a) *What links can be found between specific psychological components and specific cancers?*

17.4   Interventions

Interventions that deal directly with physiology are less widely studied than those dealing with the psychosomatic model. Issues such as the therapeutic use of conditioning and hypnotic suggestions are barely studied at all. This chapter discusses possible research questions in the area of psychological interventions with cancer clients.

17.4.1 Conditioning

Studies on conditioning have always focused primarily on psychological influences. Research has proven that conditioning also influences physiology (discussed in the corresponding section). How those results can be used to enhance psychotherapeutic work with cancer clients has yet to be determined.

Questions for further study:
a)   *How can conditioning and reconditioning be used in cancer therapy?*
b)   *How can negative conditioning be prevented?*

17.4.2 Hypnotic Suggestions

Although many studies have been conducted on the effects of suggestions, many questions remain. There is still controversy regarding the use of "towards" and "away from" suggestions (as discussed in the chapter on hypnotic suggestions). Further study in this area is needed to increase the effectiveness of hypnotic suggestions.

Research suggests that the effects of hypnotic suggestions on psychology and physiology seem to be unlimited. The use of hypnotic suggestions to produce psychological change indicates that suggesting that a problem should disappear actually does make it disappear in some cases. The physiological effects of suggestions on a tumor itself have barely been studied. To really bring forward the field of complementary psychological cancer treatment (CPCT), there is a need to study the effects of hypnotic suggestions on tumors.

Questions for further study:
a)   *What would happen physiologically if the procedure for removing warts with hypnotic suggestions were applied to cancer?*

b)   *What could happen if the procedure for hypnotically creating warts with suggestions were applied to cancer?*

c)   *To what extent can we suggest that a tumor disappear? Are "cancer-be-gone" suggestions possible?*

d)   *How are tumors affected by suggestions for reducing the blood flow to them? (Or for changing temperature or direct medication, or depriving tumor cells of what they need.)*

f)   *What is the difference between the physiological effects of using "towards" vs. "away from" suggestions?*

g)   *Does the depth of the trance, stage of cancer, or client's personality influence the therapeutic choice between "towards" or "away from" suggestions?*

h)   *Can taped hypnotic sessions played during surgery enhance healing from cancer?*

17.4.3   Imagery

Studies on imagery are not yet conclusive with regard to what elements or sub-modalities produce the greatest effect. Some authors (Simonton and Achterberg) have suggested that some symbols are preferred over others in imagery, although more study is needed to fully apply this in complementary psychological cancer treatment (CPCT).

Questions for further study:

a)   *What are the effects of different primary colors on tumors during imagery?*

b)   *What colors seem to influence tumors the most?*

c)   *What metaphorical images (animals, objects, situations, etc.) are best suited for cancer imagery?*

d)   *What are the effects of imagery that switches the oncogenes to the "off" position? (Rossman 2003[869]).*

17.4.3.1 Fighting or Cooperative Imagery

In complementary cancer therapy, imagery almost exclusively takes on the role of combating the cancer. When imagery is used for psychological issues, it is almost exclusively cooperative imagery.

Contrary to some diseases, cancer is not a foreign invader of the body, but a growth from the inside. Some researchers therefore suggest that cancer conveys some kind of message to the client. Fighting the cancer is fighting the self, while at the same time shooting the messenger without receiving the message. If this is the case, cooperative imagery would be a better choice.

In the literature, very little can be found on cooperative imagery for cancer clients. The existing scientific literature does not mention the use of this type of imagery at all. Some alternative approaches mention it, but lack specificity.

Another benefit of cooperative imagery is that clients cannot fail, as they can when the fight is lost. Without the possibility of failure, there is less chance of experiencing the distressing emotions of having failed.

Questions for further study:
It is well known that imagery has an effect on physiology, but the most effective type of imagery has yet to be discovered.
a) What are the differences in the effects on physiology when using fighting or cooperative imagery?
b) What are the differences in the effects on psychological well-being when using fighting or cooperative imagery?
c) Is there a difference in the rate of cancer recurrence depending on whether the therapist uses fighting or cooperative imagery?
If a metaphorical battle is won, the enemy can retreat, grow stronger, and return for another battle. If no battle occurs, but there is cooperation and agreement, there is no chance of a returning battle.

17.4.3.2 Symbolic Modeling

In the section on organ language (17.2.2 Organ Language), I discussed the possible values of metaphorical meaning of the client's language. Interventions can be performed to address the unconscious metaphors (or images) clients have created.

Hejmadi et al. (1991[870]) noticed an increase in the pace of healing when the clients' own metaphors were used in the imagery processes. They used receptive imagery to determine the starting point of the intervention, and guided imagery to shift the image towards healing. Instead of forcing an image on the client, they worked from "within."

Working with the metaphor (or image) that a client already possesses is called "Autogenic Metaphor Resolution – AMR" (Hejmadi et al. 1991[871]), or "Symbolic Modeling" (Dilts et al. 1999[872]; Lawley et al. 2000[873]). This same process is sometimes referred to as "active imagery" in hypnotic literature. Although this specific approach is relatively new, Simonton et al. (1978[874]) already made use of the clients' own metaphors in their imagery, but never defined it as such. More research is needed on the applications and effects of this type of imagery.

> *Questions for further study:*
> a)   *What is the difference in effect when using the client's metaphor during imagery processes vs. an image constructed by the therapist?*
> b)   *What happens physiologically if the client's metaphor for their cancer is changed?*

17.4.4 Regression

Regression is a therapeutic intervention in which clients are taken back in time to experience a previous timeframe. The best-known example of regression is when clients are regressed to childhood. At that time, they only experience childhood; they play with the toys they liked, and do not seem to know what they learned later in life. When clients are regressed, physiological changes can be observed. Erickson (1937[875]) reported a case in which a client was regressed to a time when he was unconscious after a homicidal attack. Although it had happened two years earlier, the client collapsed and showed no reflexes, as if he were unconscious again.

Another physiological change caused by regression was reported by Moody (1946[876]). The client was regressed to a traumatic experience. Within a few minutes, scars and hemorrhages began to appear, and lasted several hours. The scars and hemorrhages appeared in the same places where the client had been tied up during the real event. Ford (1948[877]) studied a client who had experienced homonymous hemianopsia (partial loss of vision in one or both eyes) four years earlier. During the regression, the client's homonymous hemianopsia returned. Kuper (1945[878]) showed that a client who was epileptic could be regressed to a time prior to his first attack. During that regression, his EEG was normal, similar to that of a non-epileptic client.

Grue (1951[879]) and Gidro-Frank (1948[880]) observed changes in the Babinski reflex during regression. This is the automatic curling of the toes when a person is stroked on the soles of their feet. When children under the age of six months are stroked, their toes curl outwards. After six months, they curl inwards. The Babinski reflex corresponded to the regressed age, not the biological age.

Although these studies are not related to complementary psychological cancer treatment (CPCT), they do provide some interesting examples of how regression creates extreme physiological changes.

After observing the dramatic effects of regression, Barrios (1961[881]) concluded that the study of regression might be of interest with regard to psychological cancer treatment.

Questions for further study:

a) *What would happen to the immune system and the tumor if the client were regressed, for a short time, to a time long before the onset of the cancer?*

b) *What would happen if the client were regressed to a time prior to the onset of the cancer, and remained in that regressive trance for a prolonged period of time (several weeks or months)?*

c) *What would happen to the cancer and the immune system upon the client's return to the present after a pre-cancer regression?*

18

Conclusions

This study has highlighted many individual psychological elements that are somehow associated with cancer. For the sake of clarity, I have discussed them separately, but in reality they cannot be separated. They are omnipresent and interact with each other at all times. For example, clients' coping styles cannot be regarded as separate from their beliefs or emotions.

18.1 General Conclusions

18.1.1 Psychotherapy Plays an Important Role in Cancer Treatment

Based on this study, one can conclude that psychotherapy plays an important role in the treatment of cancer.

There are currently no psychological interventions that can actually cure a client. The lack of evidence to suggest that psychological interventions can cure clients should not result in the rejection of such interventions by therapists or clients. There are a multitude of interventions available to help clients regain their physical health. Even if they only help marginally, it is still worth it !

Such psychological interventions either work directly to influence physiology, or indirectly through psychological elements.

Clients no longer have to be passive in their treatments - they can become active participants in their healing processes. By seeking professional help, clients can assist their own physiology in its healing process. Clients who are actively involved in their healing processes increase their psychological well-being and positively affect their physiology.

*"Nobody made a greater mistake than he who did nothing because
he could only do a little."*
- Edmund Burke-

18.1.2 There is Much Information, But Less Hard Data

There is much more scientific research available on the psychological influences on health than is generally believed. Everyone agrees that the psychology of cancer clients influences their health. However, hard data indicating that psychological interventions can increase clients' cure rates is lacking. The absence of such hard data is due to the problems caused by using a scientific model to gain evidence for the effects of psychotherapeutic interventions. Although the field of psychotherapy has evolved tremendously over the last couple of decades, it still uses a "black box" approach. Hard data in psychotherapy would have to prove that the same intervention would work for the same problem in every client for every therapist. Such evidence is non-existent (so far). The pursuit of such hard data in psychotherapy should be abandoned and replaced with a pragmatic approach.

Another problem when seeking evidence of the effects of psychological interventions is that not only the psychology of the client needs to be considered, but also the beliefs of the therapist, and the relationship between the two.

Available research papers and books rarely provide detailed descriptions of the actual interventions used. This prevents the appropriate validation of such studies and, more importantly, limits the practical psychotherapeutic applications of the findings.

Different psychotherapeutic disciplines seem to put more effort into promoting their own ideas than combining the effective interventions into an all-encompassing psychological therapeutic program. To gain acceptance for the field of complementary psychological cancer treatment (CPCT), all therapists need to acknowledge the value inherent in other approaches.

My initial goal was to distill a complementary psychological cancer treatment (CPCT) program from the existing literature. Unfortunately, there is currently no such therapeutic program. My ongoing research will focus on the development of such an all-encompassing complementary psychological cancer treatment program.

18.1.3   One Should Use "Complementary" as a Descriptive Term

Traditional cancer care often has an aversion to psychological treatment to assist health. They generally accept that psychological treatment helps to increase psychological well-being, but the possibility of it being used to aid the physical healing process is often rejected.

This rejection is partly due to bad communication from working psychological therapists. Some of these therapists promote "alternative" therapies. By definition, "alternative" means that such therapies are used *instead* of regular medicine. Such therapists thus communicate that they reject traditional cancer treatment. This is not only inconsiderate, but also inaccurate. It led to the generalization that every therapist promoting non-medical interventions was "alternative," and should therefore be banned. This is not correct.

As discussed in the introductory sections, medicine has much to offer clients. This study indicates that other therapeutic disciplines also have much to offer, both psychologically and physiologically. To clearly distinguish between the treatments I describe and so-called "alternative" therapies, I propose using the term "complementary" treatment. Although the terms "alternative" and "complementary" are often used interchangeably (even among therapists, who should know better), there is a huge difference between them.

"Complementary" practitioners work in cooperation with the medical team on those issues that do not fall within the physicians' specialties. They acknowledge the value of the medical team, and assist clients in aligning their psychology towards healing. The medical staff and complementary therapists should form one team. Physicians are specialized in curing the body, and psychological therapists are specialized in helping the mind to heal. Each "complements" the other.

Therapists who reject the medical approach (for whatever reason) should continue using the term "alternative treatment" to describe their approach. Those therapists who work in conjunction with the medical team, and provide additional psychological treatment, should use the proper descriptive term "complementary." Only through constant use of this proper term can these approaches become accepted and integrated into mainstream cancer care, which is necessary. Medical practitioners can only fully obey their Hippocratic oath if they accept and support complementary psychological cancer treatment (CPCT).

"To keep the good of the patient as the highest priority."
- Hippocratic oath -

18.1.4   There is Always Hope

This study has shown that there is always hope of improving psychological and physiological well-being. Therefore, I would like to finish this chapter with my most important conclusion. If you only remember one thing, remember this:

Even if the situation seems hopeless, there are still many
things you can do to increase your psychological as well as
physiological health.

18.2   "Fundamental Image": A New Psychosomatic Model

The section on directly influencing physiology has shown that interventions such as imagery, hypnotic suggestions, and language influence physiology directly, without having to "go through" the psychological elements. This cannot be explained using the current psychosomatic model. Therefore, a revised model is needed.

The original psychosomatic model consisted of a sequential chain of psychological elements that ended up influencing physiology. Interventions were used to change a specific psychological process, which also influenced all subsequent elements, including the physiological result at the end of the chain.

The following diagram illustrates the simplified model, including the interventions.

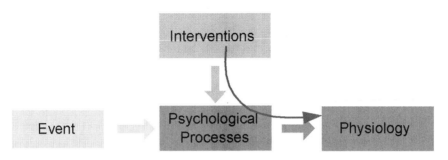

The interventions discussed in the section on direct psychological influences on physiology do not seem to fit into this model. Those interventions seem to influence physiology without going through the psychological elements.

Therefore, I suggest that an intermediate element exists between the "psychological elements" and "physiology," which I call the "Fundamental Image." The fundamental image can be defined as a (deep) unconscious image, represented by all of the senses, that guides the client's psychology and physiology.

Each psychological process influences, and is influenced by, the fundamental image. Physiology is directly guided by the fundamental image. The fundamental image acts as the core that influences every psychological process, as well as one's entire physiology.

Interventions can be grouped into those that influence the psychological elements (appraisal, coping, emotions or behavior), or those that influence the fundamental image itself. The first type influences the fundamental image and physiology through the psychological elements. The second type of psychological intervention alters the fundamental image itself, without going through the psychological elements, and thereby affects physiology more directly.

This leads to the following (simplified) diagram.

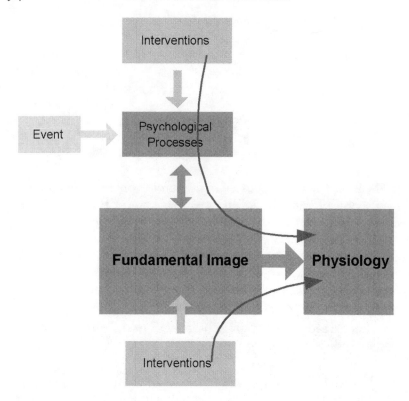

The fundamental image can also be used to gain information from clients. Clients' own images (or metaphors) about their state of health, or about their psychology, stem from this fundamental image. The therapist can use these images as a diagnostic tool, or as a starting point for an intervention to alter the fundamental image directly from "within" (17.4.3.2 Symbolic Modeling).

The fundamental image also formulates language. Language created by the fundamental image is especially interesting in the case of organ language (17.2.2 Organ Language). Observing a client's language patterns can help the therapist gain insight into the client's fundamental image. When clients utter organ language, they reinforce their fundamental image (because they also pick up their own patterns), and thus affect their own health. This illustrates that language functions both as a diagnostic tool and an intervention for addressing the client's fundamental image.

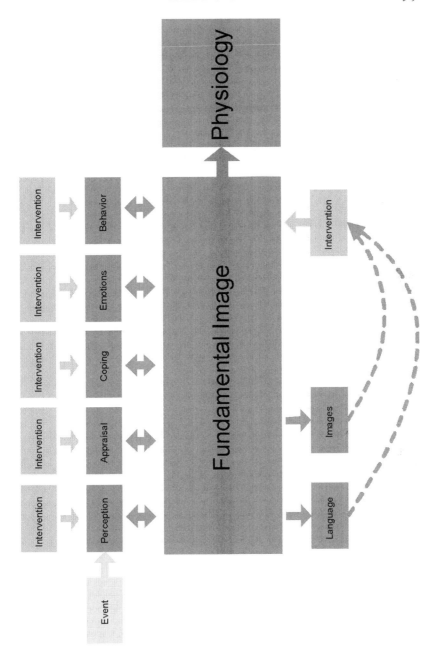

The following diagram is the full model, including the fundamental image and the interventions. It represents the functional location of the fundamental image, the psychological elements, and the interventions.

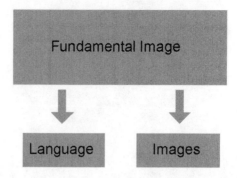

The Fundamental Image: The revised psychosomatic model

The psychological elements (perception, appraisal, coping, emotions and behavior) do not influence each other directly, as proposed by the original psychosomatic model. They influence each other via the fundamental image. The psychological elements influence this image, and at the same time are influenced by it. For example, appraisal does not directly influence coping, but appraisal does influence the fundamental image, and that image influences coping. At the same time, the fundamental image also influences the other psychological elements, such as perception, emotions, and behavior.

This new model, based on the existence of a (conscious or unconscious) fundamental image, also includes the effects observed in studies of regression (17.4.4 Regression) and Dissociative Identity Disorder (17.1 Mind-Body Connection). With this model, regression and changing alters can be explained as a replacement of the fundamental image. An entirely different fundamental image results instantaneously in radical changes in psychology and physiology.

This revised model explains how psychological interventions can influence physiology, either directly or indirectly, via the psychological elements. At the same time, this model explains the dramatic changes noticed during regression or with changing alters.

Health is therefore not created by the outcome of the psychological elements, as the previous model indicates, but as a result of the fundamental image, as indicated by this new model.

19

About the author

Rob A.A. van Overbruggen Ph.D., uses his expert knowledge of Neurolinguistics and Hypnotherapy to help clients use their minds to influence the cancer process.

Rob was born in 1972, in a small town in the south of The Netherlands. His early education was in the field of Software Engineering, where he learned to identify patterns and distil commonalities from different viewpoints. To satisfy his desire to understand the mind, he began studying Neuro Linguistic Programming, Time Line Therapy, and Hypnotherapy in 1993. A few years later, he decided to study psychological influences on the cancer process. After 12 years of study, he has finished with his dissertation: Healing Psyche - Patterns and Structure of Complementary Psychological Cancer Treatment (CPCT). In his dissertation, he identified overlapping patterns from different psychological approaches to cancer therapy. He identified the psychological patterns that influence the cancer process.

Rob holds a Doctorate in Clinical Hypnotherapy, and is an internationally licensed Hypnotherapist, NLP, and TLT Trainer. He is the founder and director of Mexion, a company specializing in therapy and training. He is the director of therapeutic research for Healing Psyche, and is responsible for maintaining the quality of licensed hypnotherapists in The Netherlands.

Rob A.A. van Overbruggen Ph.D., lives in Rotterdam, The Netherlands, where he runs a successful therapy practice and continues his research. His dissertation formed the foundation of his complementary psychological cancer treatment (CPCT) program. This program is designed for therapists to use it with their clients to aid in their healing processes. It includes guidelines for therapists, a self-help CD set for patients, a patient workbook, and the general public edition of his original dissertation. The Healing Psyche website supports this program by providing online tools for therapists to use in their psychological work with cancer patients.

Rob can be contacted via www.healingpsyche.com.

Appendix

20

Diagnostic Belief list

The purpose of this diagnostic belief list is to help the therapist to quickly determine whether the client possesses unhealthy beliefs. If the client acknowledges such unhealthy beliefs, the therapist should work on changing them. This composition is based on Simonton et al. (1978[882]; 1992[883]), LeShan (1977[884]; 1989[885]) and McDermott et al. (1996[886])

About Me
- I cannot do anything about it.
- I cannot get better.
- I will die very soon.
- I am hopeless.
- I deserve to suffer.
- I am worthless.
- I cannot ask for love.
- I do not deserve to live.
- I cannot control my feelings.
- I cannot control my thoughts.
- I am responsible for my illness.
- I have no influence over my health.
- I cannot stand this situation.
- I will never be happy again.
- I am responsible for other people's happiness.
- I cannot ask my physician those questions.

About Cancer
- Cancer is synonymous with death.
- Cancer is something that strikes from without and there is no hope of controlling it.

- Cancer is a strong and powerful enemy and is able to destroy the entire body.
- When a health problem has lasted for years, it will also take years to resolve it.

About Treatment
- The treatment is drastic and has many undesirable effects.
- Pain can only be treated with medication and surgery.
- The disease will progress and become worse.

21

Healthy Beliefs

U nlike unhealthy beliefs, the following beliefs support clients in their well-being. Such beliefs can be installed in clients.

Mind-Body
- Mind and body are one and the same. Changes in the body are reflected in the mind, and changes in the mind are reflected in the body.
- Physiological processes, such as the immune system and the endocrine system, can be modified by voluntary means.
- With imagery, I can change physiological processes.
- I listen to my body - it knows how to heal, and it tells me what to do.
- Pain and illness are messages from my body, telling me what to do.

Cancer
- Cancer also conveys a hidden message. Understanding this message will help me to improve my quality of life.
- The immune system influences cancer growth and healing.
- Psychological factors and emotional responses to stress play a crucial role in modulating the immune system.
- Physicians are very successful in curing cancer.
- There are always cancer cells present in the body, but the immune system prevents them from doing any harm.

Personal
- I believe that my goals are achievable.
- I have whatever it takes to reach my goals.
- I deserve to get well.

- Life is to be celebrated.
- I am valuable and have something to contribute to this world.
- What I am doing is something to be proud of.
- I accept myself as I am.
- I want to be healthy.
- I have many choices of how to respond.
- It is possible for me to be healthy and feel well.

Healing
- People can overcome cancer, even if it seems impossible.
- Everyone's healing journey is unique. I do not know how my personal healing process will manifest itself.
- Health is a continuous, ongoing process.
- Beliefs influence emotions, and emotions significantly influence health.
- Changing limiting beliefs improves one's quality of life and promotes healing.
- I can easily learn to change my beliefs.
- Stress promotes disease; relaxation promotes health.
- Resolving unwanted emotions releases one's healing energy and influences health.
- My active participation will help to increase my quality of life.
- My body is designed to be healthy and well. It was built to be able to recognize health and well-being, as well as to heal itself.
- My body has already healed itself from different illnesses many times before, so it knows what to do.
- I can support my body in getting well.
- Psychological factors play a crucial role in healing.
- Events have changed my life, but that does not mean that my life has changed for the worse. I will decide how my life has been changed.
- While there may be moments of uncertainty, there will always be reasons for hope.
- Healing is a normal and natural process. The body can restore itself, even from cancer.
- Many people have healed from cancer, sometimes even without medical attention.

22

Imagery Scripts

22.1   Fighting Imagery

Script adapted from Simonton et al. (1978[887])

- Sit back, relax, and close your eyes.
- Imagine yourself in a pleasant and relaxed state.
- Imagine the cancer cells as weak and confused.
- Imagine the treatment coming into your body.
- If you are receiving radiation treatment, picture it as a beam of millions of bullets of energy hitting any cancer cells in its path.
- Imagine the healthy cells repairing themselves, and the cancer cells dying.
- If you are receiving chemotherapy, picture that drug coming into your body and entering your bloodstream. Picture the drug acting like a poison.
- Imagine the healthy cells recognizing the poison and staying away from it. The cancer cells absorb the poison and die.
- Imagine the body's own strong, vast army of white blood cells easily finding and destroying the cancer cells.
- Imagine the cancer shrinking, and the dead cancer cells being flushed out of your body.
- Imagine the cancer shrinking until it is gone, while your energy and strength increase.
- Imagine yourself reaching your goals in life, and having strong reasons to live.
- Open your eyes.

22.2   Cooperating Imagery

Adapted from Simonton et al. (1992[888])

- Sit back and relax.

- Imagine that your body is cooperating with your chosen treatment in order to heal itself.
- Imagine that your cancer is a messenger, communicating a message sent from a loving source to you.
- Imagine that you become aware of the ways in which you need to change in order to become more of who you are.
- Imagine one step you can take to act on this message in order to change.
- Decide to take action and take the first step.
- Imagine what it will feel like as you begin to regain your natural state of health.
- Imagine the cancer leaving your body, having served as a messenger that brought about needed changes in your life.
- Open your eyes.

When using this cooperative imagery, Simonton et al. suggest that the client write down the actions he is going to take immediately after the imagery session.

23

Healing Psyche Online Resources

To accompany this dissertation, I have developed a website: http://www.healingpsyche.com. This site is intended to provide a platform for therapists working with cancer clients on a psychological basis. Therapists can find information on Complementary Psychological Cancer Treatment (CPCT) protocols and interventions. Clients can find information and resources to support them in their healing process.

One of these resources is a set of questionnaires that can be used by clients to gain insight into their healing process. The results of these questionnaires can be used by the therapist. It allows the therapist to go straight to the most problematic issues. When these are resolved, that will boost the client's healing process.

One of the resource tools is the "stressor inventory." This questionnaire was created by integrating several of the questionnaires discussed in this dissertation, and lists events that clients have experienced in their lives. The questionnaire asks clients what triggers they have perceived, and on what dates. The dates are used to quantify the triggers during a certain timeframe. After completing the questionnaire, clients can choose to print out several different reports, grouped by timeframe. These reports include the Homes and Rahe "Life Change Units," and the Cochrane and Roberts "points."

The data gathered will be analyzed for further development of Complementary Psychological Cancer Treatments (CPCT). Although it is not mandatory to include the type of disease, that would help enormously in the development of treatment programs. Please direct clients to these tools and ask them to include as much information as possible about their disease.

FREE Companying Audio Program

Thank you for reading this book all the way through. I hope you enjoyed it and learned many new things. Based on my research, I created a very special audio program to accompany this book and this program is for sale during my seminars. This is a very advanced audio program that liberates your life from those limiting thoughts and emotions. People who have bought and used this program noticed marvellous results.

This is what other people said about this program:

- *"I finally can sleep well again" – Will*

- *"I do not know what happened, but I feel more relaxed now" – Malou*

- *"It is an intensive program, but I am glad I followed through, thank you Rob" – Richard*

- *"I already noticed the first shifts in the first week." - Joyce*

This program was previously exclusively sold at my seminars, but I would like you to benefit from it too, even if we have never met.

So I decided to GIVE you this for FREE, just as a present from me to you for having read my book.

Here is how to get your free audio program
Go to: **HTTP://WWW.HEALINGPSYCHE.COM**
And click on: **REGISTER**
Fill in your name and email address and the program will be sent to you and remember...
Your Health is in Your Hands

Rob van Overbruggen Ph.D.

24

Bibliography

(Endnotes)

[1] Siegel, Bernie S (1986) <u>Love, Medicine and Miracles</u>, New York: Harper and Row

[2] Greco, P.J. & Eisenberg, J.M. (1993) 'Changing physicians' practices,' <u>New England Journal of Medicine</u>, 329(17):1271-3

[3] O'Regan, Brendan (ed) & Hirshberg, Caryle (ed) (1993) <u>Spontaneous Remission - An Annotated Bibliography</u>: Inst. of Noetic Sciences

[4] Garssen, Bert (2004) 'Psychological factors and cancer development - Evidence after 30 years of research,' <u>Clinical Psychology Review</u>

[5] Spiegel, David (2002) 'Effects of psychotherapy on Cancer Survival,' <u>Nature Reviews</u>, 2:338-389

[6] Answer: Place one of the coins in the horizontal row of 4, on top of the coin that intersects both the horizontal and vertical rows.

[7] Preamble to the Constitution of the World Health Organization as adopted by the International Health Conference, New York, 19-22 June, 1946; signed on 22 July, 1946, by the representatives of 61 States (Official Records of the World Health Organization, no. 2, p. 100) and entered into force on 7 April 1948.

[8] Temoshok, Linda & Dreher, Henry (1992), <u>Type C Connection, The - The Mind-Body Link to cancer and your Health</u>, Random House

[9] National Institutes Of Health (1995), <u>Alternative Medicine - Expanding Medical Horizons A Report to the National Institutes of Health on Alternative Medical Systems and Practices in the United States</u>

[10] Green, Elmer & Green, Alice M. (1977), <u>Beyond Biofeedback</u>, New York: Delacorte

[11] Pelletier, Kenneth R. (1992), <u>Mind as a Healer, Mind as a Slayer</u>, New York: Delacorte

[12] Cohen, S. & Smith, A.P. & Tyrrell, D.A.J. (1991), 'Psychological Stress and Susceptibility to the Common Cold,' New England Journal of Medicine, 325:606-612

[13] 'Breast Cancer: How Your Mind Can Help Your Body,' American Psychological Association Practice Directorate, 1997

[14] Eysenck, Hans Jurgen & Grossarth-Maticek, Ronald (1991) 'Creative novation behaviour therapy as a prophylactic treatment for cancer and coronary heart disease - Part II effects of treatment,' Behaviour Research and Therapy, 29:17-31

[15] Grossarth-Maticek, Ronald & Bastiaan, Ronald Jan & Kanazir, Dusan T. (1985) 'Psychosocial factors as strong predictions of mortality from cancer, ischemic heart disease and stroke - Yugoslav Prospective Study,' J. of Psychosomatic Research, Vol. 29, pp. 167-176.

[16] Grossarth-Maticek, Ronald & Eysenck, Hans Jurgen (1995) 'Self-regulation and mortality from cancer, coronary heart disease, and other causes - A prospective study,' Personality and Individual Differences, 19(6):781-795

[17] Eugene Pendergrass, 1959, then President of the American Cancer Society, in an address to the Society

[18] Bahnson, Claus Bahne (1980), 'Stress and cancer - State of the Art,' Psychosomatics, 21(12):975-980 in Lerner, Michael (1994), Choices in Healing, Cambridge: MIT Press

[19] Gendron, Enquiries into nature, knowledge, and the cure of cancers, in LeShan, Lawrence (1989), Cancer as a Turning Point: Penguin Putman

[20] Burrows, J.A., 'A Practical Essay On Cancer,' 1783 in Simonton, O. Carl & Simonton - Matthews, Stephanie & Creighton, James L (1978), Getting Well Again, New York: Bantam Books

[21] Nunn, T.h. 'Cancer of the breast,' J &A Churchill 1822 in Simonton, O. Carl & Simonton - Matthews, Stephanie & Creighton, James L (1978), Getting Well Again, New York: Bantam Books

[22] Walshe, Walter Hoyle, 'Nature and Treatment of Cancer,' 1846, in LeShan, Lawrence (1989) Cancer as a Turning Point: Penguin Putman

[23] Claus Bahne Bahnson 'Stress and cancer: The state of the art,' Psychosomatics 21(12):975 1980 in Lerner, Michael (1994) 'Choices in Healing,' Cambridge: MIT Press

[24] Parker, Willard, Cancer : a study of ninety-seven cases of cancer of the female breast, 1885, in Pelletier, Kenneth R. (1992), Mind as a Healer,

Mind as a Slayer, New York: Delacorte

[25] Paget, Sir James, Surgical Pathology, Longman's Green, in LeShan, Lawrence (1989), Cancer as a Turning Point: Penguin Putman

[26] Watson, Thomas, Sir, in LeShan, Lawrence (1989), Cancer as a Turning Point: Penguin Putman

[27] Snow, Herbert (1893), Cancer and the cancer process, J &A Churchill, in Simonton, O. Carl & Simonton - Matthews, Stephanie & Creighton, James L (1978), Getting Well Again, New York: Bantam Books

[28] Snow, Herbert (1893), Cancer and the cancer process, J &A Churchill, in LeShan, Lawrence (1989), Cancer as a Turning Point: Penguin Putman

[29] Evans, Elida (1926), Psychological Study of Cancer, Dodd, Mead & Company

[30] (2004) Kanker, wat moet je ervan weten? KWF Kankerbestrijding

[31] (2004) Kanker, wat moet je ervan weten? KWF Kankerbestrijding

[32] Chopra, Deepak (1989)'Quantum Healing - Exploring the frontiers of mind-body medicine, New York: Bantam

[33] Dollinger, Malin & Rosenbaum, Ernest H. & Cable, Greg (1997) Everyone's Guide to cancer therapy - How cancer is Diagnosed, Treated and Managed Day to Day, Toronto: Summerville House Books

[34] Dollinger, Malin & Rosenbaum, Ernest H. & Cable, Greg (1997) Everyone's Guide to cancer therapy - How cancer is Diagnosed, Treated and Managed Day to Day, Toronto: Summerville House Books

[35] Riley, Vernon (1975) Mouse Mammary Tumors: Alteration of incidence as apparent function of stress in Simonton, O. Carl & Simonton - Matthews, Stephanie & Creighton, James L (1978) Getting Well Again, New York: Bantam Books

[36] Glasser, Ronald (1976) The body is the hero in Simonton, O. Carl & Simonton - Matthews, Stephanie & Creighton, James L (1978) Getting Well Again, New York: Bantam Books

[37] West, P.M. (1954) Origin and development of the psychological approach to the cancer problem, University of California Press, 17-26

[38] Barrios, A.A. (1961) Hypnosis as a possible means for curing cancer: unpublished

[39] Rossi, E (1986) Psychobiology of Mind Body Healing, New York: W.W. Norton

[40] Elizabeth Arias, Ph.D.; Robert N. Anderson, Ph.D.; Hsiang-Ching Kung, Ph.D.; Sherry L. Murphy, B.S.; Kenneth D. Kochanek, M.A. (2003) Deaths: Final Data for 2001, Division of Vital Statistics

[41] Steward, FJ (1925) 'Cancer of the Breast, Recurrence Thirty-One Years After Operation' British Medical Journal 1, 156 in O'Regan, Brendan (ed) & Hirshberg, Caryle (ed) (1993) Spontaneous Remission - An annotated Bibliography: Inst. of Noetic Sciences

[42] American Cancer Society (2002) SEER Cancer Statistics Review, 1973-1993.

[43] American Cancer Society (2002) SEER Cancer Statistics Review, 1973-1998.

[44] Cancer Facts & Figures 2004, American Cancer Society

[45] Blumberg, E.M. & West, R.M. & Ellis, F.W. (1954) 'Possible relationship between psychological factors and human cancer,' Psychosomatic Medicine, 16:277-290

[46] Folkman, S (1997) 'Positive psychological states and coping with severe stress,' Social Science and Medicine, 45:1207-1221

[47] Selye, Hans (1956) Stress Of Life, New York: McGraw-Hill

[48] Selye, Hans (1956) Stress Of Life, New York: McGraw-Hill

[49] Lazarus, Richard S. (1966) Psychological Stress and the Coping Process, New York: McGraw-Hill

[50] Vingerhoets, AJJM & Rigter, H (ed.) (1994) Stress en Gezondheid, Tilburg: Tilburg University Press

[51] Published at the Dept. of Medical Oncology, University of Newcastle upon Tyne

[52] Basowitz, H & Persky, H & Korchin, S.J. & Grinker, R.R. (1955) Anxiety and Stress, New York: McGraw-Hill

[53] Reid, D (1948) 'Sickness and stress in operational flying,' British J. of Social Medicine, 2:123-131

[54] Fritz, C.E. (1957) 'Disaster compared in six American communities,' Human Organization, 16:6-9

[55] Lazarus, Richard S. & Baker, R.W. & Broverman, M. & Mayer, J. (1957) 'Personality and psychological stress,' J. of Personality, 25:559-577

[56] Vingerhoets, A.J.J.M. & Rigter, H. (ed.) (1994) Stress en Gezondheid, Tilburg: Tilburg University Press

[57] Howard, Pierce J (1994) Owner's manual for the brain, Texas: Bard Press

[58] Thompson, G (1988) The Psychobiology of Emotions, New York: Plenum

[59] Plutchik, R (ed.) & Kellerman, H (ed.) (1989) The emotions: Theory, Research, and Experience - Measurement of Emotions, San Diego: Academic Press

[60] Lazarus, Richard S. (1991) Emotion and Adaptation, New York: Oxford University Press

[61] Folkman, S. (1997) 'Positive psychological states and coping with severe stress,' Social Science and Medicine, 45:1207-1221

[62] Wolff, H.G. (1953) Stress and disease, Illinois: Charles C. Thomas in Monat, Alan (ed.) & Lazarus, Richard S. (ed.) (1977) Stress and Coping - Anthology, New York: Columbia University Press

[63] Selye, Hans (1956) Stress Of Life, New York: McGraw-Hill

[64] Holmes, T.H. & Rahe, R.H. (1967) 'Social readjustment rating scale,' J. of Psychosomatic Research, 11:213-218

[65] Holmes, T.H. & Rahe, R.H. (1967) 'Social readjustment rating scale,' J. of Psychosomatic Research, 11:213-218

[66] Brown, George W. (ed.) & Harris, Tirril O. (ed.) (1989) Life events and illness, New York: Guilford Press

[67] Cochrane, R. & Robertson, A. (1973) 'Life Events Inventory - A Measure of the Relative Severity of Psycho-Social Stressors,' J. of Psychosomatic Research

[68] Rahe, Richard H. & Bennett, L. & Romo, M. & Arthur, R.J. (1973) 'Subjects' recent life changes and coronary heart disease in Finland,' Am. J. Psychiatry, 130:1222-1226

[69] Mattila, V.J. & Salokangas, R.K (1977) 'Life changes and social group in relation to illness onset,' J. of Psychosomatic Research, 21:167-174

[70] Holmes, T.H. & Rahe, R.H. (1967) 'Social readjustment rating scale,' J. of Psychosomatic Research, 11:213-218

[71] Brown, George W. (ed.) & Harris, Tirril O. (ed.) (1989) Life events and illness, New York: Guilford Press

[72] Symington, T. & Currie, A.R. & Curran, R.S. & Davidson, J.N. (1955) Reaction of the adrenal cortex in conditions of stress, Boston: Little, Brown and company Hill in Monat, Alan (ed.) & Lazarus, Richard

S. (ed.) (1977) Stress and Coping - Anthology, New York: Columbia University Press

[73] Shannon, T.X. & Isbell, G.M. (1963) 'Stress in dental patients: Effect of local anesthetic procedures - Technical Report No SAM-TDR-63-29; US Air Force School of Aerospace Medicine,' Texas: Brooks Air Force Base

[74] Epstein, S (1967) Towards a unified theory of anxiety, in B.A. Maher (ed.) Progress in Experimental Personality Research, Vol. 4, New York, Academic Press.

[75] Brinbaum, R.M. (1964) Autonomic reaction to threat and confrontation conditions of psychological stress - unpublished doctoral dissertation, Berkely: University of California Press

[76] Nomikos, M.S. & Opton, E.M. & Averil, J.R. & Lazarus, Richard S. (1968) 'Surprise versus suspense in the production of stress reaction,' J. of Personality and Social Psychology, 8:204-208

[77] Lazarus, Richard S. & Averil, J.R. & Opton, E.M. (1970) Towards a cognitive theory of emotion, San Diego: Academic Press in Monat, Alan (ed.) & Lazarus, Richard S. (ed.) (1977) Stress and Coping - Anthology, New York: Columbia University Press

[78] Lazarus, Richard S. & Deese, J. & Osler, S. (1951) Review of research on effects of psychological stress upon performance, Research Bulletin: Human Resource Research Center, 51-28 in Monat, Alan (ed.) & Lazarus, Richard S. (ed.) (1977) Stress and Coping - Anthology, New York: Columbia University Press

[79] Arnold, M.B. (1960) Emotion and Personality – Vol. 1 + 2, New York: Columbia University Press in Monat, Alan (ed.) & Lazarus, Richard S. (ed.) (1977) Stress and Coping - Anthology, New York: Columbia University Press

[80] Lazarus, Richard S. (1966) Psychological Stress and the Coping Process, New York: McGraw-Hill in Monat, Alan (ed.) & Lazarus, Richard S. (ed.) (1977) Stress and Coping - Anthology, New York: Columbia University Press

[81] Appley, M.H. (1962) 'Motivation, threat perception, and the induction of psychological stress,' Proc. of the 16th International Congress of Psychology, 880-881 in Monat, Alan (ed.) & Lazarus, Richard S. (ed.) (1977) Stress and Coping - Anthology, New York: Columbia University Press

[82] Goldstein, M.J. (1959) 'Relationship between coping and avoiding behavior and response to fear-arousing propaganda,' J. of Abnormal and Social Psychology, 58:247-252 in Monat, Alan (ed.) & Lazarus, Richard S. (ed.) (1977) Stress and Coping - Anthology, New York: Columbia University Press

[83] Eckerman, W.C. (1964) 'Relationship of need achievement to production, job satisfaction, and psychological stress,' Dissertation Abstracts, 24:3446 in Monat, Alan (ed.) & Lazarus, Richard S. (ed.) (1977) Stress and Coping - Anthology, New York: Columbia University Press

[84] Selye, Hans (1956) Stress of Life, New York: McGraw-Hill

[85] Lazarus, Richard S. (1991) Emotion and Adaption, New York: Oxford University Press

[86] Volgyesi, F.A. (1954) 'School for Patients - Hypnosis therapy and psychoprophylaxis,' British Journal of Medical Hypnosis, 5:8-17

[87] Beecher, H.K. (1959) Measurement of subjective responses - Quantitative effects of drugs, New York: Oxford University Press Rossi, E. (1986) Psychobiology of Mind Body Healing, New York: W.W. Norton

[88] Evans, F. (1985) Expectancy, therapeutic instructions, and the placebo response in Tursky, B (ed.) & Schwartz, G. (ed.) (1985) Placebo - Theory, research, and mechanism, New York: Guilford Press

[89] Beecher, H.K. (1961) 'Surgery as placebo,' J. American Medical Association, 176:1102-1107

[90] Brehm, M.F. & Back, K.W. & Bogdonoff, M.D. (1964) 'Physiological effect of cognitive dissonance under stress and deprivation,' J. of Abnormal and Social Psychology, 69:303-310 in Monat, Alan (ed.) & Lazarus, Richard S. (ed.) (1977) Stress and Coping - Anthology, New York: Columbia University Press;

[91] Wrightsman, L.S. (1960) 'Effects of waiting with others on changes in level of felt anxiety,' J. of Abnormal and Social Psychology, 61:216-222 in Monat, Alan (ed.) & Lazarus, Richard S. (ed.) (1977) Stress and Coping - Anthology, New York: Columbia University Press

[92] Wolf, S. (1950) 'Effects of suggestion and conditioning on the action of chemical agents in human subjects - The pharmacology of placebo's,' J. of Clinical Investigation, 29;100-109

[93] Rossi, E. (1986) Psychobiology of Mind Body Healing, New York: W.W. Norton

[94] Goleman Ph.D., Daniel (ed.) (1993) Mind Body Medicine - How to use your Mind for Better Health, New York: Consumer Reports Books

[95] Fielding, J.W.L. & Fagg, S.L. & Jones, B.G. & Et Alia, (1983) 'An interim report of a prospective, randomized, controlled study of adjuvant chemotherapy in operable gastric cancer - British stomach cancer group,' World J Surg, 7:390-399

[96] Cannon, Walter Bradford (1942) 'Voodoo Death,' Am. Anthropologist, 44:169-181 in Rossi, E. (1986) 'Psychobiology of Mind Body Healing,' New York: W.W. Norton

[97] Cannon, Walter Bradford (1963) Wisdom of the body 2nd, New York: W.W. Norton in Rossi, E. (1986) Psychobiology of Mind Body Healing, New York: W.W. Norton

[98] Simmons, Leo W. (1947) SUN CHIEF The Autobiography of a Hopi Indian, New Haven: Yale University Press

[99] Simonton, O. Carl & Simonton - Matthews, Stephanie & Creighton, James L. (1978) Getting Well Again, New York: Bantam

[100] Oosterwijk, Mieke (2004) Cognitieve strategieen van borstkankerpatienten en de relatie met aanpassing - Longitudinale studie, University of Maastricht

[101] Folkman, Susan (1997) 'Positive psychological states and coping with severe stress,' Social Science and Medicine, 45:1207-1221

[102] Mechanic, D. (1962) Students under stress, New York: Free Press of Glencoe in Monat, Alan (ed.) & Lazarus, Richard S. (ed.) (1977) Stress and Coping - Anthology, New York: Columbia University Press

[103] Folkman, S. (1997) 'Positive psychological states and coping with severe stress,' Social Science and Medicine, 45:1207-1221

[104] Folkman, S. (1997) 'Positive psychological states and coping with severe stress,' Social Science and Medicine, 45:1207-1221

[105] Menninger, Karl (1954) 'Regulatory Devices of the Ego Under Major Stress,' J. of the American Psychoanalytic Association, 1:67-106

[106] Gendron, (1759) Enquiries into nature, knowledge, and the cure of cancers, in Simonton, O. Carl & Simonton - Matthews, Stephanie & Creighton, James L (1978) Getting Well Again, New York: Bantam

[107] Simonton, O. Carl & Simonton - Matthews, Stephanie & Creighton, James L (1978) Getting Well Again, New York: Bantam

[108] Ramirez, A.J. & Craig, TKC & Watson, J.P. & Fentiman, IS & North, W.R.S. & Rubens, R.D. (1989) 'Stress and relapse of breast cancer,' British Medical Journal, 298:291-293

[109] Geyer, S (1991) 'Life events prior to manifestation of breast cancer - a limited prospective study covering eight years before diagnosis,' J. of Psychosomatic Research, 35:355-363

[110] Forsen, A (1991) 'Psychosocial stress as a risk for breast cancer,' Psychotherapy and Psychosomatics, 55:176-185

[111] Cooper, Cary L. & Faragher, E.B. (1993) 'Psychosocial Stress and Breast Cancer - the inter-relationship between stress events, coping strategies and personality,' Psychological Medicine, 23:653-662

[112] Chen, C.C. & David, A.S. & Nunnerley, H & Michell, M & Dawson, J.L. & Berry, H & Dobbs, J & Fahy, T (1995) 'Adverse Life events and breast cancer - case-control study,' British Medical Journal, 311:1527-1530

[113] Goodkin, Karl & Antoni, Michael H. & Blaney, P.H. (1986) 'Stress and hopelessness in the promotion of cervical intraepithelial neoplasia to invasive squamous cell carcinoma of the cervix,' J. of Psychosomatic Research, 30:67-76

[114] Garssen, Bert (2001) Psychosociale factoren en het beloop van kanker - een literatuuroverzicht, tsg, 365-371

[115] Snow, Herbert (1893) Cancer and the cancer process, London: J &A Churchill

[116] Evans, Dr, Elida (1926) Psychological Study of Cancer, New York: Dodd, Mead & Company

[117] Greene Jr, W.A. (1954) 'Psychological factors and reticuloendothelial disease I - Preliminary observations on a group of males with lymphomas and Leukemia,' Psychosomatic Medicine, 16:220-230

[118] LeShan, Lawrence & Worthington, R.E. (1956) 'Some recurrent life history patterns observed in patients with malignant disease,' J. Nerv Ment. Disorders, 124:460-465

[119] LeShan, PhD, Lawrence (1977) You can fight for your life, New York: M. Evans

[120] Pennebaker, J.W. & Kiecolt-Glaser PhD, Janice K. & Glaser, Ronald (1988) 'Disclosure of traumas and immune function: Health implications for psychotherapy,' J. of Consulting and Clinical Psychology, 56;2;239-245

[121] Holland, Jimmy C (1990) Behavioral and Psychological Risk Factors in Cancer - Human Studies, New York: Oxford University Press

[122] LeShan, PhD, Lawrence (1989) Cancer as a Turning Point, Penguin Putman

[123] Cooper, Cary L. & Faragher, E.B. (1993) 'Psychosocial Stress and Breast Cancer - the inter-relationship between stress events, coping strategies and personality,' Psychological Medicine, 23:653-662

[124] Glaser, Ronald & Kiecolt-Glaser PhD, Janice K. (1994) Stress-Associated Immune Modulation and Its Implications for Reactivation of Latent Herpes viruses, Ohio State University Medical Center

[125] Martikainen, P & Valkonen, T (1996) 'Mortality after death of a spouse - Rates and causes of death in a large Finnish cohort,' Am. J. of Public Health, 86:1087-1093

[126] Booth, Gary (1969) 'General and organic specific object relationships in cancer,' Ann. N.Y, Acad. Sci, 164; 568-577

[127] Greer, Steven & Morris, T. (1975) 'Psychological attributes of women who develop breast cancer - A controlled study,' J. of Psychosomatic Research, 19; 147-153

[128] Holmes, T.H. & Rahe, Richard H. (1967) 'Social readjustment rating scale,' J. of Psychosomatic Research, 11:213-218

[129] Brown, G.W. & Harris, T (1979) College life events and difficulty schedule, the - directory of severity for longer term difficulties, University of London

[130] Kissen, David M. (1967) 'Psychosocial factors, personality and lung cancer in men aged 55-64,' British J. Med. Psychology, 40:29

[131] LeShan, Lawrence & Worthington, R.E. (1956) 'Some recurrent life history patterns observed in patients with malignant disease,' J. Nerv Ment. Disorders, 124:460-465

[132] Simonton, O. Carl & Simonton - Matthews, Stephanie (1975) 'Belief Systems and management of emotional aspects of malignancy,' J. of Transpersonal Psychology, 7 no. 1: 29-48

[133] Blumberg, E.M. & West, R.M. & Ellis, F.W. (1954) 'Possible relationship between psychological factors and human cancer,' Psychosomatic Medicine, 16:277-290

[134] Jansen, M.A. & Muenz, L.R. (1984) 'Retrospective study of personality variables associated with fibrocystic disease and breast cancer, A,' J. of Psychosomatic Research, 28;35-42

[135] Stavraky, K.M & Donner, A.P. & Kincade, J.E. & Stewart, M.A. (1988) 'Effect of psychosocial factors on lung cancer mortality at one year,' J Clin. Epidemiology, 41:75-82

[136] Kune, G.A. & Kune, S. & Watson, L.F. & Bahnson, Claus Bahne (1991) 'Personality as a risk factor in large bowel cancer - data from the Melbourne Colorectal Cancer Study,' Psychological Medicine, 21(1):29-41

[137] Petitto, J.M. (1993) 'Genetic differences in social behavior - Relation to NK function and tumor development,' Neuropsychopharmacology, 8:35

[138] LeShan, PhD, Lawrence & Worthington, R.E. (1956) 'Personality as a factor in the pathogenesis of cancer - Review of the literature,' British J. Med. Psychology, 29:49-56

[139] Brémond, A & Kune, G.A. & Bahnson, Claus Bahne (1986) 'Psychosomatic factors in breast cancer patients - Results of a case control study,' J. of Psychosomatic Obstetrics and Gynecology, 5;127-136

[140] Temoshok, Linda (1987) 'Personality, Coping Style, Emotion and Cancer - Towards an Integrative Model,' Cancer Surveys, 6(3)545-567

[141] Simonton, O. Carl & Simonton - Matthews, Stephanie (1978) Getting Well Again, New York: Bantam

[142] Bahnson, Claus Bahne & Bahnson, M.B. (1966) 'Role of ego defenses - Denial and repression in the etiology of malignant neoplasm,' Ann. N.Y, Acad. Sci, 125; 827-845

[143] Bahnson, M.B. & Bahnson, Claus Bahne (1969) 'Ego defenses in cancer patients,' Ann. N.Y, Acad. Sci, 14;164(2):546-59

[144] Temoshok, Linda (1987) 'Personality, Coping Style, Emotion and Cancer - Towards an Integrative Model,' Cancer Surveys, 6(3)545-567

[145] LeShan, Lawrence (1989) Cancer as a Turning Point, Penguin Putman

[146] Evans, Dr, Elida (1926) Psychological Study of Cancer, New York: Dodd, Mead & Company

[147] Greene Jr., W.A. (1954) 'Psychological factors and reticuloendothelial disease I - Preliminary observations on a group of males with lymphomas and leukemia,' Psychosomatic Medicine, 16:220-230

[148] LeShan, PhD, Lawrence (1977) You Can Fight for Your Life, New York: M. Evans

[149] LeShan, PhD, Lawrence (1989) Cancer as a Turning Point, Penguin Putman

[150] Bahnson, Claus Bahne & Bahnson, M.B. (1966) 'Role of ego defenses - Denial and repression in the etiology of malignant neoplasm,' Ann. N.Y, Acad. Sci, 125; 827-845

[151] Bahnson, M.B. & Bahnson, Claus Bahne (1969) 'Ego defenses in cancer patients,' Ann. N.Y, Acad. Sci, 14;164(2):546-59

[152] Newton, Bernhauer W. (1982) 'Use of Hypnotherapy in the Treatment of Cancer Patients,' American Journal of Clinical Hypnosis, 25(2-3):104-113

[153] LeShan, PhD, Lawrence (1989) Cancer as a Turning Point, Penguin Putman

[154] LeShan, PhD, Lawrence (1989) Cancer as a Turning Point, Penguin Putman

[155] LeShan, PhD, Lawrence (1977) You Can Fight for Your Life, New York: M. Evans

[156] LeShan, PhD, Lawrence (1989) Cancer as a Turning Point, Penguin Putman

[157] Visintainer, M.A. (1982) 'Tumor rejection in rats after inescapable or escapable shock,' Science, 216:437

[158] Sklar, Lawrence S. & Anisman, Hymie (1981) 'Stress and cancer,' Psychological Bulletin, 89;369-406

[159] Greer, S. & Silverfarb, Peter M (1982) 'Psychological Concomitants of Cancer - Current State of Research,' Psychological Medicine, 12:567-568

[160] Temoshok, Linda (1987) 'Personality, coping style, emotion and cancer,' Cancer Survivor, 6:545

[161] Peterson, C. & Maier, S.F. & Seligman, M.E.P. (1987) Learned helplessness - A theory for the age of personal control, New York: Oxford University Press

[162] Shavit, Yehuda (1990) 'Stress-Induced Immune Modulation in Animals - Opiates and Endogenous Opiod Peptides,' Academic Press, 789-790 in Ader, Robert & Cohen, Nicholas & Felten, David (1990) PsychoNeuroImmunology, San Diego: Academic Press

[163] Wiedenfeld, S.A. & O'Leary, A & Bandura, A & Brown, S & Levine, S & Raska, K (1990) 'Impact of perceived self-efficacy in coping with stressors on components of the immune system,' J. of Personality and Social Psychology, 59(5):1082-1094

[164] Blancy, N.T. & Feaster, D. & Goodkin, K. (1992) 'Active coping style is associated with natural killer cell cytotoxicity in asymptomatic HIV-1 seropositive homosexual men,' J. of Psychosomatic Research, 36-635-650

[165] Peterson, C. & Bossio, Lisa M. (1993) Healthy Attitudes - Optimism, Hope and Control, New York: Consumer Reports Books

[166] Grossarth-Maticek, Ronald & Eysenck, Hans Jurgen (1995) 'Self-Regulation and Mortality from Cancer, Coronary Heart Disease, and Other Causes - A Prospective Study,' Personality and Individual Differences, 6:781-795

[167] Goodkin, Karl & Antoni, Michael H. & Servin, B.U. & Fox, B.H. (1993) 'Partially testable, predictive model of psychosocial factors in the etiology of cervical cancer - I biological psychological and social aspects,' Psycho-Oncology, 2:79-98

[168] Visser, Adriaan P. & Vingerhoets, A.J.J.M. & Goodkin, Karl & Peters, L. & Doornbosch, M. (1998) 'Voorstadia van baarmoederhalskanker - Spelen ook psychosociale en gedragsfactoren een rol?,' Medisch Contact, 295-297

[169] Andersen, M. Robyn & Urban, Nicole (1999) 'Participation in decision-making regarding follow-up care improves quality of life among breast-cancer survivors,' An. of Behavioral Medicine, 21

[170] Martin, Dr, Paul (1999) Healing Mind - The Vital Links Between Brain and Behavior, Immunity and Disease, St. Martin's Griffin

[171] Cunningham, Alastair J. & Phillips, Cathy & Lockwood, Gina A. & Hedley, David W. & Edmonds, Claire V.I. (2000) 'Association of

involvement in psychological self-regulation with longer survival in patients with metastatic cancer: an exploratory study,' Advances in Mind Body Medicine, 16(4):287-294.

[172] Cunningham, Alastair J. & Edmonds, Claire V.I. & Phillips, Cathy & Soots, K.I. & Hedley, David W. & Lockwood, Gina A. (2000) 'Prospective, longitudinal study of the relationship of psychological work to duration of survival in patients with metastatic cancer,' Psycho-Oncology, 9(4):323-339

[173] Cunningham, Alastair J. & Phillips, Cathy & Stephen, J & Edmonds, Claire V.I. (2002) 'Fighting for Life - A Qualitative Analysis of the Process of Psychotherapy-Assisted Self-Help in Patients With Metastatic Cancer,' Integrative Cancer Therapies, 1;2;146-161

[174] Simonton, O. Carl & Simonton - Matthews, Stephanie (1978) Getting Well Again, New York: Bantam;

[175] Simonton, O. Carl & Simonton - Matthews, Stephanie (1978) Getting Well Again, New York: Bantam

[176] Cunningham, Alastair J. & Edmonds, Claire V.I. & Phillips, Cathy & Soots, K.I. & Hedley, David W. & Lockwood, Gina A. (2000) 'Prospective, longitudinal study of the relationship of psychological work to duration of survival in patients with metastatic cancer,' Psycho-Oncology, 9(4):323-39

[177] Greer, S. & Morris, T. & Pettingale, K.W. (1979) 'Psychological responses to breast cancer - effect and outcome,' Lancet, 13:785-787

[178] Greer, S. & Morris, T. & Pettingale, K.W. & Haybittle, J.L. (1990) 'Psychological response to breast cancer and 15-year outcome,' Lancet, 335:49-50

[179] Dean, C. & Surtees, P.G. (1989) 'Do psychological factors predict survival in breast cancer?' J. of Psychosomatic Research, 33:561-569

[180] Butow, P.N. & Coates, A.S. & Dunn, S.M. (1999) 'Psychosocial predictors of survival in metastatic melanoma,' J Clin Oncology, 17:2256-2263

[181] Butow, P.N. & Coates, A.S. & Dunn, S.M. (2000) 'Psychosocial predictors of survival - Metastatic breast cancer,' Ann. Oncology, 11:469-474

[182] Oosterwijk, Mieke (2004) Cognitieve strategieen van borstkankerpatienten en de relatie met aanpassing - longitudionale studie, University of Maastricht

[183] Cooper, Cary L. & Faragher, E.B. (1993) 'Psychosocial Stress and Breast Cancer,' Psychological Medicine, 23:653

[184] Bleiker, Eveline M.A. & Ploeg, Henk. van der & Hendriks, Jan H.C.L. & Ader, Herman J (1996) 'Personality Factors and Breast Cancer Development - a Prospective Longitudinal Study,' J. Nat. Cancer Institute, 88-20:1480-1482

[185] Temoshok, Linda (1985) 'Biopsychological Studies on Cutaneous Malignant Melanoma - Psychosocial Factors Associated with prognostic indicators, Progression, Psychophysiology, and tumor-Host Response,' Social Science and Medicine, 20(8):833-840 in Lerner, Michael (1994) Choices in Healing, Cambridge: MIT Press;

[186] Pert, C.B. (1997) Molecules of Emotion - Why You Feel the Way You Feel, New York: Simon and Schuster; 285

[187] Moyers, Bill (1993) Healing and the Mind, New York: Bantam

[188] Temoshok, Linda (1985) 'Biopsychological Studies on Cutaneous Malignant Melanoma - Psychosocial Factors Associated with prognostic indicators, Progression, Psychophysiology, and tumor-Host Response,' Social Science and Medicine, 20(8):833-840 in Lerner, Michael (1994) Choices in Healing, Cambridge: MIT Press;

[189] Pert, Candace B. (1997) Molecules of Emotion - Why You Feel the Way You Feel, New York: Simon and Schuster

[190] Blumberg, E.M. & West, R.M. & Ellis, F.W. (1954) 'Possible relationship between psychological factors and human cancer,' Psychosomatic Medicine, 16:277-290

[191] LeShan, PhD, Lawrence & Worthington, R.E. (1956) 'Loss of cathexes as a common psychodynamic characteristic of cancer patients - An attempt at statistical validation of a clinical hypothesis,' Psychological Report, 2:183-193

[192] LeShan, PhD, Lawrence (1977) You can fight for your life, New York: M. Evans

[193] Goldfarb, O. Charles & Driessen, J. & Cole, D. (1967) 'Psychophysiological aspects of malignancy,' Am. J. Psychiatry, 123:1545-1551

[194] Kissen, David M. (1966) 'Significance of personality in lung cancer in men,' Ann. N.Y, Acad. Sci, 125:820-826

[195] Dattore, P.J. & Shontz, F.C. & Coyne, L (1980) 'Premorbid personality differentiation of cancer and noncancer groups: a test of the hypothesis

of cancer proneness,' J. of Consulting and Clinical Psychology, 48(3):388-94

[196] Watson, M & Pettingale, K.W. & Greer, Steven (1984) 'Emotional control and autonomic arousal in breast cancer patients,' J. of Psychosomatic Research, 28;467-474

[197] Greer, S. & Morris, T. (1975) 'Psychological attributes of women who develop breast cancer - A controlled study,' J. of Psychosomatic Research, 19; 147-153

[198] Greer, S. & Morris, T. (1978) 'Study of psychological factors in breast cancer - Problems of,' Social Science and Medicine, 12:129-134

[199] Bagley, C (1979) 'Control of the emotions, remote stress and the emergence of breast cancer,' Int J Clin Psychol, 6(2):213-220

[200] Tarlau, M & Smalheiser, I (1951) 'Personality patterns in patients with malignant tumors of the breast and cervix - Exploratory study,' Psychosomatic Medicine, 13;117-121

[201] Reznikoff, M. (1955) 'Psychological factors in breast cancer - a preliminary study of some personality trends in patients with cancer of the breast,' Psychosomatic Medicine, 18;2;96-108

[202] Schonfield, J (1975) 'Psychological and life-experience differences between Israeli women with benign and cancerous breast lesions,' J. of Psychosomatic Research, 19;229-234

[203] Brémond, A & Kune, G.A. & Bahnson, Claus Bahne (1986) 'Psychosomatic factors in breast cancer patients - Results of a case control study,' J. of Psychosomatic Obstetrics and Gynecology, 5;127-136

[204] Weihs, K.L. & Enright, T.M. & Simmens, S.J. & Reiss, D (2000) 'Negative affectivity, restriction of emotions, and site of metastases predict mortality in recurrent breast cancer,' J. of Psychosomatic Research, 49:59-68

[205] Ganz, Bernhard J (1991) 'Psychosocial issues in lung cancer patients (part 1),' Chest, 99:216-223

[206] Thomas, Caroline B. & Duszynski, Karen R. & Shaffer, J. W (1974) 'Closeness to parents and the family constellation in a - prospective study of five disease states: suicide, mental illness, malignant tumor, hypertension and coronary heart disease,' John Hopkins Medical Journal, 134 No 5: 251-270

[207] Bieliauskas, Linus A & Garron, David C (1982) 'Psychological depression and cancer,' Gen. Hospital Psychiatry 4: 187-195 in brown

[208] Jensen, M.R. (1987) 'Psychobiological factors predicting the course of breast cancer,' J. of Personality, 55:317-342 in Visser, Adriaan & Remie, Margot & Garssen, Bert (2000) Psychosociale begeleiding en onderzoek bij kanker en aids, Utrecht: Helen Dowling Instituut;

[209] Weihs, K & Simmens, S & Reiss, D (1996) 'Survival in recurrent breast cancer patients predicted by patient coping style,' Tilburg: Katolieke Universiteit Brabant in Visser, Adriaan & Remie, Margot & Garssen, Bert (2000) Psychosociale begeleiding en onderzoek bij kanker en aids, Utrecht: Helen Dowling Instituut;

[210] Weihs, K & Enright, T.M. & Simmens, S & Reiss, D (2000) 'Negative affectivity, restriction of emotions, and site of metastases predict mortality in recurrent breast cancer,' J. of Psychosomatic Research, 49:59-68

[211] Gross, J. (1989) 'Emotional expression in cancer onset and progression,' Social Science and Medicine, 28:1239-1248

[212] Cooper, Cary L. & Faragher, E.B. (1993) 'Psychosocial Stress and Breast Cancer,' Psychological Medicine, 23:653

[213] Garssen, Bert (2000) Rol van psychologische factoren bij het ontstaan en beloop van kanker, Utrecht: Helen Dowling Instituut

[214] Garssen, Bert (2001) Psychosociale factoren en het beloop van kanker - een literatuuroverzicht, tsg, 365-371

[215] Reynolds, P & Hurley, S & Torres, M & Jackson, J & Boyd, P & Chen, V.W. (2000) 'Use of coping strategies and breast cancer survival - Results from the black/white cancer survival study,' Am. Jo of Epidemiology, 152:940-949

[216] Hislop, T.G. & Waxler, N.E. & Coldman, A.J. & Elwood, J.M. & Kan, L (1987) 'Prognostic significance of psychosocial factors in women with breast cancer,' J. Chronic Disease, 40:729-735

[217] Pert, C.B. (1997) Molecules of Emotion - Why You Feel the Way You Feel, New York: Simon and Schuster

[218] Garssen, Bert (2002) 'Psycho-oncology and cancer - linking psychosocial factors with cancer development,' Ann. Oncology, 13:171-175

[219] Bleiker, Eveline M.A. (1995) Personality factors and breast cancer - A prospective study of the relationship between psychological factors and the development of breast cancer, Vrije Universiteit Amsterdam, 261

[220] Wirsching, M. & Hoffmann, F & Stierlin, H & Weber, G & Wirsching, B (1985) 'Prebioptic psychological characteristics of breast cancer patients,' Psychotherapy and Psychosomatics, 43:69-76

[221] Watson, M & Pettingale, K.W. & Greer, Steven (1984) 'Emotional control and autonomic arousal in breast cancer patients,' J. of Psychosomatic Research, 28;467-474

[222] Grossarth-Marticek, R & Bastiaan, Ronald Jan & Kanazir, Dusan (1985) 'Psychosocial factors as strong predictions of mortality from cancer, ischemic heart disease and stroke - Yugoslav Prospective Study,' J. of Psychosomatic Research, Vol. 29, pp. 167-176.

[223] Temoshok, Linda & Dreher, Henry (1992) Type C Connection, The - The Mind-Body Link to cancer and your Health, Random House

[224] Bleiker, Eveline M.A. & Ploeg, Henk. van der & Hendriks, Jan H.C.L. & Ader, Herman J (1996) 'Personality Factors and Breast Cancer Development - a Prospective Longitudinal Study,' J. Nat. Cancer Institute, 88-20:1480-1482

[225] Hislop, T.G. & Waxler, N.E. & Coldman, A.J. & Elwood, J.M. & Kan, L (1987) 'Prognostic significance of psychosocial factors in women with breast cancer,' J. Chronic Disease, 40:729-735

[226] Waxler-Morrison, N & Hislop, T.G. & Mears, B & Kan, L (1991) 'Effects of social relationships on survival for woman with breast cancer - a prospective study,' Social Science and Medicine, 33:177-183

[227] Reynolds, P & Kaplan, G.A. (1990) 'Social connections and risk for cancer - Prospective evidence from the Alameda Country study,' Behavioral Medicine, 16:101-110

[228] Maunsell, E & Brisson, J & Dechenes, L (1995) 'Social support and survival among women with breast cancer,' Cancer, 76:631-637

[229] Pert, C.B. (1997) Molecules of Emotion - Why You Feel the Way You Feel, New York: Simon and Schuster;

[230] Gilbar, Ora (1996) 'The connection between the psychological condition of breast cancer patients and survival - A follow-up after eight years,' Gen. Hospital Psychiatry, 18;4;266-270

[231] Weihs, K.L. & Enright, T.M. & Simmens, S.J. & Reiss, D (2000) 'Negative affectivity, restriction of emotions, and site of metastases predict mortality in recurrent breast cancer,' J. of Psychosomatic Research, 49:59-68

[232] LeShan, PhD, Lawrence & Worthington, R.E. (1956) 'Loss of cathexes as a common psychodynamic characteristic of cancer patients - An attempt at statistical validation of a clinical hypothesis,' Psychological Report, 2:183-193

[233] LeShan, PhD, Lawrence (1977) You Can Fight for Your Life, New York: M. Evans

[234] Goldfarb, O. Charles & Driessen, J. & Cole, D. (1967) 'Psychophysiological aspects of malignancy,' Am. J. Psychiatry, 123:1545-1551

[235] Greer, S. & Morris, T. (1975) 'Psychological attributes of women who develop breast cancer - A controlled study,' J. of Psychosomatic Research, 19; 147-153

[236] Greer, S. & Morris, T. (1978) 'Study of psychological factors in breast cancer - Problems of,' Social Science and Medicine, 12:129-134

[237] Scherg, H & Cramer, I & Blohmke, M (1981) 'Psychosocial factors and breast cancer - a critical re-evaluation of established hypothesis,' Cancer Detect Prevention, 4(1-4):165-171

[238] Watson, M & Pettingale, K.W. & Greer, Steven (1984) 'Emotional control and autonomic arousal in breast cancer patients,' J. of Psychosomatic Research, 28;467-474

[239] Jansen, M.A. & Muenz, L.R. (1984) 'Retrospective study of personality variables associated with fibrocystic disease and breast cancer, A,' J. of Psychosomatic Research, 28;35-42

[240] Brémond, A & Kune, G.A. & Bahnson, Claus Bahne (1986) 'Psychosomatic factors in breast cancer patients - Results of a case control study,' J. of Psychosomatic Obstetrics and Gynecology, 5;127-136

[241] Simonton, O. Carl & Simonton - Matthews, Stephanie (1975) 'Belief Systems and management of emotional aspects of malignancy,' J. of Transpersonal Psychology, 7 no 1: 29-48

[242] Cooper, Cary L. & Faragher, E.B. (1993) 'Psychosocial Stress and Breast Cancer,' Psychological Medicine, 23:653

[243] Garssen, Bert (2002) 'Psycho-oncology and cancer - linking psychosocial factors with cancer development,' Ann. Oncology, 13:171-175

[244] Garssen, Bert (2004) 'Psychological factors and cancer development - Evidence after 30 years of research,' Clinical Psychology Review

[245] Schmale, A.H. & Iker, H (1971) 'Hopelessness as a predictor of cervical cancer,' Social Science and Medicine, 5:95-100

[246] Temoshok, Linda (1987) 'Personality, coping style, emotion and cancer,' Cancer Survivor, 6:545

[247] Goldfarb, O. Charles & Driessen, J. & Cole, D. (1967) 'Psychophysiological aspects of malignancy,' Am. J. Psychiatry, 123:1545-1552

[248] Thomas, Caroline B. & Duszynski, Karen R. & Shaffer, J. W (1974) 'Closeness to parents and the family constellation in a prospective study of five disease states: suicide, mental illness, malignant tumor, hypertension and coronary heart disease,' John Hopkins Medical Journal, 134 No 5: 251-270

[249] Bahnson, Claus Bahne (1980) 'Stress and cancer - State of the Art,' Psychosomatics, 21(12):975-980

[250] Jensen, M.R. (1987) 'Psychobiological factors predicting the course of breast cancer,' J. of Personality, 55:317-342

[251] Everson, S.A. & Goldberg, D.E. & Kaplan, G.A. & Cohen, R.D. & Pukalla, E & Tuomilehto, J & Salonen, J.T. (1996) 'Hopelessness and risk of mortality and incidence of myocardial infarction and cancer,' Psychological Medicine, 58:113-121

[252] Schulz, R. & Bookwala, J. & Knapp, J.E. & Scheier, M. & Williamson, G.M. (1996) 'Permission, age and cancer mortality,' Psychology of Aging, 11:304-309

[253] Molassiotis, A. & Vandenakker, O.B.A. & Milligan, D.W. & Goldman, J.M. (1997) 'Symptom distress, coping style and biological variables as predictors of survival after bone marrow transplantation,' J. of Psychosomatic Research, 42:275-285

[254] Watson, M. & Haviland, J.S. & Greer, S. & Davidson, J.N. & Bliss, J.M. (1998) 'Does psychological response influence survival from breast cancer?' Psycho-Oncology, 7:284

[255] Garssen, Bert (2000) Rol van psychologische factoren bij het ontstaan en beloop van kanker, Utrecht: Helen Dowling Instituut

[256] Garssen, Bert (2001) Psychosociale factoren en het beloop van kanker - een literatuuroverzicht, tsg, 365-371

[257] Watson, M. & Haviland, J.S. & Greer, Steven & Davidson, J. & Bliss, J.M. (1999) 'Influence of psychological response on survival in breast cancer,' Lancet, 16;354:1331-1336

[258] Greer, S. & Morris, T. & Pettingale, K.W. (1979) 'Psychological responses to breast cancer - effect and outcome,' Lancet, 13:785-787

[259] Greer, S. & Silverfarb, Peter M. (1982) 'Psychological Concomitants of Cancer - Current State of Research,' Psychological Medicine, 12:567-568

[260] Greer, S. (1991) 'Psychological response to cancer and survival,' Psychological Medicine, 21:43-49

[261] Greer, S. & Morris, T. & Pettingale, K.W. & Haybittle, J.L. (1990) 'Psychological response to breast cancer and 15-year outcome,' Lancet, 335:49-50

[262] Everson, S.A. & Goldberg, D.E. & Kaplan, G.A. & Cohen, R.D. & Pukalla, E. & Tuomilehto, J. & Salonen, J.T. (1996) 'Hopelessness and risk of mortality and incidence of myocardial infarction and cancer,' Psychosomatic Medicine, 58:113-121

[263] Grossarth-Maticek, Ronald & Bastiaan, Ronald Jan & Kanazir, Dusan (1985) 'Psychosocial factors as strong predictions of mortality from cancer, ischemic heart disease and stroke - Yugoslav Prospective Study,' J. of Psychosomatic Research, Vol. 29, pp. 167-176.

[264] Bartrop, R.W. & Luckhurst, E. & Lazarus, L. & Kiloh, L.G. & Penny, R. (1977) 'Depressed lymphocyte function after bereavement,' Lancet, 1:834-839

[265] Jasmin, C. & Le, M.G. & Marty, P & Herzberg, R (1990) 'Evidence for a link between certain psychological factors and the risk of breast cancer in a case-control study - Psycho-Oncologic Group (P.O.G.).,' Ann. Oncology, 1(1):22-29

[266] Cooper, Cary L. & Faragher, E.B. (1993) 'Psychosocial Stress and Breast Cancer - the inter-relationship between stress events, coping strategies and personality,' Psychological Medicine, 23:653-662

[267] Glaser, Ronald & Kiecolt-Glaser PhD, Janice K. & Speicher, C.E. & Holliday, J.E. (1985) 'Stress, Loneliness, and Changes in Herpes Virus Latency,' J. of Behavioral Medicine, 8(3):249-260

[268] Kiecolt-Glaser PhD, Janice K. (1984) 'Stress and the transformation of lymphocytes by Epstein-Bar Virus,' J. of Behavioral Medicine, 7(1): 1-12

[269] Reynolds, P & Kaplan, G.A. (1990) 'Social connections and risk for cancer - Prospective evidence from the Alameda County study,' Behavioral Medicine, 16:101-110

[270] Berkman, L.F. & Syme, S.L. (1979) 'Social Networks, Host Resistance and Mortality - A nine-year follow up study of Alameda County residents,' Am. Jo of Epidemiology, 109:186-204)

[271] Ell, K & Nishimoto, R & Mediansky, L & Mantell, J & Hamovitch, M (1992) 'Social relations, social support and survival among patients with cancer,' J. of Psychosomatic Research, 36:531-541

[272] Spiegel, David (1997) 'Psychosocial aspects of breast cancer treatment,' Seminars in Oncology, 24(1), Suppl 1 (February):S1-36-S1-47

[273] Maunsell, E. & Brisson, J. & Dechenes, L (1995) 'Social support and survival among women with breast cancer,' Cancer, 76:631-637

[274] Waxler-Morrison, N. & Hislop, T.G. & Mears, B. & Kan, L. (1991) 'Effects of social relationships on survival for woman with breast cancer - a prospective study,' Social Science and Medicine, 33:177-183

[275] LeShan, Lawrence (1989) Cancer as a Turning Point, Penguin Putman

[276] LeShan, PhD, Lawrence & Worthington, R.E. (1956) 'Loss of cathexes as a common psychodynamic characteristic of cancer patients - An attempt at statistical validation of a clinical hypothesis,' Psychological Report, 2:183-193

[277] LeShan, PhD, Lawrence (1977) You Can Fight for Your Life, New York: M. Evans

[278] Kissen, David M. (1967) 'Psychosocial factors, personality and lung cancer in men aged 55-64,' British J. Med. Psychology, 40:29

[279] Kune, G.A. & Kune, S. & Watson, L.F. & Bahnson, Claus Bahne (1991) 'Personality as a risk factor in large bowel cancer - data from the Melbourne Colorectal Cancer Study,' Psychological Medicine, 21(1):29-41

[280] Thomas, Caroline B. & Duszynski, Karen R. & Shaffer, J. W (1974) 'Closeness to parents and the family constellation in a prospective study of five disease states: suicide, mental illness, malignant tumor,

hypertension and coronary heart disease,' John Hopkins Medical Journal, 134 No 5: 251-270

[281] Shaffer, J.W. & Duszynski, Karen R. & Thomas, Caroline B. (1982) 'Family attitudes in youth as a possible precursor of cancer among physicians - a search for explanatory mechanisms,' J. of Behavioral Medicine, 5:143-163

[282] Bahnson PhD, Claus Bahne (1980) 'Stress and cancer - State of the Art,' Psychosomatics, 21(12):975-980

[283] Lerner, Michael (1994) Choices in Healing, Cambridge: MIT Press

[284] Hamer, Ryke Geert (1999) Vermächtnis einer NEUEN MEDIZIN teil 1 - Die 5 biologischen Naturgesetze: Krebs, Leukamie, Epilepsie, Koln, Germany: Amici di Dirk Verlag

[285] Hamer, Ryke Geert (1999) Vermächtnis einer NEUEN MEDIZIN teil 2 - Die 5 biologischen Naturgesetze: Psychosen, Syndrome, Krebs bei kindern tieren, pflanzen, Koln, Germany: Amici di Dirk Verlag

[286] Lerner, Michael (1994) Choices in Healing, Cambridge: MIT Press

[287] Gendron, (1759) Enquiries into nature, knowledge, and the cure of cancers

[288] Thomas, Caroline B. & Duszynski, Karen R. & Shaffer, J.W. (1973) 'Closeness to parents and the family constellation in a prospective study of five disease states: suicide, mental illness, malignant tumor, hypertension and coronary heart disease,' John Hopkins Medical Journal, 134 No 5: 251-270

[289] Persky, V.W. & Kempthorne-Rawson, J. & Shekelle, R.B. (1987) 'Personality and risk of cancer,' Psychosomatic Medicine, 49(5):435-49

[290] Simonton, O. Carl & Simonton - Matthews, Stephanie & Creighton, James L. (1978) Getting Well Again, New York: Bantam

[291] Simonton, O. Carl & Simonton - Matthews, Stephanie & Creighton, James L. (1978) Getting Well Again, New York: Bantam

[292] Simonton, O. Carl & Simonton - Matthews, Stephanie & Sparks, T.F. (1980) 'Psychological Intervention and Survival Time of Patients with Metastatic Breast cancer,' Psychosomatics, 21:226-233

[293] Spiegel, David & Spira, James (1991) Supportive-expressive group therapy - A treatment manual of psychosocial intervention for women with recurrent breast cancer, Stanford: Psychosocial treatment laboratory, Stanford Univ. of Med.

294 Spiegel, David (1993) Brief Supportive-Expressive Group Therapy for Women with Primary Breast Cancer - a treatment manual, Stanford: Psychosocial treatment laboratory, Stanford Univ. of Med.

295 Spiegel, David & Spira, James (1991) Supportive-expressive group therapy - A treatment manual of psychosocial intervention for women with recurrent breast cancer, Stanford: Psychosocial treatment laboratory, Stanford Univ. of Med.

296 Spiegel, David (1993) Brief Supportive-Expressive Group Therapy for Women with Primary Breast Cancer - a treatment manual, Stanford: Psychosocial treatment laboratory, Stanford Univ. of Med.

297 Spiegel, David & Bloom, J.R. (1983) 'Group therapy and hypnosis reduce metastatic breast carcinoma pain,' Archives of General Psychiatry, 38:527-533

298 Spiegel, David (1991) Psychological Treatment Manual for Patients with Cancer, unpublished

299 Spiegel, David & Spira, J. (1991) Supportive-expressive group therapy - A treatment manual of psychosocial intervention for women with recurrent breast cancer, Stanford: Psychosocial treatment laboratory, Stanford Univ. of Med.

300 Vries, de, Marco J. & Schilder, Johannes N. & Mulder, Cornelis L. & Vrancken, Adriana M.E. & Remie, Margot E. & Garssen, Bert (1997) 'Phase II study of psychotherapeutic intervention in advanced cancer,' Psycho-Oncology, 6:129-137

301 Spiegel, David & Kraemer, H.C. & Bloom, J.R. & Gottheil, E. (1989) 'Effect of psychosocial Treatment on Survival of Patients with Metastatic Breast Cancer,' Lancet, Vol. II (8668):888-891

302 Deurzen, Emmy. van (1990) Existential Therapy, Open Univ Pr.

303 Frankl, Victor E. (1959) Man's Search For Meaning, New York: Washington Square Press

304 Spiegel, David & Bloom, J.R. & Yalom, I.D. (1981) 'Group support for patients with metastatic cancer - A randomized prospective outcome study,' Archives of General Psychiatry, 38:527-533

305 Grossarth-Maticek, Ronald & Kanazir, Dusan T. & Schmidt, P & Vetter, H (1982) 'Psychosomatic factors in the progress of cancerogenesis, Theoretical models and empirical results,' Psychotherapy and Psychosomatics, 38;284-302

306 Grossarth-Marticek, R. & Schmidt, P. & Vetter, H. & Arundt, S. (1984) Psychotherapy research in oncology in Steptoe, A. (ed.)& Mathews, A. (ed.)(1984) Health Care and Human Behavior, San Diego: Academic Press

307 Grossarth-Marticek, R. & Eysenck, H.J. (1991) 'Creative novation behaviour therapy as a prophylactic treatment for cancer and coronary heart disease - Part I: description of treatment,' Behav Res Ther, 29:1-16

308 Grossarth-Maticek, Ronald & Bastiaan, Ronald Jan & Kanazir, Dusan T. (1985) 'Psychosocial factors as strong predictions of mortality from cancer, ischemic heart disease and stroke - Yugoslav Prospective Study,' J. of Psychosomatic Research, Vol. 29, pp. 167-176.

309 Grossarth-Maticek, Ronald & Eysenck, Hans Jurgen (1995) 'Self-regulation and mortality from cancer, coronary heart disease, and other causes - A prospective study,' Personality and Individual Differences, 19(6):781-795

310 Simonton, O. Carl (1992) Healing Journey - The Simonton Center Program for Achieving Physical, Mental and Spiritual Health, New York: Bantam

311 Eysenck, H.J. & Grossarth-Marticek, R (1991) 'Creative novation behaviour therapy as a prophylactic treatment for cancer and coronary heart disease - Part II effects of treatment,' Behav Res Ther, 29:17-31

312 LeShan, Lawrence (1977) You Can Fight for Your Life, New York: M. Evans

313 LeShan, Lawrence (1989) Cancer as a Turning Point, Penguin Putman

314 LeShan, Lawrence (1989) Cancer as a Turning Point, Penguin Putman

315 LeShan, Lawrence (1989) Cancer as a Turning Point, Penguin Putman

316 Temoshok, Linda & Dreher, Henry (1992) Type C Connection, The - The Mind-Body Link to Cancer and Your Health, Random House

317 Temoshok, Linda & Dreher, Henry (1993) 'Type C Connection - Noetic Sciences Review,' Noetic Sciences Review, 25:21-26

318 Spiegel, David & Glafkides, M.S. (1983) 'Effects of group confrontation with death and dying,' Int. J. of Group Psychotherapy, 33:433-447

[319] Spiegel, David & Kraemer, H.C. & Bloom, J.R. & Gottheil, E. (1989) 'Effect of psychosocial Treatment on Survival of Patients with Metastic Breast Cancer,' Lancet, Vol. II (8668):888-891

[320] Spiegel, David (1991) 'Psychosocial Intervention and Survival Time of Patients with Metastatic Breast Cancer,' Advances in Mind Body Medicine, 7(3) 10-19

[321] Levy, Sandra M. (1987) 'Correlations of Stress with sustained depression of NK cell activity and prognosis in breast cancer,' J. Clin. Oncology, 5:348

[322] Fawzy, F.I. & Cousins, Norman & Fawzy, N.W. & Kemeny, Margaret E. & Elashof, R & Morton, D.L. (1990) 'Structured psychiatric intervention for cancer patients. - Part I: Changes over time in methods of coping and affective disturbance,' Archives of General Psychiatry, 47:729-735

[323] Melia, T. (1987) Wellness Community Lives Up To, LACMA Physician

[324] http://www.ecap-online.org/

[325] Siegel, Bernie S. (1989) Peace, Love, and Healing, Harper & Row

[326] Official Commonweal website: http://www.commonweal.org/

[327] Official Commonweal website: http://www.commonweal.org/ programs/cancer-help.html

[328] Benson, Herbert & Klipper, Miriam Z. (1975) Relaxation Response, New York: William Morrow

[329] Official website (2004) Mind Body Medical Institute; http://www. mbmi.org/

[330] Fawzy, F.I. & Fawzy, N.W. & Hyun, C.S. (1993) 'Malignant Melanoma - Effects of an early structured psychiatric intervention, coping and affective state on recurrence and survival 6 years later,' Archives of General Psychiatry, 50:681-689

[331] Fawzy, F.I. & Kemeny, M.E. & Fawzy, N.W. & Elashof, R & Morton, D. & Cousins, Norman & Fahey, J.L. (1990) 'Structured psychiatric intervention for cancer patients. - Part II: Changes over time in immunological measures,' Archives of General Psychiatry, 47:729-735

[332] Fawzy, F.I. & Cousins, Norman & Fawzy, N.W. & Kemeny, M.E. & Elashof, R & Morton, D. (1990) 'Structured psychiatric intervention for cancer patients. - Part I: Changes over time in methods of coping and affective disturbance,' Archives of General Psychiatry, 47:729-735

333 Fawzy, F.I. & Fawzy, N.W. & Hyun, C.S. (1993) 'Malignant Melanoma - Effects of an early structured psychiatric intervention, coping and affective state on recurrence and survival 6 years later,' Archives of General Psychiatry, 50:681-689

334 Vries, de, Marco J. & Schilder, Johannes N. & Mulder, Cornelis L. & Vrancken, Adriana M.E. & Remie, Margot E. & Garssen, Bert (1997) 'Phase II study of psychotherapeutic intervention in advanced cancer,' Psycho-Oncology, 6:129-137

335 Fawzy, F.I. & Canada, A.L. & Fawzy, N.W. (2003) 'Malignant melanoma - of a brief, structured psychiatric intervention on survival and recurrence at 10-year follow-up,' Archives of General Psychiatry, 60(1):100-3

336 Baalen, van, Daan C. & Vries, de, Marco J. (1987) Spontaneous regression of cancer - A clinical, pathological and psycho-social study, Rotterdam: Erasmus University

337 Solano, L. & Costa, M. & Salvati, S. & Coda, R. & Aiuti, F. & Mezzaroma, I. & Bertini, M. (1993) 'Psychosocial factors and clinical evolution in HIV-1 infection - a longitudinal study,' J. of Psychosomatic Research, 37(1):39-51

338 Eells, Tracy D (2000) 'Can Therapy Affect Physical Health?' J Psychother Pract Res, 2:100-104

339 Carter, Stephan K. (1976) 'Immunotherapy of cancer in men,' American Scientist, 64:418-423 in Brown, P. & Fromm, E. (1984) 'Hypnosis and behavioral medicine, London: Lawrence Erlbaum publishers.

340 Simonton, O. Carl & Simonton - Matthews, Stephanie & Creighton, James L. (1978) Getting Well Again, New York: Bantam

341 Simonton, O. Carl (1992) Healing Journey - The Simonton Center Program for Achieving Physical, Mental and Spiritual Health, New York: Bantam

342 Peynovska, Rumy & Fisher, Jackie & Oliver, David & Mathew, V.M. (2005) 'Efficacy of Hypnotherapy as a Supplement Therapy in Cancer Intervention,' European Journal of Clinical Hypnosis, 6:1

343 Newton, Bernhauer W. (1982) 'Use of Hypnotherapy in the Treatment of Cancer Patients,' American Journal of Clinical Hypnosis, 25(2-3):104-113

344 Simonton, O. Carl & Simonton - Matthews, Stephanie & Creighton, James L (1978) Getting Well Again, New York: Bantam

[345] LaBaw, Wallace & Holton, Charlene & Tewell, Karen & Eccles, Doris (1975) 'Use of self-hypnosis by children with cancer,' American Journal of Clinical Hypnosis, 17:233-238

[346] Dempster, C.R. & Balson, P. & Whalen, B.T. (1976) 'Supportive hypnotherapy during the radical treatment of malignancies,' J. of Clin. and Experimental Hypnosis, 24(1):1-9

[347] Simonton, O. Carl & Simonton - Matthews, Stephanie & Creighton, James L. (1978) Getting Well Again, New York: Bantam

[348] Grosz, Hanus J. (1979) 'Hypnotherapy in the management of terminally ill cancer patients,' J. of the Indiana Medical Association, 72:126-129

[349] Grosz, Hanus J. (1979) 'Hypnotherapy in the management of terminally ill cancer patients,' J. of the Indiana Medical Association, 72:126-129

[350] Coates, A. & Gebski, V. & Signorini, D. & Murray, P. & McNeil, D. & Byrne, M. & Forbes, J.F. (1992) 'Prognostic value of quality-of-life scores during chemotherapy for advanced breast cancer - Australian New Zealand Breast Cancer Trials Group,' J. of Clinical Oncology, 12:1833-1838

[351] LeShan, Lawrence (1989) Cancer as a Turning Point, Penguin Putman

[352] LeShan, Lawrence (1989) Cancer as a Turning Point, Penguin Putman

[353] Berland, Warren (1995) 'Unexpected Cancer Recovery - Why Patients Believe They Survive,' Advances in Mind Body Medicine, 11:5-19

[354] Simonton, O. Carl & Henson, Reid (1992) Healing Journey - The Simonton Center Program for Achieving Physical, Mental and Spiritual Health, New York: Bantam

[355] Simonton, O. Carl & Simonton - Matthews, Stephanie & Creighton, James L. (1978) Getting Well Again, New York: Bantam

[356] Rosenthal, R. (1966) Experimenter effects in behavioral research, New York: Appleton Century

[357] Rosenthal, R. & Jacobson, L. (1968) Pygmalion in the Classroom, New York: Holt, Rinehart and Winston

[358] LeShan, Lawrence (1989) Cancer as a Turning Point, Penguin Putman

359 LeShan, Lawrence (1989) <u>Cancer as a Turning Point,</u> Penguin Putman

360 Frank, Jerome (1973) <u>Persuasion and healing: a comparative study of psychotherapy,</u> Johns Hopkins University, Baltimore

361 Newton, Bernhauer W. (1982) 'Use of Hypnotherapy in the Treatment of Cancer Patients,' <u>American Journal of Clinical Hypnosis,</u> 25(2-3):104-113

362 Simonton, O. Carl & Simonton - Matthews, Stephanie & Creighton, James L. (1978) <u>Getting Well Again,</u> New York: Bantam

363 Simonton, O. Carl & Simonton - Matthews, Stephanie & Creighton, James L. (1978) <u>Getting Well Again,</u> New York: Bantam

364 LeShan, Lawrence (1989) <u>Cancer as a Turning Point,</u> Penguin Putman

365 Spiegel, David & Spira, James (1991) 'Supportive-expressive group therapy - A treatment manual of psychosocial intervention for women with recurrent breast cancer,' Stanford: Psychosocial treatment laboratory, <u>Stanford Univ. School of Med.</u>

366 Brown, George W. (ed.) & Harris, Tirril O. (ed.) (1989) <u>Life Events and Illness,</u> New York: Guilford Press

367 Holmes, T.H. & Rahe, Richard H. (1967) 'Social readjustment rating scale,' <u>J. of Psychosomatic Research,</u> 11:213-218

368 Cochrane , R. & Robertson, A. (1973) 'Life Events Inventory - A Measure of the Relative Severity of Psycho-Social Stressors,' <u>J. of Psychosomatic Research</u>

369 See appendix "Healing Psyche Online Resources"

370 Richardson, J.L. & Shelton, R.C. & Krailo, M. & Levine, A.M. (1990) 'Effect of compliance with treatment on survival among patients with hematological malignancies,' <u>J. of Clinical Oncology,</u> 8:356-364

371 Spiegel, David (1995) 'Essentials of psychotherapeutic intervention for cancer patients,' <u>Support Care Cancer,</u> 3252-256

372 Helgeson, V.S. & Cohen, S. & Schulz, R. & Yasko, J. (1999) 'Education and peer discussion group interventions and adjustment to breast cancer,' <u>Archives of General Psychiatry,</u> 56:340-347

373 Fritz, C.E. & Marks, E.S (1954) 'NORC studies of human behavior in disaster,' <u>J. of Social Issues,</u> 10:26-41 in Monat, Alan (ed.) & Lazarus,

Richard S. (ed.) (1977) Stress and Coping - Anthology, New York: Columbia University Press

374 Elliott, R. (1966) 'Effects of uncertainty about the nature and advent of a noxious stimulus (shock) upon heart rate,' J. of Personality and Social Psychology, 3:353-357 in Monat, Alan (ed.) & Lazarus, Richard S. (ed.) (1977) Stress and Coping - Anthology, New York: Columbia University Press

375 Elliott, R (1966) 'Effects of uncertainty about the nature and advent of a noxious stimulus (shock) upon heart rate,' J. of Personality and Social Psychology, 3:353-357 in Monat, Alan (ed.) & Lazarus, Richard S (ed.) (1977) Stress and Coping - Anthology, New York: Columbia University Press

376 Fritz, C.E. & Marks, E.S (1954) 'NORC studies of human behavior in disaster,' J. of Social Issues, 10:26-41 in Monat, Alan (ed.) & Lazarus, Richard S. (ed.) (1977) Stress and Coping - Anthology, New York: Columbia University Press

377 Malmo, R.B. & Smith, A.A. & Kohlmeyer, W.A. (1956) 'Motor manifestation of conflict in interview - A case study,' J. of Abnormal and Social Psychology, 52:268-271 in Monat, Alan (ed.) & Lazarus, Richard S. (ed.) (1977) Stress and Coping - Anthology, New York: Columbia University Press

378 Roher, J.H. (1959) 'Studies of human adjustment to polar isolation and implications of those studies for living in fallout shelters,' : Disaster Research Group; D. Anthropology and Psychology; Na Ac Sc; Monat, Alan (ed.) & Lazarus, Richard S. (ed.) (1977) Stress and Coping - Anthology, New York: Columbia University Press

379 Vingerhoets, AJJM & Rigter, H. (ed.) (1994) Stress en Gezondheid, Tilburg: Tilburg University Press

380 Rice, P.L. (1999) Stress and Health, Pacific Grove: Brooks Cole

381 Hill, R & Hansen, D.A. (1962) 'Families in disaster,' in Monat, Alan (ed.) & Lazarus, Richard S. (ed.) (1977) Stress and Coping - Anthology, New York: Columbia University Press

382 Feather, N.T. (1965) 'Relationship of expectation of success to need achievement and test anxiety,' J. of Personality and Social Psychology, 1:118-126 in Monat, Alan (ed.) & Lazarus, Richard S. (ed.) (1977) Stress and Coping - Anthology, New York: Columbia University Press

383 Postman, L. & Brown, D. (1952) 'Perceptual consequences of success and failure,' J. of Abnormal and Social Psychology, 47:213-221 in Monat, Alan (ed.) & Lazarus, Richard S. (ed.) (1977) 'Stress and Coping - Anthology,' New York: Columbia University Press

384 Feather, N. T. (1966) 'Effects of prior success and failure on expectations of success and subsequent performance,' J. of Personality and Social Psychology, 3:237-299 in Monat, Alan (ed.) & Lazarus, Richard S. (ed.) (1977) Stress and Coping - Anthology, New York: Columbia University Press

385 Kalish, H. & Garmezy, N. & Rodnick, E. & Bleke, R. (1958) 'Effects of anxiety and experimentally induced stress on verbal learning,' J. of General Psychology, 59:87-95 in Monat, Alan (ed.) & Lazarus, Richard S. (ed.) (1977) Stress and Coping - Anthology, New York: Columbia University Press

386 Harleston, B. W. (1962) 'Test anxiety and performance in problem-solving situations,' J. of Personality, 30:557-573 in Monat, Alan (ed.) & Lazarus, Richard S. (ed.) (1977) Stress and Coping - Anthology, New York: Columbia University Press

387 Feather, N. T. (1965) 'Relationship of expectation of success to need achievement and test anxiety,' J. of Personality and Social Psychology, 1:118-126 in Monat, Alan (ed.) & Lazarus, Richard S. (ed.) (1977) Stress and Coping - Anthology, New York: Columbia University Press

388 Ellis, PhD, Albert & Grieger, Russell (1977) RET - Handbook of Rational Emotive Therapy, New York: Springer

389 Simonton, O. Carl & Simonton - Matthews, Stephanie & Creighton, James L. (1978) Getting Well Again, New York: Bantam Books

390 Arizona State University, (1999) Manual for the threat appraisal scale (TAS) - Program for prevention research

391 Simonton, O. Carl (1992) Healing Journey - The Simonton center program for achieving physical, mental and spiritual health, New York: Bantam

392 Ellis, PhD, Albert & Grieger, Russell (1977) RET - Handbook of Rational Emotive Therapy, New York: Springer

393 Spiegel, David & Spira, James (1991) Supportive-expressive group therapy - A treatment manual of psychosocial intervention for women with recurrent breast cancer, Stanford: Psychosocial treatment laboratory, Stanford Univ. School of Med.

[394] Spiegel, David (1993) <u>Brief Supportive-Expressive Group Therapy for Women with Primary Breast Cancer - a treatment manual</u>, Stanford: Psychosocial treatment laboratory, Stanford Univ. School of Med.

[395] See appendix, "Diagnostic Belief List."

[396] McDermott, Ian & O'Connor, Joseph (1996) <u>NLP & Health</u>, London: Thornson's Publications

[397] Bandura, A. (1977) 'Self-Efficacy - Towards a unifying theory of behavior change,' <u>Psychological Rev.</u>, 84:191-215

[398] Itano, J. & Tanabe, P. & Lum, J. & Lamkin, L. & Rizzo, E. & Weiland, M. & Sato, P. (1983) 'Compliance and noncompliance in cancer patients,' <u>Prog. Clin. Biol. Res</u>, 120:483-495

[399] Marcus, A.C. & Crane, L.A. & Kaplan, C.P. & Reading, A.E. & Savage, E. & Gunning, J. & Bernstein, G. & Berek, J.S. (1992) 'Improving adherence to screening, follow-up among women with abnormal Pap smears - Results from a large clinic-based trial of three intervention strategies,' <u>Med. Care</u>, 30:216-230

[400] Spiegel, David (1997) 'Psychosocial aspects of breast cancer treatment,' <u>Seminars in Oncology</u>, 24(1), Supplement 1 (February):S1-36-S1-47

[401] Ayres, A. & Hoon, P.W. & Franzoni, J.B. & Matheny, K.B. & Cotanch, P.H. & Takayanagi, S. (1994) 'Influence of mood and adjustment to cancer on compliance with chemotherapy among breast cancer patients,' <u>J. of Psychosomatic Research</u>, 83:393-402

[402] Simmel, M.L. (1967) 'Body percept in physical medicine and rehabilitation, the,' <u>J. of Health and Social Behavior</u>, 8:60-64

[403] Moss, D (1978) <u>Brain, body, and world - Perspectives on body-image</u>, New York: Oxford University Press

[404] Trestman, Robert Lee (1981) <u>Imagery, Coping and Physiological Variables in Adult Cancer Patients - PhD dissertation</u>, Knoxville: University of Tennessee;

[405] Simonton, O. Carl & Simonton - Matthews, Stephanie & Creighton, James L. (1978) <u>Getting Well Again</u>, New York: Bantam

[406] Achterberg, Jeanne (1985) <u>Imagery In Healing - Shamanism in modern medicine</u>, Boston: New Science Library 188-189

[407] Achterberg, Jeanne (1984) <u>Imagery and disease - image-CA, image-</u>

SP, image-DB: a diagnostic tool for behavioral medicine, Inst. for Personality & Ability Testing

[408] Trestman, Robert Lee (1981) Imagery, Coping and Physiological Variables in Adult Cancer Patients - PhD dissertation,' Knoxville: University of Tennessee in Achterberg, Jeanne (1985) Imagery In Healing - Shamanism in modern medicine, Boston: New Science Library 188-189

[409] Shorr, J.E. (1972) Psycho-imagination therapy, Intercontinental Medical Book Corporation

[410] Achterberg, Jeanne A. & Lawlis, G. Frank (1978) Imagery of cancer: An evaluation tool for the process of disease, Champaign, Ill, Institute for Personality and Ability Testing.

[411] Simonton, O. Carl & Simonton - Matthews, Stephanie & Creighton, James L. (1978) Getting Well Again, New York: Bantam

[412] Simonton (2003) Personal communication

[413] Gardner, G. Gail & Lubman, Alison (1983) 'Hypnotherapy for children with cancer: some current issues,' American Journal of Clinical Hypnosis, 25, 135-142

[414] Simonton, O. Carl & Simonton - Matthews, Stephanie & Creighton, James L. (1978) Getting Well Again, New York: Bantam

[415] Achterberg, Jeanne (1984) Imagery and disease - image-CA, image-SP, image-DB: a diagnostic tool for behavioral medicine, Inst. for Personality & Ability Testing

[416] Simonton, O. Carl & Simonton - Matthews, Stephanie & Creighton, James L. (1978) Getting Well Again, New York: Bantam

[417] Simonton, O. Carl & Henson, Reid (1992) Healing Journey - The Simonton center program for achieving physical, mental and spiritual health, New York: Bantam Books

[418] Achterberg, Jeanne & Lawlis, Frank (1978) Imagery of Cancer, Inst. of Personality Testing

[419] Achterberg, Jeanne & Lawlis, Frank (1978) Imagery of Cancer, Inst. of Personality Testing

[420] Dilts, Robert & Hallbom, Tim & Smith, Suzi (1990) Beliefs - Pathways to Health and Well Being, Metamorphous Press

[421] Farrelly, Frank & Brandsma, Jeff (1974) Provocative Therapy, Capitola: Meta Publications

422 Maultsby, Maxie C. & Hendricks, A. (1974) You and Your Emotions, Lexington, KY: Rational Self-Help Aids

423 Maultsby, Maxie C. & Hendricks, A. (1974) You and Your Emotions, Lexington, KY: Rational Self-Help Aids

424 Dilts, Robert (1990) Changing Belief Systems with NLP, Capitola: Meta Publications

425 Dilts, Robert & Hallbom, Tim & Smith, Suzi (1990) Beliefs - Pathways to Health and Well Being, Metamorphous Press

426 James, Tad & Woodsmall, Wyatt (1988) Time Line Therapy and the Basis of Personality, Capitola: Meta Publications

427 Simonton, O. Carl & Simonton - Matthews, Stephanie & Creighton, James L. (1978) Getting Well Again, New York: Bantam

428 Ellis, PhD, Albert & Grieger, Russell (1977) RET - Handbook of Rational Emotive Therapy, New York: Springer

429 Simonton, O. Carl & Henson, Reid (1992) Healing Journey - The Simonton center program for achieving physical, mental and spiritual health, New York: Bantam

430 Simonton, O. Carl (2003) Personal Communication

431 Ellis, PhD, Albert (1971) Growth through Reason - Verbatim cases in rational Emotive Therapy, Hollywood: Wilshire Book Company

432 Ellis, PhD, Albert & Grieger, Russell (1977) RET - Handbook of Rational Emotive Therapy, New York: Springer

433 Ellis, PhD, Albert & Harper PhD, Robert A. (1961) A New Guide to Rational Living, Hollywood: Wilshire Book Company

434 Ellis, PhD, Albert (1971) Growth through Reason - Verbatim cases in rational Emotive Therapy, Hollywood: Wilshire Book Company

435 Ellis, PhD, Albert & Grieger, Russell (1977) RET - Handbook of Rational Emotive Therapy, New York: Springer

436 Simonton, O. Carl & Henson, Reid (1992) Healing Journey - The Simonton center program for achieving physical, mental and spiritual health, New York: Bantam

437 Watzlawick PhD, Paul (1976) How Real is Real - Confusion, Disinformation, Communication, Random House Books

438 Bandler, Richard & Grinder, John (1982) Reframing - Neuro Linguistic Programming and the Transformation of Meaning, Moab, UT: Real

People Press

439 Erickson, Milton H. & Rossi PhD, Ernest L. (1985) <u>Seminars, Workshops and Lectures, Vol. 2 - Life Reframing in Hypnosis</u>, New York: Irvington Publishers

440 Dilts, Robert (1999) <u>Sleight of Mouth - The Magic of Conversational Belief Change</u>, Capitola: Meta Publications

441 Donovan, M. (1980) 'Relaxation with guided imagery: a useful technique,' <u>Cancer Nurse</u>, 3:27-32

442 Simonton, O. Carl & Simonton - Matthews, Stephanie & Creighton, James L. (1978) <u>Getting Well Again</u>, New York: Bantam

443 Achterberg, Jeanne (1985) <u>Imagery in Healing - Shamanism and Modern Medicine</u>, New Science Library

444 Rossman M.D., Martin (2000) <u>Guided Imagery for Self-Healing - An Essential Resource for Anyone Seeking Wellness</u>, CA, San Raphael: New World Library

445 Rossman M.D., Martin (2003) <u>Fighting Cancer from Within - How to Use the Power of Your Mind for Healing</u>, Henry Holt & Co.

446 Dilts, Robert & Hallbom (M.S.W), Tim & Smith (M.S), Suzi (1990) <u>Beliefs - Pathways to Health & Well Being</u>, Portland, Oregon: Metamorphous Press

447 Cameron Bandler, Leslie (1978) <u>They Lived Happily Ever After</u>, Capitola: Meta Publications

448 Bandler, Richard & Grinder, John (1979) <u>Frogs Into Princes - Neuro Linguistic Programming</u>, Moab, UT: Real People Press

449 Dilts, Robert & Grinder, John & Bandler, Richard & DeLozier, Judith (1980) <u>Neuro Linguistic Programming: Volume 1 - The study of the structure of subjective experience</u>, Capitola: Meta Publications

450 Dilts, Robert & Hallbom (M.S.W), Tim & Smith (M.S), Suzi (1990) <u>Beliefs - Pathways to Health & Well Being</u>, Portland, Oregon: Metamorphous Press

451 Dilts, Robert (1990) <u>Changing Belief Systems with NLP</u>, Capitola: Meta Publications

452 Dilts, Robert (1994) <u>Strategies of Genius Vol. III</u>, Capitola: Meta Publications

[453] Grinder, John & DeLozier, Judith (1987) Turtles all the Way Down - Prerequisites to Personal Genius, Grinder & DeLozier Associates

[454] Dilts, Robert & Hallbom (M.S.W), Tim & Smith (M.S), Suzi (1990) Beliefs - Pathways to Health & Well Being, Portland, Oregon: Metamorphous Press

[455] Dilts, Robert (1990) Changing Belief Systems with NLP, Capitola: Meta Publications

[456] Dilts, Robert (1994) Strategies of Genius Vol. III, Capitola: Meta Publications

[457] Dilts, Robert & DeLozier, Judith (2000) Encyclopedia of Systemic NLP and NLP New Coding, NLP University Press

[458] James, Tad & Woodsmall, Wyatt (1988) Time Line Therapy and the Basis of Personality, Capitola: Meta Publications

[459] Andreas, Connirae & Andreas PhD, Steve (1987) Change your Mind and Keep the Change, Moab, UT: Real People Press

[460] James, Tad & Woodsmall, Wyatt (1988) Time Line Therapy and the Basis of Personality, Capitola: Meta Publications

[461] Dilts, Robert & Epstein, Todd (1991) Tools for Dreamers - Strategies for Creativity and the Structure of Innovation, Capitola: Meta Publications

[462] Bandler, Richard (1993) Time for a Change, Capitola: Meta Publications

463 Dilts, Robert & Hallbom (M.S.W), Tim & Smith, Suzi (1999) NLP Health Certification Training manual 1999,

[464] See appendix "Healthy Beliefs"

[465] Olness, Karen (1981) 'Imagery (self-hypnosis) as adjunct therapy in childhood cancer - Clinical experience with 25 patients,' American Journal of Pediatric Hematology/Oncology, 3:313-321

[466] Brown, Daniel P. & Fromm, Erika (1987) Hypnosis and Behavioral Medicine, New Jersey: Lawrence Erlbaum Associates Publishers

[467] Brown, Daniel P. & Fromm, Erika (1987) Hypnosis and Behavioral Medicine, New Jersey: Lawrence Erlbaum Associates Publishers

[468] Hartland, John (1971) 'Further observations on the use of 'ego-strengthening' techniques,' American Journal of Clinical Hypnosis, 14:1-8

469 Olness, Karen (1981) 'Imagery (Self-hypnosis) as adjunct therapy in childhood cancer: Clinical experience with 25 patients' American Journal of Pediatric Hematology/Oncology, 3, 313-321

470 Finkelstein, Selig & Howard, Marcia Greenleaf (1982) 'Cancer Prevention - A Three year pilot study,' American Journal of Clinical Hypnosis

471 Hammond, D. Corydon (1990) Handbook of Hypnotic Suggestions and Metaphors, W. W. Norton

472 Simonton, O. Carl & Simonton - Matthews, Stephanie & Creighton, James L. (1978) Getting Well Again, New York: Bantam

473 Spiegel, David (1993) Brief Supportive-Expressive Group Therapy for Women with Primary Breast Cancer - a treatment manual, Stanford: Psychosocial treatment laboratory, Stanford Univ. School of Med.

474 Bugental, J. F. T (1973) 'Confronting the existential meaning of 'my death' through group exercises,' Interpersonal Development, 4:148-163

475 Bugental, J. F. T (1973) 'Confronting the existential meaning of 'my death' through group exercises,' Interpersonal Development, 4:148-163

476 James, Tad (1998) Manual Accelerated Master Practitioner Training - Spring 1998, Irvine, Honolulu: Advanced Neuro Dynamics

477 Bateson, Gregory (1972) Steps to an Ecology Of Mind - The new information sciences can lead to a new understanding of man, Ballentine

478 Dilts, Robert (1990) Changing Belief Systems with NLP, Capitola: Meta Publications

479 Dilts, Robert (1990) Changing Belief Systems with NLP, Capitola: Meta Publications

480 McDermott, Ian & O'Connor, Joseph (1996) NLP & Health, London: Thornson's Publications

481 Simonton, O. Carl & Simonton - Matthews, Stephanie & Creighton, James L. (1978) Getting Well Again, New York: Bantam

482 Temoshok, Linda & Dreher, Henry (1992) Type C Connection, The - The Mind-Body Link to Cancer and Your Health, Random House

483 Baalen, van, Daan C. & Vries, de, Marco J. & Gondrie, Marjolein T. (1987) Psycho-Social Correlates of 'spontaneous' regression in cancer – Monograph, Department of general pathology, Medical faculty,

Erasmus University Rotterdam, The Netherlands,

[484] Temoshok, Lydia & Dreher, Henry (1992) Type C Connection - The Behavioral Links to Cancer and your Health, Random House Books

[485] Temoshok, Lydia & Dreher, Henry (1992) Type C Connection - The Behavioral Links to Cancer and your Health, Random House Books

[486] Temoshok, Lydia & Dreher, Henry (1992) Type C Connection - The Behavioral Links to Cancer and your Health, Random House Books

[487] Temoshok, Lydia & Dreher, Henry (1992) Type C Connection - The Behavioral Links to Cancer and your Health, Random House Books

[488] Temoshok, Lydia & Dreher, Henry (1992) Type C Connection - The Behavioral Links to Cancer and your Health, Random House Books

[489] Temoshok, Lydia & Dreher, Henry (1992) Type C Connection - The Behavioral Links to Cancer and your Health, Random House Books

[490] Derks, Drs, Lucas A.C. & Hollander, Jaap (1996) Essenties van NLP - Sleutels tot Persoonlijke Verandering, Utrecht: Sevire Uitgevers B.V.

[491] Derks, Drs, Lucas A.C. (1999) The Social Panorama and its Exploration, Crownhouse Publishing

[492] Hellinga, Gerben (1999) Lastige Lieden - Inleiding over persoonlijkh eidsstoornissen, Boom Amsterdam

[493] Baalen, van, Daan C. & Vries, de, Marco J. (1987) Spontaneous regression of cancer - A clinical, pathological and psycho-social study, Rotterdam: Erasmus University

[494] Schilder, Johannes N (1992) 'Psychosociale veranderingen bij spontane regressie van kanker - Een kwalitatieve studie bij zeven patienten,' Gedrag & Gezondheid, 24(4):165-173

[495] Cunningham, Alastair J. & Watson, Kimberly (2004) 'How Psychological Therapy may Prolong Survival in Cancer Patients: New Evidence and a Simple Theory,' Integrative Cancer Therapies, 214-229(16)

[496] Grossarth-Maticek, Ronald & Bastiaan, Ronald Jan & Kanazir, Dusan T. (1985) 'Psychosocial factors as strong predictions of mortality from cancer, ischemic heart disease and stroke - Yugoslav Prospective Study,' J. of Psychosomatic Research, Vol. 29, pp. 167-176.

[497] Grossarth-Maticek, Ronald & Eysenck, Hans Jurgen (1991) 'Creative novation behaviour therapy as a prophylactic treatment for cancer

and coronary heart disease - Part I: description of treatment,' Behav. Research and Therapy, 29:1-16

[498] Eysenck, Hans Jurgen & Grossarth-Maticek, Ronald (1991) 'Creative novation behaviour therapy as a prophylactic treatment for cancer and coronary heart disease - Part II: Effects of treatment,' Behav. Research and Therapy, 29:17-31

[499] Grossarth-Maticek, Ronald & Eysenck, Hans Jurgen (1995) 'Self-regulation and mortality from cancer, coronary heart disease, and other causes - A prospective study,' Personality and Individual Differences, 19(6):781-795

[500] Temoshok, Lydia & Dreher, Henry (1992) Type C Connection - The Behavioral Links to Cancer and your Health, Random House Books

[501] Borysenko, Joan (1984) Minding the Body, Mending the Mind, New York: Bantam

[502] Dilts, Robert & Hallbom, Tim & Smith, Suzi (1990) Beliefs - Pathways to Health and Well Being, Metamorphous Press

[503] Bowers, J.E. & Kemeny, Margaret E. & Taylor, S.E. & Fahey, J.L. (2003) 'Finding positive meaning and its association with natural killer cell cytotoxicity among participants - in a bereavement-related disclosure intervention,' An. of Behavioral Medicine, 25(2):146-55

[504] LeShan, Lawrence (1959) 'Psychological States as factors in the development of Neoplastic Disease - A critical Review,' J. Nat. Cancer Institute, 22

[505] LeShan, Lawrence (1977) You Can Fight for Your Life, New York: M. Evans

[506] LeShan, Lawrence (1989) Cancer as a Turning Point, Penguin Putman

[507] Hawley, G. (1989) 'Role of holistic variables in the attribution of cancer survival,' Dissertation Abstracts International, 50:11b

[508] Huebscher, R (1992) 'Spontaneous remission of cancer - An example of health promotion,' Nurse Practitioner Forum, 3(4): 228-235

[509] Schilder, Johannes N. (1992) 'Psychossociale veranderingen bij spontane regressie van kanker - Een kwalitatieve studie bij zeven patiënten,' Gedrag & Gezondheid, 24(4):165-173

[510] Roud, P.C. (1985) 'Psychological variables associated with the exceptional survival of "terminally ill" cancer patients - Doctoral

dissertation, University of Massachusetts,' University Microfilms International, 8517148

511 Shanfield, S.B. (1980) 'On surviving cancer - Psychological considerations,' Comprehensive Psychiatry, 21(2):128-134

512 Ikemi, Yujiro & Nakagawa, S. & Nakagawa, T. & Sugita, M. (1975) 'Psychosomatic consideration on cancer patients who made a narrow escape from death,' Dynamic psychiatry, 8:77-92

513 Ikemi, Yujiro & Ikemi, A (1986) 'An oriental point of view in psychosomatic medicine,' Psychotherapy and Psychosomatics, 45(3):118-126

514 Cunningham, Alastair J. & Watson, Kimberly (2004) 'How Psychological Therapy may Prolong Survival in Cancer Patients: New Evidence and a Simple Theory,' Integrative Cancer Therapies, 214-229(16)

515 Cskiszenthihalyi, Mihaly (1990) Flow - The Psychology of Optimal Experience, New York: HarperCollins

516 Simonton, O. Carl & Simonton - Matthews, Stephanie & Creighton, James L. (1978) Getting Well Again, New York: Bantam Books

517 James, Tad & Woodsmall, PhD, Wyatt (1988) Time Line Therapy and the Basis of Personality, Capitola: Meta Publications

518 Simonton, O. Carl & Henson, Reid (1992) Healing Journey - The Simonton center program for achieving physical, mental and spiritual health, New York: Bantam

519 Covey, Stephen R. (1989) 7 Habits of Highly Effective People - Powerful Lessons in Personal Change, New York: Fireside

520 Dilts, Robert (1994) Strategies of Genius, Vol. III, Capitola: Meta Publications

521 Dilts, Robert (1996) Visionary Leadership Skills - Creating a World to Which People Want To Belong, Capitola: Meta Publications

522 Jones, Laurie Beth (1998) Path, The - Creating Your Mission Statement for Work and for Life, Hyperion

523 Dilts, Robert (1994) Strategies of Genius Vol. III, Capitola: Meta Publications

524 Dilts, Robert (1996) Visionary Leadership Skills - Creating a World to Which People Want To Belong, Capitola: Meta Publications

525 Covey, Stephen R. (1989) 7 Habits of Highly Effective People -

Powerful Lessons in Personal Change, New York: Fireside

[526] Spiegel, David & Yalom, I.D. (1978) 'Support group for dying patients,' Int. J. of Group Psychotherapy, 28:233-245

[527] Spiegel, David (1990) 'Facilitating emotional coping during treatment,' Cancer, 66(Supplement 6):1422-14226

[528] Simonton, O. Carl (1992) Healing Journey - The Simonton center program for achieving physical, mental and spiritual health, New York: Bantam

[529] Simonton, O. Carl (1992) Healing Journey - The Simonton center program for achieving physical, mental and spiritual health, New York: Bantam

[530] Spiegel, David & Bloom, J.R. & Yalom, I.D. (1981) 'Group support for patients with metastatic cancer - A randomized prospective outcome study,' Archives of General Psychiatry, 38:527-533

[531] Spiegel, David & Glafkides, M.S. (1983) 'Effects of group confrontation with death and dying,' Int. J. of Group Psychotherapy, 33:433-447

[532] Spiegel, David (1990) 'Facilitating emotional coping during treatment,' Cancer, 66(Supplement 6):1422-14226

[533] Kübler-Ross, Elisabeth (1975) Death, the final stage of growth, New Jersey: Prentice Hall

[534] Kübler-Ross, Elisabeth (1975) Death, the final stage of growth, New Jersey: Prentice Hall

[535] Kübler-Ross, Elisabeth (1975) Death, the final stage of growth, New Jersey: Prentice Hall

[536] Kübler-Ross, Elisabeth (1975) Death, the final stage of growth, New Jersey: Prentice Hall

[537] Simonton, O. Carl & Henson, Reid (1992) Healing Journey - The Simonton center program for achieving physical, mental and spiritual health, New York: Bantam Books

[538] Simonton, O. Carl & Henson, Reid (1992) Healing Journey - The Simonton center program for achieving physical, mental and spiritual health, New York: Bantam Books

[539] McDermott, Ian & O'Connor, Joseph (1996) NLP & Health, London: Thornson's Publications

[540] Spiegel, David (1993) 'Brief Supportive-Expressive Group Therapy for Women with Primary Breast Cancer - a treatment manual,' Stanford:

Psychosocial treatment laboratory, <u>Stanford Univ. School of Med.</u>

[541] LeShan, Lawrence (1989) <u>Cancer as a Turning Point</u>, Penguin Putman

[542] Grosz, Hanus J. (1979) 'Hypnotherapy in the management of terminally ill cancer patients,' <u>J. of the Indiana Medical Association</u> 72:126-129 in Brown, Daniel P & Fromm, Erika (1987) <u>Hypnosis and Behavioral Medicine</u>, New Jersey: Lawrence Erlbaum associates publishers

[543] LeShan, Lawrence (1989) <u>Cancer as a Turning Point</u>, Penguin Putman

[544] LeShan, Lawrence (1989) <u>Cancer as a Turning Point</u>, Penguin Putman

[545] Ferrell, B.R. & Cronin, Nash C. & Warfield, C. (1992) 'The role of patient controlled analgesia in the management of cancer pain,' <u>J. of Pain and Symptom Management,</u> 7:149 154

[546] Owen, H. & Plummer, J. (1997) 'Patient controlled analgesia - Current concepts in acute pain management,' <u>CNS Drugs,</u> 8: 203 218

[547] Ellis, J.A. & Blouin, R. & Lockett, J. (1999) 'Patient controlled analgesia - Optimizing the experience,' <u>Clinical Nursing Research</u>, (3):283-294

[548] Thomas, V.J. & Rose, F.D. & Heath, M.L. & Flory, P (1993) 'A multidimensional comparison of nurse and patient controlled analgesia in the management of acute postsurgical pain,' <u>Medical Science Research</u>, 21: 379 381

[549] Vingerhoets, A.J.J.M. (2000) 'Patient en Stress,' <u>Verpleegkunde</u>, 4:214-223)

[550] Cousins, Norman (1979) <u>Anatomy of an Illness</u>, New York: W.W. Norton

[551] Lerche, Davis Jeanie (1999) 'Breast cancer patients thrive when they are involved in decision making,' <u>WebMD Medical News</u>, 1728.52585

[552] Baalen, van, Daan C. & Vries, de, Marco J. (1987) <u>Spontaneous' regression of cancer - A clinical, pathological and psycho-social study,</u> Rotterdam: Erasmus University

[553] Berland, Warren (1994) <u>Unexpected Cancer Recovery - Dissertation,</u> Saybrook Institute

[554] Cunningham, Alastair J. & Phillips, Cathy & Lockwood, Gina A. & Hedley, David W. & Edmonds, Claire V.I. (2000) 'Association of involvement in psychological self-regulation with longer survival in

patients with metastatic cancer: an exploratory study,' Advances in Mind Body Medicine, 16(4):287-294.

555 McDermott, Ian & O'Connor, Joseph (1996) NLP & Health, London: Thornson's Publications

556 Simonton, O. Carl & Simonton - Matthews, Stephanie & Creighton, James L. (1978) Getting Well Again, New York: Bantam Books

557 Simonton, O. Carl & Henson, Reid (1992) Healing Journey - The Simonton center program for achieving physical, mental and spiritual health, New York: Bantam Books

558 LeShan, Lawrence (1989) Cancer as a Turning Point, Penguin Putman

559 LeShan, Lawrence (1977) You Can Fight for Your Life, New York: M. Evans

560 Pelletier, Kenneth R. (1992) Mind as a Healer, Mind as a Slayer, New York: Delacorte

561 O'Regan, Brendan (ed) & Hirshberg, Caryle (ed.) (1993) Spontaneous Remission - An Annotated Bibliography, Inst. of Noetic Sciences

562 Hutschnecker, A.A. (1953) Will to Live, Thomas Y. Crowell Company

563 Samuels, M. & Samuels, N. (1975) Seeing with the Mind's Eye, Random House

564 Simonton, O. Carl & Henson, Reid (1992) Healing Journey - The Simonton center program for achieving physical, mental and spiritual health, New York: Bantam

565 Simonton, O. Carl & Simonton - Matthews, Stephanie & Creighton, James L. (1978) Getting Well Again, New York: Bantam Books

566 Contrary to the earlier discussion, I will be using 'patient' within this chapter to describe relationships with physicians.

567 Spiegel, David & Spira, James (1991) Supportive-expressive group therapy - A treatment manual of psychosocial intervention for women with recurrent breast cancer, Stanford: Psychosocial treatment laboratory, Stanford Univ. School of Med.

568 Spiegel, David (1993) Brief Supportive-Expressive Group Therapy for Women with Primary Breast Cancer - a treatment manual, Stanford: Psychosocial treatment laboratory, Stanford Univ. School of Med

[569] Temoshok, Linda & Dreher, Henry (1992) The type C Connection - The Mind-Body Link to Cancer and your Health, Random House

[570] Spiegel, David & Spiegel, H. (1978) Trance and Treatment - Clinical Uses of Hypnosis, New York: Basic Books

[571] Spiegel, David & Spira, James (1991) Supportive-expressive group therapy - A treatment manual of psychosocial intervention for women with recurrent breast cancer, Stanford: Psychosocial treatment laboratory, Stanford Univ. School of Med.

[572] Spiegel, David (1993) 'Brief Supportive-Expressive Group Therapy for Women with Primary Breast Cancer - a treatment manual,' Stanford: Psychosocial treatment laboratory, Stanford Univ. School of Med.

[573] Spiegel, David & Spira, James (1991) 'Supportive-expressive group therapy - A treatment manual of psychosocial intervention for women with recurrent breast cancer,' Stanford: Psychosocial treatment laboratory, Stanford Univ. School of Med.

[574] Alder, Harry (1996) NLP for managers - How to achieve excellence at work, London: Piatkus

[575] Knight, Sue (1997) NLP at Work, Nicholas Brealey Publishing

[576] Temoshok, Linda & Dreher, Henry (1992) The type C Connection - The Mind-Body Link to cancer and your Health, Random House

[577] Temoshok, Linda & Dreher, Henry (1992) The type C Connection - The Mind-Body Link to cancer and your Health, Random House

[578] Ikemi, Yujiro (1978) 'Premorbid psychological factors as related to cancer incidence,' J. of Behavioral Medicine, 1, 45-133 in Brown, Daniel P. & Fromm, Erika (1987) Hypnosis and Behavioral Medicine, New Jersey: Lawrence Erlbaum associates publishers

[579] Oliver, G.W. (1982) 'Cancer patient and her family, a - a case study,' American Journal of Clinical Hypnosis, 25(2-3):156-160

[580] Romo, M. (1984) 'Stress and Cancer,' Comp. Ther., 10(1):3-6 in Cooper, Cary L. (1984) Psychosocial stress and cancer, New York: John Wiley & Sons

[581] Simonton, O. Carl & Simonton - Matthews, Stephanie & Creighton, James L. (1978) Getting Well Again, New York: Bantam

[582] Berland, Warren (1995) 'Unexpected Cancer Recovery - Why Patients Believe They Survive,' Advances in Mind Body Medicine, 11:5-19

[583] Cousins, Norman (1979) <u>Anatomy of an Illness</u>, New York: W.W. Norton

[584] Brown, Daniel P. & Fromm, Erika (1987) <u>Hypnosis and Behavioral Medicine</u>, New Jersey: Lawrence Erlbaum Associates Publishers

[585] Newton, Bernauer W. (1982) 'The use of hypnosis in the treatment of cancer patients,' <u>American Journal of Clinical Hypnosis</u>, 25:104-113

[586] Taylor, Shelly E. & Kemeny, Margaret E. & Reed, Geoffrey M. & Bowers, Julienne E. & Gruenewald, Tara L. (2000) 'Psychological resources, positive illusions, and health,' <u>American Psychologist</u>, 55(1) 99-109

[587] Cole, D.C. & Mondloch, M.V. & Hogg-Johnson, S. (2002) 'Listening to injured workers: how recovery expectations predict outcomes - a prospective study,' <u>Canadian Medical Association Journal (CMAJ)</u>, 166(6):749-54.

[588] Idler, E.L. & Kasl, S. (1991) 'Health perceptions and survival - do global evaluations of health status really predict mortality?' <u>J Gerontol</u>, 46:S55-S65

[589] Baalen, van, Daan C. & Vries, de, Marco J. (1987) <u>Spontaneous regression of cancer - A clinical, pathological and psycho-social study</u>, Rotterdam: Erasmus University

[590] Simonton, O. Carl & Henson, Reid (1992) <u>Healing Journey - The Simonton center program for achieving physical, mental and spiritual health</u>, New York: Bantam;

[591] Simonton, O. Carl & Simonton - Matthews, Stephanie & Creighton, James L. (1978) <u>Getting Well Again</u>, New York: Bantam

[592] Achterberg, Jeanne (1985) <u>Imagery in Healing - Shamanism and Modern Medicine</u>, New Science Library

[593] Rossman M.D., Martin (2000) <u>Guided Imagery for Self-Healing - An Essential Resource for Anyone Seeking Wellness</u>, C.A., San Raphael: New World Library

[594] Rossman M.D., Martin (2003) <u>Fighting Cancer from Within - How to Use the Power of Your Mind for Healing</u>, Henry Holt & Co

[595] Simonton, O. Carl & Simonton - Matthews, Stephanie & Creighton, James L. (1978) <u>Getting Well Again</u>, New York: Bantam Books

[596] Antoni, Michael H. & Lehman, J.M. & Kilbourn, K.M. & Boyers, A.E. & Culver, J.L. & Alferi, S.M. & Yount, S.E. & McGregor, B.A. & Arena,

P.L. & Carver, C.S. (2001) 'Cognitive-behavioral stress management intervention decreases the prevalence of depression and enhances benefit finding among women under treatment for early-stage breast cancer,' Health Psychology, 20:20-32

[597] Cruess, D.G. & Antoni, Michael H. & McGregor, B.A. & Kilbourn, K.M. & Boyers, A.E. & Alferi, S.M. & Carver, C.S. & Kumar, M. (2001) 'Cognitive-behavioral stress management reduces serum cortisol by enhancing benefit finding among women being treated for early stage breast cancer,' Psychosomatic Medicine, 62(3):304-308

[598] Simonton, O. Carl & Simonton - Matthews, Stephanie & Creighton, James L. (1978) Getting Well Again, New York: Bantam Books

[599] Robbins, Anthony (1987) Unlimited Power - The Way to Peak Personal Achievement, Ballentine

[600] Robbins, Anthony (1992) Awaken The Giant Within - How to Take Immediate Control of Your Destiny, Simon & Schuster

[601] Pert, Candace B. (1997) Molecules of Emotion - Why You Feel the Way You Feel, New York: Simon and Schuster

[602] Spielberger, C.D. (1988) State-Trait Anger Expression Inventory STAXI - Professional Manual, Odessa: PAR

[603] Watson, M. & Greer, Steven (1983) 'Development of a questionnaire measure of emotional control,' J. of Psychosomatic Research, 27(4):299-305

[604] Grossarth-Maticek, Ronald (1979) Soziales verhalten und die Krebserkrankung, Beltz: Weinheim und Basel

[605] Grossarth-Maticek, Ronald & Bastiaan, Ronald Jan & Kanazir, Dusan T. (1985) 'Psychosocial factors as strong predictions of mortality from cancer, ischemic heart disease and stroke - Yugoslav Prospective Study,' J. of Psychosomatic Research, Vol. 29, pp. 167-176.

[606] Spielberger, C.D. (1988) Rationality/Emotional Defensiveness (R/ED) Scale - Preliminary Test Manual, Tampa: University of South Florida

[607] Ploeg, Henk. van der & Kleijn, W.C. & Mook, J & Donge, M & Pieterse, A.M.J. & Leer, J.W. (1989) 'Rationality and antiemotionality as a risk factor for cancer - Concept differentiation,' J. of Psychosomatic Research, 33(2):217-225

[608] Swan, G.E. & Carmelli, D & Dame, A & Rosenman, R.H. & Spielberger, C.D. (1991) 'Rationality/Emotional Defensiveness Scale,'

The - I. Internal structure and stability,' J. of Psychosomatic Research, 35(4-5):545-54

609 Bleiker, Eveline M.A. & Ploeg, Henk. van der & Hendriks, Jan H.C.L. & Leer, J.W. & Kleijn, W.C. (1993) 'Rationality, emotional expression and control: psychometric characteristics of a questionnaire for research in psycho-oncology,' J. of Psychosomatic Research, 37(8):861-72

610 Pert, Candace B. (1997) Molecules of Emotion - Why You Feel the Way You Feel, New York: Simon and Schuster

611 Vingerhoets, A.J.J.M. (ed.) & Bussel, F.J. van (ed.) & Boelhouwer, A.J.W. (ed.) (1997) The (non)expression of emotions in health and disease, Tilburg: Tilburg University Press

612 Pennebaker, J.W. & Kiecolt-Glaser PhD, Janice K. & Glaser, Ronald (1988) 'Disclosure of traumas and immune function - Health implications for psychotherapy,' J. of Consulting and Clinical Psychology, 56;2;239-245

613 Smyth, J.M. (1998) 'Written emotional expression - Effect sizes, outcome types, and moderating variables,' J. of Consulting and Clinical Psychology, 66:174 184

614 Smyth, J.M. & Stone, A.A. & Hurewitz, A. & Kaell, A. (1999) 'Effects of writing about stressful experiences on symptom reduction in patients with asthma or rheumatoid arthritis,' J. American Medical Association, 281:1304 1309

615 Antoni, Michael H. (1997) Emotional Disclosure in the Face of Stress, Tilburg: Tilburg University Press

616 Esterling, B. & Antoni, Michael H. & Kumar, M. & Schneiderman, N. (1990) 'Emotional repression, trauma disclosure responses and Epstein-Barr viral capsid antigen titers,' Psychosomatic Medicine, 52:397-410

617 Pennebaker, J.W. (1997) Health Effects of the Expression (and Non-Expression) of Emotions through Writing, Tilburg: Tilburg University Press in Vingerhoets, A.J.J.M. (ed.) & Bussel, F.J. van (ed.) & Boelhouwer, A.J.W. (ed.) (1997) The (non)expression of emotions in health and disease,' Tilburg: Tilburg University Press

618 Spiegel, David (1995) 'Essentials of psychotherapeutic intervention for cancer patients,' Support Care Cancer, 3252-256

619 Spiegel, David (1995) 'Essentials of psychotherapeutic intervention for cancer patients,' Support Care Cancer, 3252-256

620 Temoshok, Linda & Dreher, Henry (1992) The Type C Connection

- The Mind-Body Link to Cancer and your Health, Random House

621 Staps, Ton & Yang, W. (1991) Psycho-energetische therapie, Nijmegen: Intro

622 Yang, W. (1997) The Role of Non-Expression of Emotions in Counseling - Psycho-Energetic Therapy, Tilburg: Tilburg University Press in Vingerhoets, A.J.J.M. (ed.) & Bussel, F.J. van (ed.) & Boelhouwer, A.J.W. (ed.) (1997) The (non)expression of emotions in health and disease, Tilburg: Tilburg University Press

623 Labott, S.M. & Martin, R.B. (1987) 'Stress moderating effects of weeping and humor, the,' J. of Human Stress, 13: 159-164

624 Vingerhoets, A.J.J.M. & Scheirs, J.G.M. (2001) Crying and Health, Brunner-Routledge, 227-247 in Vingerhoets, A.J.J.M. & Cornelius, R.R. (2001) Adult Crying - a Biopsychosocial Approach, Sussex: Brunner-Routledge

625 Bolstad, Dr, Richard (2004) 'The Crying Game,' Anchor Point

626 Stavraky, K.M. & Buck, C.N. & Lott, J.S. & Worklin, J.M. (1968) 'Psychological factors in the outcome of human cancer,' J. of Psychosomatic Research, 12:251-259

627 Temoshok, Linda & Dreher, Henry (1992) The Type C Connection - The Mind-Body Link to Cancer and Your Health, Random House

628 Temoshok, Linda & Dreher, Henry (1992) The Type C Connection - The Mind-Body Link to Cancer and Your Health, Random House

629 Temoshok, Linda & Dreher, Henry (1992) The Type C Connection - The Mind-Body Link to Cancer and Your Health, Random House

630 Fiore, Neil A. (1986) Road Back to Health, New York: Bantam

631 Spiegel, David (1993) Brief Supportive-Expressive Group Therapy for Women with Primary Breast Cancer - a treatment manual, Stanford: Psychosocial treatment laboratory, Stanford Univ. School of Med.

632 Simonton, O. Carl & Henson, Reid (1992) Healing Journey - The Simonton center program for achieving physical, mental and spiritual health, New York: Bantam

633 Cohen, M.M. & Wellisch, D.K. (1974) 'Living in Limbo - Psychosocial intervention in families with a cancer patient,' Am. Journal of Psychotherapy, 34:561-571

634 Spiegel, David & Bloom, J.R. & Gottheil, E. (1983) 'Family environment of patients with metastatic carcinoma,' J. of Psychosocial

Oncology, 1:33-44

[635] Temoshok, Linda & Dreher, Henry (1992) The Type C Connection - The Mind-Body Link to Cancer and Your Health, Random House

[636] Temoshok, Linda & Dreher, Henry (1992) The Type C Connection - The Mind-Body Link to Cancer and Your Health, Random House

[637] Pennebaker, J.W. & Kiecolt-Glaser, PhD, Janice K. & Glaser, Ronald (1988) 'Disclosure of traumas and immune function - Health implications for psychotherapy,' J. of Consulting and Clinical Psychology, 56;2;239-245

[638] Pennebaker, J.W. (1990) Opening Up - The Healing Power of Expressing Emotions, New York: William Morrow

[639] Pennebaker, J.W. (1997) Health Effects of the Expression (and Non-Expression) of Emotions through Writing, Tilburg: Tilburg University Press

[640] Temoshok, Linda & Dreher, Henry (1992) The Type C Connection - The Mind-Body Link to Cancer and Your Health, Random House

[641] Baalen, van, Daan C. & Vries, de, Marco J. (1987) 'Spontaneous' regression of cancer - A clinical, pathological and psycho-social study, Rotterdam: Erasmus University

[642] Pert, Candace B. (1997) Molecules of Emotion - Why You Feel the Way You Feel, New York: Simon and Schuster

[643] Rossi, E. (1986) Psychobiology of Mind Body Healing, New York: W.W. Norton

[644] Sachar, Edward J. & Cobb, Jeremy C. & Shor, Ronald E. (1966) 'Plasma cortisol changes during hypnotic trance,' Archives of General Psychiatry, 14:482-490

[645] Katz, J. & Gallagher, T. & Hellman, L. & Sachar, Edward J. & Weiner, H. (1969) 'Psychoendocrine considerations in cancer of the breast,' Ann. N.Y. Acad. Sci., 164:509-516

[646] Spiegel, David (1993) Brief Supportive-Expressive Group Therapy for Women with Primary Breast Cancer - a treatment manual, Stanford: Psychosocial treatment laboratory, Stanford Univ. School of Med.

[647] Simonton, O. Carl & Simonton - Matthews, Stephanie & Creighton, James L. (1978) Getting Well Again, New York: Bantam Books

[648] Kiecolt-Glaser PhD, Janice K. & Williger, D. & Stout, J. & Messick, G. & Sheppard, S. & Ricker, D. & Romisher, S.C. & Briner, W. &

Bonnell, G. & Glaser, Ronald (1985) 'Psychosocial enhancement of immunocompetence in a geriatric population,' Health Psychology, 4(1):25-41

649 Fawzy, F.I. & Cousins, Norman & Fawzy, N.W. & Kemeny, Margaret E. & Elashof, R. & Morton, D.L. (1990) 'Structured psychiatric intervention for cancer patients. - Part I: Changes over time in methods of coping and affective disturbance,' Archives of General Psychiatry, 47:729-735

650 Fawzy, F.I. & Kemeny, Margaret E. & Fawzy, N.W. & Elashof, R. & Morton, D.L. & Cousins, Norman & Fahey, J.L. (1990) 'Structured psychiatric intervention for cancer patients. - Part II: Changes over time in immunological measures,' Archives of General Psychiatry, 47:729-735

651 Simonton, O. Carl & Simonton - Matthews, Stephanie & Creighton, James L. (1978) Getting Well Again, New York: Bantam Books

652 Simonton, O. Carl & Simonton - Matthews, Stephanie & Sparks, T.F. (1980) 'Psychological Intervention and Survival Time of Patients with Metastatic Breast Cancer,' Psychosomatics, 21:226-233

653 Benson, Herbert & Klipper, Miriam Z. (1975) Relaxation Response, New York: William Morrow

654 Borysenko, Joan (1984) Minding the Body, Mending the Mind, New York: Bantam

655 Meares, Ainslie (1982) 'Stress, meditation and regression of cancer,' Practitioner, 226:1607-1609

656 Benson, Herbert & Klipper, Miriam Z. (1975) Relaxation Response, New York: William Morrow

657 Goleman PhD, Daniel (1978) The Varieties of the Meditative Experience, Halsted

658 Chopra, Deepak(1987) Creating Health - How to Wake Up the Body's Intelligence, : Houghton-Mifflin

659 Meares, Ainslie (1979) 'Mind and Cancer,' Lancet, 1

660 Meares, Ainslie (1982) 'A form of intensive meditation associated with the regression of cancer, ' American Journal of Clinical Hypnosis, 25:114-121

661 Meares, Ainslie (1983) 'Psychological mechanisms in the regression of cancer,' Med. Journal of Australia, 1(12):583-584

[662] Meares, Ainslie (1983) 'Psychological mechanisms in the regression of cancer,' Med. Journal of Australia, 1(12):583-584

[663] Meares, Ainslie (1978) 'Vivid Visualization and Dim Visual Awareness in the Regression of Cancer in Meditation,' J. of Am. Soc. of Psychosomatic Dental Medicine, 25:85-88

[664] Meares, Ainslie (1979) 'Mind and Cancer,' Lancet, 1

[665] Meares, Ainslie (1982) 'A form of intensive meditation associated with the regression of cancer,' American Journal of Clinical Hypnosis, 25:114-121

[666] Meares, Ainslie (1982) 'Stress, meditation and regression of cancer,' Practitioner, 226:1607-1609

[667] Lebaw, Wallace & Holton, Charlene & Tewell, Karen & Eccles, Doris (1975) 'Use of self-hypnosis by children with cancer,' American Journal of Clinical Hypnosis, 17:233-238

[668] Newton, Bernhauer W. (1982) 'Use of Hypnotherapy in the treatment of Cancer Patients,' American Journal of Clinical Hypnosis, 25(2-3):104-113

[669] Kiecolt-Glaser PhD, Janice K. & Glaser, Ronald & Strain, E.C. & Stout, J.C. & Tarr, K. & Holliday, J.E. & Speicher, C.E. (1986) 'Modulation of cellular immunity in medical students,' J. of Behavioral Medicine, 9:311-320

[670] Glaser, Ronald & Kiecolt-Glaser PhD, Janice K. (1992) 'PsychoNeuroImmunology - Can psychological interventions modulate immunity?' J. of Consulting and Clinical Psychology, 60:569-575

[671] Silvertsen, I. & Dahlstrom, A.W. (1921) 'Relation of muscular activity to carcinoma - Preliminary report,' J. of Cancer Research, 6;365-378 in Simonton, O. Carl & Simonton - Matthews, Stephanie & Creighton, James L. (1978) Getting Well Again, New York: Bantam Books

[672] Silvertsen, I. & Hastings, W.H. (1938) 'Preliminary report on influence of food and function on incidence of mammary gland tumor in 'A' stock albino mice,' Minnesota Med, 21:873-75 in Simonton, O. Carl & Simonton - Matthews, Stephanie & Creighton, James L. (1978) Getting Well Again, New York: Bantam Books

[673] Rusch, H.P. & Kline, B.E. (1944) 'Effect of exercise on the growth of a mouse tumor,' Cancer Research, 4:116-118

[674] Hoffman, S. & Paschikis, K.E. & Cantarow, A. (1960) 'Exercise, fatigue, and tumor growth,' Fed. Proc., March 19(abs) 396

[675] Hoffman, S. & Paschikis, K.E. & DeBiar, D.A. & Cantarow, A. & Williams, T.L. (1962) 'Influence of exercise on the growth of transplanted rat tumors,' Cancer Research, June: 22; 597-599

[676] Thompson, H.J. & Westerlind, K.C. & Snedden, J. & Briggs, S. & Singh, M. (1995) 'Exercise intensity dependent inhibition of 1-methyl-1-nitrosourea induced mammary carcinogenesis in female F-344 rats,' Carcinogenesis, 16:1783-1786

[677] Westerlind, K.C. & McCarty, H.L. & Schultheiss, P.C. & Story, R. & Reed, A.H. & Baier, M.L. & Strange, R. (2003) 'Moderate exercise training slows mammary tumour growth in adolescent rats,' Eur. J. of Cancer Prevention, 12:281-287

[678] Zielinski, Mark R. & Muenchow, Melissa & Wallig, Matthew A. & Horn, Peggy L. & Woods, Jeffrey A. (2004) 'Exercise delays allogeneic tumor growth and reduces intratumoral inflammation and vascularization,' J. of Appl. Physiol., 96: 2249-2256

[679] Selye, Hans (1956) Stress of Life, New York: McGraw-Hill in Simonton, O. Carl & Simonton - Matthews, Stephanie & Creighton, James L. (1978) Getting Well Again, New York: Bantam Books

[680] Simonton, O. Carl & Simonton - Matthews, Stephanie & Creighton, James L. (1978) Getting Well Again, New York: Bantam Books

[681] Simonton, O. Carl & Simonton - Matthews, Stephanie & Creighton, James L. (1978) Getting Well Again, New York: Bantam Books

[682] Simonton, O. Carl & Henson, Reid (1992) Healing Journey - The Simonton center program for achieving physical, mental and spiritual health, New York: Bantam

[683] Simonton, O. Carl & Simonton - Matthews, Stephanie & Creighton, James L. (1978) Getting Well Again, New York: Bantam Books

[684] Simonton, O. Carl & Simonton - Matthews, Stephanie & Creighton, James L. (1978) Getting Well Again, New York: Bantam Books

[685] Simonton, O. Carl & Simonton - Matthews, Stephanie & Creighton, James L. (1978) Getting Well Again, New York: Bantam Books

[686] Simonton, O. Carl & Simonton - Matthews, Stephanie & Creighton, James L. (1978) Getting Well Again, New York: Bantam Books

[687] Simonton, O. Carl & Henson, Reid (1992) Healing Journey - The Simonton center program for achieving physical, mental and spiritual health,' New York: Bantam

[688] Fox, E. (1938) 'Sermon on the Mount,' : Harper & Row

[689] Dilts, Robert & Hallbom (M.S.W), Tim & Smith (M.S), Suzi (1990) Beliefs - Pathways to Health & Well Being, Portland, Oregon: Metamorphous Press

[690] Dilts, Robert (1990) Changing Belief Systems with NLP, Capitola: Meta Publications

[691] Dilts, Robert (1994) Strategies of Genius Vol. III, Capitola: Meta Publications

[692] James, Ardie & James, Tad (1993) Lost secrets of ancient Hawaiian Huna, Honolulu: Advanced Neuro Dynamics

[693] James, Tad & Woodsmall, PhD, Wyatt (1988) Time Line Therapy and the Basis of Personality, Capitola: Meta Publications

[694] James, Tad (2000) Manual Accelerated NLP Trainers Training 2000, Honolulu: Advanced Neuro Dynamics

[695] James, Tad & Woodsmall, PhD, Wyatt (1988) Time Line Therapy and the Basis of Personality, Capitola: Meta Publications

[696] James, Tad (2000) Manual Accelerated NLP Trainers Training 2000, Honolulu: Advanced Neuro Dynamics

[697] Spiegel, David & Bloom, J.R. & Yalom, I.D. (1981) 'Group support for patients with metastatic cancer - A randomized prospective outcome study,' Archives of General Psychiatry, 38:527-533

[698] James, Tad & Woodsmall, PhD, Wyatt (1988) Time Line Therapy and the Basis of Personality, Capitola: Meta Publications

[699] James, Tad & Woodsmall, PhD, Wyatt (1988) Time Line Therapy and the Basis of Personality, Capitola: Meta Publications

[700] Cousins, Norman (1979) Anatomy of an Illness - as perceived by the patient, New York: W.W. Norton

[701] Dillon, K.M. & Minchoff, B. & Baker, K.H. (1985) 'Positive emotional states and enhancement of the immune system,' Int. J. of Psychiatry in Medicine, 15(1):13-18

[702] Berk, Lee S. & Felten, David & Tan, S.A. & Bittman, Barry B. & Westengard, James (2001) 'Modulation of Neuroimmune Parameters During the Eustress of Humor-Associated Mirthful Laughter,' Alternative Therapies, 2:62-76

[703] Levy, Sandra M. & Lee, J. & Bagley, C. & Lippman, M.E. (1988)

'Survival hazards analysis in first recurrent breast cancer patients - seven year follow-up,' Psychosomatic Medicine, 51:1-9

[704] Futterman, A.D. & Kemeny, Margaret E. & Shapiro, Debbie & Fahey, J.L. (1994) 'Immunological and physiological changes associated with induced positive and negative moods,' Psychosomatic Medicine, 56:499-511

[705] Blakeslee, Thomas R. & Grossarth-Maticek, Ronald (unknown) Feelings of Pleasure & Well-being as Predictors of Health Status 21 Years Later, unpublished

[706] Simonton, O. Carl & Henson, Reid (1992) Healing Journey - The Simonton center program for achieving physical, mental and spiritual health, New York: Bantam

[707] McDermott, Ian & O'Connor, Joseph (1996) NLP & Health, London: Thornson's Publications

[708] McDermott, Ian & O'Connor, Joseph (1996) NLP & Health, London: Thornson's Publications

[709] Margolis, Clorinda G. (1983) 'Hypnotic imagery with cancer patients,' American Journal of Clinical Hypnosis

[710] Simonton, O. Carl & Simonton - Matthews, Stephanie & Creighton, James L. (1978) Getting Well Again, New York: Bantam

[711] Metalnikov , S. & Chorine , V. (1926) 'Role des réflexes conditionnells dans l'imuunité,' Annales de l'Institut Pasteur, 40:893-900

[712] Smith, G. & McDaniel, S. (1983) 'Psychologically mediated effect on the delayed hypersensitivity reaction to tuberculin in Humans,' Psychosomatic Medicine, 46; 65-73

[713] Ader, Robert & Cohen, Nicholas & Felten, David (1990) PsychoNeuroImmunology, San Diego: Academic Press

[714] Buske-Kirschbaum, A. & Kirschbaum, C. & Stierle, H. & Lehnert, H. & Hellhammer, D. (1992) 'Conditioned increase in natural killer cell activity in humans,' Psychosomatic Medicine, 54:123-132

[715] Pert, Candace B. (1997) Molecules of Emotion - Why You Feel the Way You Feel, New York: Simon and Schuster

[716] Kornblith , A.B. & Herndon , J.E. & Zuckerman , E. & Cella , D.F. & Cherin, E. & Holland, Jimmy C. et al. (1998) 'Comparison of psychosocial adaptation of advanced stage Hodgkin's disease and acute leukemia survivors,' Ann. Oncology, 9:297-306 in Holland, Jimmy C.

(2002) 'History of Psycho-Oncology - Overcoming Attitudinal and Conceptual Barriers,' Psychosomatic Medicine, 64:206-221

[717] Bovbjerg, D. & Redd, W.H. & Maier, L.A. & Holland, Jimmy C. & Lesko, L. & Niedzwiecki, D. & Rubin, S.C. & Hakus, T.B. (1990) 'Anticipatory immune suppression and nausea in women receiving cyclic chemotherapy for ovarian cancer,' J. of Consulting and Clinical Psychology, 58,153-15

[718] Bellis, J.M. (1966) 'Hypnotic pseudo-sunburn,' American Journal of Clinical Hypnosis, 8:310-312

[719] Johnson, R.F.Q. & Barber, T.X. (1976) 'Hypnotic suggestions for blister formation - subjective and physiological effects,' American Journal of Clinical Hypnosis, 18:172-181

[720] Gravitz, Melvin A. (1981) 'Production of warts by suggestion as a cultural phenomenon,' American Journal of Clinical Hypnosis, 23:281-283

[721] Bennett, H.L. & Davis, H.S. (1984) 'Non-verbal response to intraoperative conversation,' Anesthesia and Analgesia, 63:185

[722] Bennett, H.L. & Davis, H.S. & Giannini, J.A. (1985) 'Non-verbal response to intraoperative conversation,' British Journal of Anaesthesia, 57:174-179

[723] Bennett, H.L. & Disbrow, E.A. (1999) Preparing for Surgery and Medical Procedures in Goleman PhD, Daniel (ed.) (1993) Mind Body Medicine - How to Use Your Mind for Better Health, New York: Consumer Reports Books

[724] Yapko, Michael (1990) Trancework - An Introduction to the Practice of Clinical Hypnosis, Bristol, PA 19007: Brunner/Mazel

[725] Hall, Howard R. (1982) 'Hypnosis and the immune system: a review with implications for cancer and the psychology of healing,' American Journal of Clinical Hypnosis 25:92-103

[726] Hammond, D. Corrydon (1990) Handbook of Hypnotic Suggestions and Metaphors, New York, W.W. Norton.

[727] Bonjour, J. (1929) 'Influence of the mind on the skin,' Brit. J. Dermat., 41:324-326

[728] Sulzberger, M.B. & Wolf, J. (1934) 'The treatment of warts by suggestion,' Med. Rec. New York, 140:552-556

[729] McDowell, M. (1949) 'Juvenile warts removed with the use of hypnotic suggestion,' Bull. Menninger Clinic, 13:4

[730] Obermayer et al. (1949) 'Treatment by suggestion of verrucae planea of the face,' Psychosomatic Medicine, 11:163-164

[731] Allington, H.V. (1952) 'Review of the psychotherapy of warts,' Archives of Dermatology and Syphiology, 66:316-326

[732] Ahser, R. (1956) 'Respectable hypnosis,' British Medical Journal, 1:309-313

[733] Schneck, J.M. (1959) Hypnosis in Modern Medicine, Charles Thomas Publisher

[734] Sinclair-Geiben, A.H.C & Chalmers, D. (1959) 'Evaluation of treatment of warts by hypnosis,' Lancet, 2:480-482w

[735] Ullman, M. & Dudek, S. (1960) 'On the psyche and warts: II. hypnotic suggestion and warts,' Psychosomatic Medicine, 22:68-76

[736] Surman, O.S. & Gottlieb, S.K. & Hackett, T.P. & Silverberg, E.L. (1973) 'Hypnosis in the treatment of warts,' Archives of General Psychiatry, 28:439-441

[737] Finkelstein, Selig & Howard, Marcia Greenleaf (1982) 'Cancer Prevention - A three-year pilot study,' American Journal of Clinical Hypnosis

[738] Spanos, N.P. & Stenstrom , R.J. & Johnston, J.C. (1988) 'Hypnosis, placebo, and suggestion in the treatment of warts,' Psychosomatic Medicine, 50:245-260

[739] Spanos, N.P. & Williams , V. & Gwynn , M.I. (1990) 'Effects of hypnotic, placebo, and salicylic acid treatments on wart regression,' Psychosomatic Medicine, 52:109-114

[740] Clawson, T.H. & Swade, R.H. (1975) 'Hypnotic control of blood flow and pain and the potential use of hypnosis in the treatment of cancer,' American Journal of Clinical Hypnosis, 17: 160-169

[741] Clawson, T.H. & Swade, R.H. (1975) 'Hypnotic control of blood flow and pain and the potential use of hypnosis in the treatment of cancer,' American Journal of Clinical Hypnosis, 17: 160-169

[742] Gravitz, Melvin A. (1981) 'Production of warts by suggestion as a cultural phenomenon,' American Journal of Clinical Hypnosis, 23:281-283

[743] LeShan, Lawrence (1977) You Can Fight for Your Life, New York: M. Evans

744 Rossi, E. (1986) Psychobiology of Mind-Body Healing, New York: W.W. Norton

745 Rossi Ph.D, Ernest L. (1986) The Psychobiology of Mind-Body Healing - New Concepts of Therapeutic Hypnosis, W. W. Norton

746 Brouwer, Yoka (1996) NLP en gezondheid, Deventer: Ank-Hermes b.v.

747 McDermott, Ian & O'Connor, Joseph (1996) NLP & Health, London: Thornson's Publications

748 Edelstien, Gerald (1981) Trauma, Trance and Transformation - A Clinical Guide to Hypnotherapy, : Brunner/Mazel

749 Dilts, Robert & Hallbom (M.S.W), Tim & Smith, Suzi (1999) NLP Health Certification Training manual 1999,

750 Merriam-Webster Online Dictionary 2004

751 Horowitz, M. (1970) Image Formation and Cognition, Appleton-Century-Crofts

752 Achterberg, Jeanne (1985) Imagery and Healing - Shamanism in Modern Medicine, Boston: New Science Library

753 Paivio, A.A. (1971) Imagery and Verbal Processes, New York: Holt, Rinehart and Winston

754 McGuigan, F.J. (1966) Thinking : Studies of Covert Language Processes, New York: Appleton and Company

755 McGuigan, F.J. (1978) Imagery and Thinking - Covert Functioning of the Motor System, New York: Plenum

756 Shannon, T.X. & Isbell, G.M. (1963) "Stress in dental patients: Effect of local anesthetic procedures," Technical Report No SAM-TDR-63-29; US Air Force School of Aerospace Medicine, Texas: Brooks Air Force Base

757 Brinbaum, R.M. (1964) "Autonomic reaction to threat and confrontation conditions of psychological stress," unpublished doctoral dissertation, Berkeley: University of California Press

758 Epstein, S. (1967) "Towards a unified theory of anxiety," in B.A. Maher (ed.) Progress in Experimental Personality Research Vol. 4, New York, Academic Press.

759 Nomikos, M.S. & Opton , E.M. & Averil, J.R. & Lazarus, Richard S. (1968) 'Surprise versus suspense in the production of stress reaction,' J. of Personality and Social Psychology, 8:204-208

760 Rossman, Martin L. (2003) Fighting Cancer from Within, Owl books

761 Achterberg, Jeanne & Dossy, Barbara & Kolkmeier, Leslie (1994) Rituals of Healing - Using Imagery for Health and Wellness, New York: Bantam Books

762 Simonton, O. Carl & Simonton - Matthews, Stephanie & Creighton, James L. (1978) Getting Well Again, New York: Bantam

763 Achterberg, Jeanne (1985) Imagery and Healing- Shamanism in Modern Medicine, Boston Shambhala

764 Rossman, Martin L. (2000) Guided Imagery for Self-Healing, Tiburon: H.J. Kramer

765 Achterberg, Jeanne (1985) Imagery and Healing - Shamanism in Modern Medicine, Boston: New Science Library

766 Dilts, Robert & Hallbom (M.S.W), Tim & Smith, Suzi (1990) Beliefs - Pathways to Health & Well-Being, Portland, Oregon: Metamorphous Press

767 Jacobson Edmond (1964) Anxiety and Tension Control, New York, J.B. Lippincottt Company in Alman, B. and Lambrou, P. (1983) Self-Hypnosis New York, Brunner/Mazel

768 Trestman, Robert Lee (1981) Imagery, Coping and Physiological Variables in Adult Cancer Patients, PhD dissertation, Knoxville: University of Tennessee

769 Achterberg, Jeanne & Lawlis, Frank (1978) Imagery and Disease - A Diagnostic Tool for Behavioral Medicine, Inst. of Personality Testing

770 Rossman, Martin L. (2000) Guided Imagery for Self-Healing, Tiburon: H.J. Kramer

771 Trestman, Robert Lee (1981) Imagery, Coping and Physiological Variables in Adult Cancer Patients, PhD dissertation, Knoxville: University of Tennessee

772 McDermott, Ian & O'Connor, Joseph (1996) NLP & Health, London: Thornson's Publications

773 McDermott, Ian & O'Connor, Joseph (1996) NLP & Health, London: Thornson's Publications

774 Newton, Bernhauer W. (1982) 'Use of hypnotherapy in the treatment of cancer patients,' American Journal of Clinical Hypnosis, 25(2-3):104-113

775 Meares, Ainslie (1982) 'A form of intensive meditation associated with the regression of cancer,' American Journal of Clinical Hypnosis, 25:114-121

776 Richardson , M.A. & Post-White, J & Grimm , E.A. & Moye , L.A. & Singletary , S.E. & Justice , B (1997) 'Coping, life attitudes, and immune responses to imagery and group support after breast cancer treatment,' Altern. Ther. Health Med., 3:62-70

777 Shapiro, Arnold (1982) 'Psychotherapy as adjunct treatment for cancer patients,' American Journal of Clinical Hypnosis

778 Simonton, O. Carl & Simonton - Matthews, Stephanie & Creighton, James L. (1978) Getting Well Again, New York: Bantam

779 Rossman, Martin L. (1987) Healing Yourself - A Step by Step Program for Better Health Through Imagery, New York: Walker & Co

780 Simonton, O. Carl & Simonton - Matthews, Stephanie & Creighton, James L. (1978) Getting Well Again, New York: Bantam

781 Siegel, Bernie S. (1986) Love, Medicine and Miracles, New York: Harper and Row

782 Borysenko, Joan (1987) Minding the Body, Mending the Mind, New York: Bantam Books

783 Gruber, B.L. & Hall, N.R & Hersh, S.E. & Dubois, E. (1988) 'Immune system and psychological changes in metastatic cancer patients while using ritualized relaxation and guided imagery - a pilot study,' Scandinavian Journal of Behavioral Therapy, 17-25-46

784 Batt, Sharon (1996) Patients No More - The Politics of Breast Cancer, Melborne: Spinifex

785 Rossi, E. (1986) Psychobiology of Mind-Body Healing, New York: W.W. Norton

786 Schneider, J. & Smith, W. & Witcher, S. (1984) Relationship of mental imagery to white blood cells (neutrophil) function in normal subjects

787 Hall H. Minnes L., Olness K. 'The psychophysiology of voluntary immunomodulation,' International Journal of Neuroscience 1993;69:221-234.

788 Frank, J. (1985) 'The effects of music therapy and guided visual imagery on chemotherapy induced nausea and vomiting' Oncol. Nurse Forum, 12:47-52

[789] Scott, D.W. & Donohue, D.C. & Mastrovito, R.C. & Hakus, T.B. (1986) 'Comparative trial of clinical relaxation and an antiemetic drug regimen in reducing chemotherapy-related nausea and vomiting,' Cancer Nurse, 9:178-188

[790] Kenner, C. & Achterberg, Jeanne (1983) 'Non-pharmacologic pain relief for burn patients,' Annual Meeting of the American Burn Association

[791] Lawlis, G.F. & Selby, D. & Hinnant, G. & McCoy, C. (1985) 'Reduction of postoperative pain parameters by presurgical relaxation instructions for spinal pain patients,' Spine, 10(7):649-65

[792] Stevens, L. (1983) An intervention study of imagery with diabetes mellitus - (doctoral), University of North Texas

[793] Olness, Karen & Conroy, M. (1985) 'A pilot study of voluntary control of transcutaneous PO by children,' Int. J. Clin. Exp. Hypn., 33:1

[794] Barber, T.X. (1969) Hypnosis - A Scientific Approach, New York: Van Nostrand

[795] Green, Elmer & Green, Alice M. (1977) Beyond Biofeedback, New York: Delacorte

[796] Jordan, C.S. & Lenington, K.T. (1979) 'Psychological correlates of eidetic imagery and induced anxiety,' Journal of Mental Imagery, 3:31-42

[797] Barber, T.X. (1978) 'Hypnosis, suggestion, and psychosomatic phenomena,' American Journal of Clinical Hypnosis, 21:12-27

[798] Ornish, Dean & Scherwitz, L.W. & Doody, R.D. (1983) 'Effects of stress management training and dietary changes in treating ischemic heart disease,' J. American Medical Association, 249:54-59

[799] Ornish, Dean (1990) 'Can lifestyle changes reverse coronary heart disease?,' Lancet, 336(8708):129?133

[800] Green, Elmer & Green, Alice (1977) Beyond Biofeedback - Pioneering research that explorers the mind's power to control the body, New York: Delta

[801] Hall, H.R. & Minnes, L. & Tosi, M. & Olness, Karen (1992) 'Voluntary modulation of neutrophil adhesiveness using a cyberphysiological strategy,' Int. J. of Neuroscience, 63:287-297

[802] Achterberg, Jeanne & Lawlis, Frank (1978) Imagery and Disease - A Diagnostic Tool for Behavioral Medicine, Inst. of Personality Testing

[803] Peavey, B. & Lawlis, G.F. & Goven, P. (1985) 'Biofeedback-assisted relaxation: effects on phagocytic capacity,' Biofeedback Self Regul., 10:33-47

[804] Gruber, B.L. & Hall, N.R & Hersh, S.E. & Dubois, E. (1988) 'Immune system and psychological changes in metastatic cancer patients while using ritualized relaxation and guided imagery - a pilot study,' Scandinavian Journal of Behavioral Therapy, 17-25-46

[805] Lawley, James & Tompkins, Penny (2000) Metaphors in Mind - Transformation through Symbolic Modeling, Developing Company Press

[806] Barrios, A.A. (1961) Hypnosis as a possible means for curing cancer, unpublished

[807] Achterberg, Jeanne & Lawlis, Frank (1978) Imagery and Disease - A Diagnostic Tool for Behavioral Medicine, Inst. of Personality Testing

[808] Achterberg, Jeanne & Dossey, Barbara & Kolkmeier, Leslie (1994) Rituals in Healing - Using Imagery for Health and Wellness, New York: Bantam Books

[809] Battino , Rubin (2001) Guided Imagery and Other Approaches to Healing, Crown House Publishing

[810] Pelletier, K. (?) Personal Communication in Rossman, Martin L.; (2000) 'Guided Imagery for Self-Healing, Tiburon, CA, HJ Kramer Book

[811] Rossman, Martin L. (2003) Fighting Cancer from Within, Owl books

[812] Margolis, Clorinda G. (1983) 'Hypnotic imagery with cancer patients,' American Journal of Clinical Hypnosis

[813] Rossman, Martin L. (2000) Guided Imagery for Self-Healing, Tiburon: H.J. Kramer

[814] Achterberg, Jeanne (1985) Imagery and Healing - Shamanism in Modern Medicine, Boston: New Science Library

[815] Simonton, O. Carl & Simonton - Matthews, Stephanie & Creighton, James L. (1978) Getting Well Again, New York: Bantam

[816] Dilts, Robert & Hallbom, Tim & Smith, Suzi (1990) Beliefs - Pathways to Health and Well-Being, Metamorphous Press

[817] Simonton, O. Carl & Simonton - Matthews, Stephanie & Creighton, James L. (1978) Getting Well Again, New York: Bantam

[818] Temoshok, Linda & Dreher, Henry (1992) The Type C Connection - The Mind-Body Link to Cancer and Your Health, Random House

[819] Rossman, Martin L. (2000) Guided Imagery for Self-Healing, Tiburon: H.J. Kramer

[820] Rossman, Martin L. (2003) Fighting Cancer from Within, Owl Books

[821] Achterberg, J.; Lawlis, G.F. (1978) Imagery of Cancer, Champaign, IL, Institute for Personality and Ability Testing in Rossman, Martin L.; (2000) Guided Imagery for Self-Healing, Tiburon, CA, HJ Kramer Book

[822] Margolis, Cornelia G. (1983) 'Hypnotic imagery with cancer patients,' American Journal of Clinical Hypnosis, 25:128-134

[823] Newton, Bernauer W. (1983) 'The use of hypnosis in the treatment of cancer patients,' American Journal of Clinical Hypnosis, 25:104-113

[824] Shapiro, Arnold (1983) 'Psychotherapy as adjunct treatment for cancer patients,' American Journal of Clinical Hypnosis, 25:150-155

[825] Rosch, P.J. (1984) 'Stress and Cancer,' Compr. Ther., 10(1):3-6 in Cooper, Cary L. (1984) Psychosocial Stress and Cancer, New York: John Wiley & Sons

[826] Derogatis, L. & Abeloff, M. & Melisaratos, N. (1979) 'Psychological coping mechanisms and survival time in metastatic breast cancer,' JAMA, 242:1504-1508.

[827] Achterberg, Jeanne (1985) Imagery and Healing - Shamanism in Modern Medicine, Boston: New Science Library 192

[828] Temoshok, Linda & Dreher, Henry (1992) The Type C Connection - The Mind-Body Link to Cancer and Your Health, Random House

[829] Rossman, Martin L. (2000) Guided Imagery for Self-Healing, Tiburon: H.J. Kramer

[830] Rossman, Martin L. (2003) Fighting Cancer from Within, Owl books

[831] Simonton, O. Carl & Simonton - Matthews, Stephanie & Creighton, James L. (1978) Getting Well Again, New York: Bantam

[832] Simonton, O. Carl & Simonton - Matthews, Stephanie & Creighton, James L. (1978) Getting Well Again, New York: Bantam

[833] Simonton, O. Carl & Henson, Reid (1992) Healing Journey - The Simonton center program for achieving physical, mental and spiritual health, New York: Bantam

[834] Simonton, O. Carl & Simonton - Matthews, Stephanie & Creighton, James L. (1978) Getting Well Again, New York: Bantam

[835] Simonton, O. Carl & Henson, Reid (1992) Healing Journey - The Simonton center program for achieving physical, mental and spiritual health, New York: Bantam

[836] Simonton, O. Carl & Simonton - Matthews, Stephanie & Creighton, James L. (1978) Getting Well Again, New York: Bantam

[837] Spiegel, David & Spiegel, H. (1978) Trance and Treatment - Clinical Uses of Hypnosis, New York: Basic Books

[838] Esdaile, James (1846) Mesmerism in India, unknown

[839] Hilgard, Josephine R. & Hilgard, Ernest R. (1975) Hypnosis in the Relief of Pain, Los Altos: William Kaufman

[840] Zeig, Jeffrey (ed.) (1982) Ericksonian Approaches to Hypnosis and Psychotherapy, Bristol, PA 19007: Brunner/Mazel

[841] Hilgard, Ernest R. & LeBaron, S. (1984) Hypnotherapy of Pain in Children with Cancer, Los Altos: William Kaufman

[842] Zilbergeld, Bernie & Edelstein, M. Gerald & Araoz, Daniel (1986) Hypnosis - Questions & Answers, W. W. Norton

[843] Rossi Ph.D, Ernest L. & Cheek, David (1988) Mind-Body Therapy - Methods of Ideodynamic Healing in Hypnosis, : W. W. Norton

[844] Goleman PhD, Daniel (ed.) (1993) Mind-Body Medicine - How to Use Your Mind for Better Health, New York: Consumer Reports Books

[845] Braun, Bennett G. (1986) The Treatment of Multiple Personality Disorder, American Psychiatric Association

[846] Chase, Truddi (1987) When Rabbit Howls, New York: E.P. Dutton; Introduction by Robert A. Phillips Jr., PhD

[847] James, Tad & Woodsmall, Wyatt (1988) Time Line Therapy and the Basis of Personality, Capitola: Meta Publications

[848] Charvet, Shelle Rose (1995) Words That Change Minds - Mastering the Language of Influence, Kendall Hunt Pub. Co.

[849] Hall M.A. PhD, L. Michael & Bodenhamer D. Min, Bobby G. (2002) Figuring Out People - Design Engineering With Meta-Programs : Crownhouse Publishing

[850] Hamer, Ryke Geert (1999) Vermächtnis Einer NEUEN MEDIZIN Teil 1 - Die 5 Biologischen Naturgesetze : Krebs, Leukamie, Epilepsie, Koln, Germany: Amici di Dirk Verlag

[851] Hamer, Ryke Geert (1999) Vermächtnis Einer NEUEN MEDIZIN Teil 2 - Die 5 Biologischen Naturgesetze : Psychosen, Syndrome, Krebs by Kindern, Tieren, Pflanzen, Koln, Germany: Amici di Dirk Verlag

[852] Hamer, Ryke Geert (1999) Vermächtnis Einer NEUEN MEDIZIN Teil 1 - Die 5 Biologischen Naturgesetze : Krebs, Leukamie, Epilepsie, Koln, Germany: Amici di Dirk Verlag

[853] Hamer, Ryke Geert (1999) Vermächtnis Einer NEUEN MEDIZIN Teil 2 - Die 5 Biologischen Naturgesetze : Psychosen, Syndrome, Krebs by Kindern, Tieren, Pflanzen, Koln, Germany: Amici di Dirk Verlag

[854] Dilts, Robert & Hallbom (M.S.W), Tim & Smith, Suzi (1999) NLP Health Certification Training Manual 1999,

[855] Dilts, Robert (2000) NLP Encyclopedia, NLP University Press

[856] Lawley, James & Tompkins, Penny (2000) Metaphors in Mind - Transformation Through Symbolic Modeling, Developing Company Press

[857] Dilts, Robert & Hallbom (M.S.W), Tim & Smith, Suzi (1999) NLP Health Certification Training Manual 1999,

[858] Dilts, Robert (2000) NLP Encyclopedia, NLP University Press

[859] Lawley, James & Tompkins, Penny (2000) Metaphors in Mind - Transformation Through Symbolic Modeling, Developing Company Press

[860] Goodkin, Karl & Antoni, Michael H. & Blaney, P.H. (1986) 'Stress and hopelessness in the promotion of cervical intraepithelial neoplasia to invasive squamous cell carcinoma of the cervix,' J. of Psychosomatic Research, 30:67-76

[861] Garssen, Bert (2000) Rol van psychologische factoren bij het ontstaan en beloop van kanker, Utrecht: Helen Dowling Instituut

[862] Martikainen, P. & Valkonen, T. (1996) 'Mortality after death of a spouse - Rates and causes of death in a large Finnish cohort,' Am. J. of Public Health, 86:1087-1093

[863] Levav, I. & Kohn, R. & Iscovich, J. & Abramson, J.H. & Tsai, W.Y. & Vigdorovich, D. (2000) 'Cancer incidence and survival following bereavement,' Am. J. of Public Health, 90:1601-1607

[864] LeShan, Lawrence (1961) 'A basic psychological orientation apparently associated with malignant disease,' Psychiatric Qtly, 36:314-330

[865] LeShan, Lawrence (1961) 'A basic psychological orientation apparently associated with malignant disease,' Psychiatric Qtly, 36:314-330

[866] Hamer, Ryke Geert (1999) Vermächtnis Einer NEUEN MEDIZIN Teil 1 - Die 5 Biologischen Naturgesetze : Krebs, Leukamie, Epilepsie, Koln, Germany: Amici di Dirk Verlag

[867] Hamer, Ryke Geert (1999) Vermächtnis Einer NEUEN MEDIZIN Teil 2 - Die 5 Biologischen Naturgesetze : Psychosen, Syndrome, Krebs by Kindern, Tieren, Pflanzen, Koln, Germany: Amici di Dirk Verlag

[868] Garssen, Bert (2002) 'Psycho-oncology and cancer - linking psychosocial factors with cancer development,' Ann. Oncology, 13:171-175

[869] Rossman, Martin L. (2003) Fighting Cancer From Within, Owl Books

[870] Hejmadi , A.V. & Lyall , P.J. (o) Autogenic Metaphor Resolution, in Grinder, J. & DeLozier, J. & Bretto , C. (1991) Leaves Before the Wind - Leading Edge Applications of NLP, Grinder, DeLozier & Associates

[871] Hejmadi , A.V. & Lyall , P.J. (o) Autogenic Metaphor Resolution, in Grinder, J. & DeLozier, J. & Bretto , C. (1991) Leaves Before the Wind - Leading Edge Applications of NLP, Grinder, DeLozier & Associates

[872] Dilts, Robert & Hallbom (M.S.W), Tim & Smith, Suzi (1999) NLP Health Certification Training Manual 1999

[873] Lawley, James & Tompkins, Penny (2000) Metaphors in Mind - Transformation Through Symbolic Modeling, Developing Company Press

[874] Simonton, O. Carl & Simonton - Matthews, Stephanie & Creighton, James L. (1978) Getting Well Again, New York: Bantam

[875] Erickson, M.H. (1937) 'Development of apparent unconsciousness during reliving of traumatic experience,' Archives of Neurology and Psychiatry, 38:1282-1288

[876] Moody, R.L. (1946) 'Bodily changes during abreaction,' Lancet, 2:934-935

[877] Ford, L.F. & Yeager, C.L. (1948) 'Changes in electroencephalogram in subjects under hypnosis,' Dis. Nerv. System, 9:190-192

[878] Kuper, H.I. (1945) 'Psychic concomitants in wartime injuries,' Psychosomatic Medicine, 7:15-21

[879] Grue, R.M. & Stephenson, C.W. (1951) 'Controlled experiments correlating electroencephalogram, pulse and plantar reflexes with hypnotic age regression and induced emotional states,' Personality

[880] Gidro-Frank, L. & Bowerbuch, M.K. (1948) 'Study of the plantar response in hypnotic age regression,' J. Nerv. Ment. Disorders, 107:443-458

[881] Barrios, A.A. (1961) Hypnosis as a Possible Means for Curing Cancer, unknown

[882] Simonton, O. Carl & Simonton - Matthews, Stephanie & Creighton, James L. (1978) Getting Well Again, New York: Bantam Books

[883] Simonton, O. Carl & Henson, Reid (1992) Healing Journey - The Simonton Center Program for Achieving Physical, Mental, and Spiritual Health, New York: Bantam Books

[884] LeShan, Lawrence (1977) You Can Fight For Your Life, New York: M. Evans

[885] LeShan, Lawrence (1989) Cancer as a Turning Point, Penguin Putman

[886] McDermott, Ian & O'Connor, Joseph (1996) NLP & Health, London: Thornson's Publications

[887] Simonton, O. Carl & Simonton - Matthews, Stephanie & Creighton, James L. (1978) Getting Well Again, New York: Bantam Books

[888] Simonton, O. Carl & Henson, Reid (1992) Healing Journey - The Simonton Center Program for Achieving Physical, Mental and Spiritual Health, New York: Bantam Books